Technosubjectivities

In *Technosubjectivities*, Ezquerra invites readers to reconsider the core concepts of psychoanalysis—unconscious, body, drive, transitional object, psychosexuality, and the conditions of symbolization—in light of virtual environments and technologically mediated experiences.

Drawing on clinical experience and contemporary culture, the author proposes an innovative psychoanalytic approach for a post-organic clinic. She argues that a new psychoanalytic field is emerging at the crossroads of hybridization, technoculture, and processes of subjectivation. The book explores how subjectivation unfolds at the intersection of human and non-human agencies, animate and inanimate objects, artificial and natural forms, and realities and virtualities. It weaves conceptual argument with detailed clinical case studies, including the encounter between a psychoanalyst and the world's first state-recognized cyborg.

This ground-breaking book is essential reading for clinicians dealing with technology-mediated lives, psychoanalysts, neuroscientists, and readers interested in philosophy, psychoanalysis, anthropology, art, technology, and the humanities—and to anyone wishing to reflect on the transformations of our time.

Laura Ezquerra is a Franco-Spanish psychoanalyst and researcher whose work explores mutations of subjectivity in the technological age. She teaches in the Master's program at the University of Alcalá (Spain) and brings extensive clinical experience from both hospital and private practice. Founder and chair of EPF/IPA committees on psychoanalysis and technosubjectivities, she publishes at the intersection of humanities, art, and neuroscience, and leads international interdisciplinary research initiatives.

The International Psychoanalytical Association Current Challenges in Psychoanalysis Series

Series Editor
Silvia Flechner

IPA Publications Committee
Natacha Delgado, Nergis Güleç, Thomas Marcacci, Carlos Moguillansky, Rafael Mondrzak, Angela M. Vuotto, Gabriela Legorreta (consultant)

Recent titles in the series include

Psychoanalysis and Severe Disorders in Young Children
Clinical and Community Work with Autism Spectrum Disorder and Child Mental Health
Nahir Bonifacino

Couple Work, Work with Couples
Éric Smadja

Narcissism
Psychoanalytic Clinicians and Researchers in Dialogue
Edited by Marianne Leuzinger-Bohleber, Stephan Hau, Rogério Lerner, Erik Stänicke and Siri Erika Gullestad

Art and Psychoanalysis
Between the Dialectics of the Other and Poetic Estrangement
Gabriela Goldstein

The Defenses in Psychoanalysis
Theoretical Concepts to Empirical Research
Anna Maria Rosso

Paths of Symbolization
Alain Gibeault

Technosubjectivities
Human, Cyborg, Robot and Avatar in Contemporary Psychoanalysis
Laura Ezquerra

Technosubjectivities

Human, Cyborg, Robot and Avatar in Contemporary Psychoanalysis

Laura Ezquerra

Routledge
Taylor & Francis Group
LONDON AND NEW YORK

Designed cover image: Getty Images

First published 2027
by Routledge
4 Park Square, Milton Park, Abingdon, Oxon OX14 4RN

and by Routledge
605 Third Avenue, New York, NY 10158

Routledge is an imprint of the Taylor & Francis Group, an informa business

British Library Cataloguing-in-Publication Data
A catalogue record for this book is available from the British Library

ISBN: 978-1-041-07476-2 (hbk)
ISBN: 978-1-041-07475-5 (pbk)
ISBN: 978-1-003-64068-4 (ebk)

DOI: 10.4324/9781003640684

Typeset in Palatino
by Taylor & Francis Books

To Beltrán and M.B.

Contents

Figures

Acknowledgments

To those who have shared with me the time and uncertainty of thinking together.

To Neil Harbisson, for his generosity and for opening a path where psyche and technology meet in unexpected ways.

To my colleagues, particularly those who form the Research Group on Technosubjectivities, whose shared reflections and commitment have nourished this project.

To my friends, who have sustained and questioned me along the way—Claudia, Borja, and many others whose conversations still echo.

And, silently, to my family, whose quiet presence has accompanied me beyond words.

It is also dedicated to those who came before—the ones whose silent strength and gestures helped to pave the way—and to those who will come after, to all who, like Neil, will keep inventing new ways of inhabiting the human.

Series Editor's Foreword

The International Psychoanalytic Association Publications Committee is honored to present a new book from the Current Challenges in Psychoanalysis series. This series delves into the evolving landscape of psychoanalytic practice, addressing contemporary issues such as trauma, cultural diversity, technological influence, and shifts in psychoanalytical dynamics. Each volume offers concise, interdisciplinary insights from leading experts, bridging classical psychoanalytic theory with modern challenges. Designed for clinicians and researchers, this series is a vital resource for those seeking to navigate and innovate within today´s complex therapeutic environment.

The Publications Committee of the International Psychoanalytic Association is pleased to announce the new book *Technosubjectivities*, authored by Laura Ezquerra.

The author develops the notion of technosubjectivities as a psychoanalytic framework for understanding how technological environments are reshaping subjectivity, psychic life and contemporary clinical practice. Rather than merely reflecting new psychic configurations, the concept of technosubjectivities designates emerging modes of subjectivation in which the boundaries between human and non-human, organic and inorganic, natural and artificial become increasingly unstable. Within this perspective, technological environments are not simply external influences but actively participate in the constitution and transformation of psychic life. The author argues that technological mediation has become a constitutive dimension of psychoanalytic encounter, reconfiguring the analytical field and transforming the roles of both analyst and patient.

The book examines clinical cases, including the psychoanalytic sessions conducted with Neil Harbisson, the first legally recognized cyborg, and other patients engaged with digital environments, avatars and virtual worlds. Key questions arise regarding symbolization, mourning, and the formation of thought in a technology-saturated environment. The author proposes that psychoanalysis should engage with technological transformations rather than resist them, helping individuals articulate emerging forms of subjectivity and navigate their techno-environments. The ethical dimension lies in distinguishing creative hybridization from algorithmic colonization, while preserving the uniqueness and singularity of human experience.

A compelling issue arises when the author explores cyborg embodiment from a psychoanalytic perspective, focusing on individuals who integrate technological devices into their bodies, not merely as prostheses but as new organs that reshape subjectivity. The psychoanalytic work conducted with Neil Harbisson, the world's first legally recognized cyborg, constitutes one of the book's central clinical axes. His antenna, implanted in his skull enables him to perceive colours through sound. The author also discusses how technological mediations – whether embodied, symbolic or environmental – transform both the body and the psyche, giving rise to a hybrid subjectivity in which technology becomes a constitutive dimension of psychic life. The text introduces the concept of "techno-transference," describing how these mediations reshape libidinal transferential and countertransferential dynamics, thereby opening new perspectives on the psychoanalytic encounter. The cyborg is presented as a privileged figure through which to rethink the transformations of contemporary subjectivity, challenging traditional boundaries between the organic and the artificial. In doing so, the book raises fundamental psychoanalytic questions concerning subjectivity, embodiment, fetishism, and the processes of symbolizations, while exploring the emergence of new forms of psychic reality within increasingly post-organic and technologically mediated environments.

This book reaffirms the relevance of psychoanalytic practice in the face of contemporary transformations, inviting analysts, researchers, and a broader audience to engage with these evolving forms of subjectivity. It highlights the importance of listening to the subject within the techno-environment and understanding the new ways in which psychic life and creativity are expressed in technologically mediated contexts.

Silvia Flechner
Series Editor
Chair, IPA Publications Committee

Prologue

When I began listening to patients whose inner world unfolded through screens, avatars, and prostheses, I realized that the way human beings related to each other and inhabited their existence had radically changed. This experience took shape over time as a result of my clinical work, in which I noticed that the human and the technological inevitably intertwined and became inextricably linked.

The psychoanalytic encounter, based on words, silences, and ultimately on the intimacy between two unconscious minds, now unfolds, in my opinion in a much vaster context, in which technical objects actively participate in the transference-countertransference dynamic. The artifact that records, connects, or translates seems to become part of the analytic field, like a new skin. The psychoanalyst's own position is then reconfigured—extended, transformed by a networked world. The analytic space seems to expand to include these new mediations as configurations through which the psyche seeks to elaborate what remains unrepresentable.

This volume proposes to explore transference, countertransference, and unconscious processes within a hybrid analytic field, reformulating key psychoanalytic concepts from within practice, and outlining the first coordinates for speaking psychoanalytically about a post-organic clinic.

To speak of technosubjectivities is to give form to these emergent ways of being. The term does not describe a pathology; it designates new configurations of the subject in which the boundary between organic and inorganic, animate and inanimate, is continuously reworked. This notion suggests a psychoanalytic horizon, in which post-organic bodies, hybrid organisms, biotechnologies, algorithmic interfaces, virtual environments, and prosthetic integrations are structural participants in psychic life.

Drawing on psychoanalytic practice and contemporary interdisciplinary research, this book provides a perspective for understanding the evolving landscape of psychic life and how it is woven into the very fabric of our subjectivity.

Above all, it is an invitation to reimagine our practice and our concepts in the face of the anthropological mutation that questions what it means to be human.

From the body as transmitter of cultural heritage to the emergence of multiple and networked bodies; from the drive's energetic origin to its technological reformulations; from the transitional object to the interface—each chapter traces a line that deepens the psychic life of our time.

The cases described present richly detailed clinical material that brings the reader into contemporary analytic practice. The book recounts an initial encounter with Neil Harbisson—legally recognized in the United Kingdom as the first cyborg in the world– and, six years later, a series of in-depth sessions that trace the unfolding of an analytic process over time. Alongside this, the volume delves into work with other patients who find fleeting yet vital support in digital images, avatars, and virtual worlds.

The cyborg, the avatar, the connected body, and the digital psychoanalyst serve as a testament to contemporary phenomena—all are, in my opinion, figures through which the psyche explores new modes of figuration, continuity and discontinuity, connection and withdrawal.

This raises fundamental questions. What happens to the processes of symbolization, mourning, and the construction of thought when the object is always available, when technology offers an apparent continuity that denies absence and interruption? How do thinking and fantasy emerge when perception itself is extended and filtered through technical mediations? These are clinical realities that, as psychoanalysts, we face every day—in the adolescent who lives through virtual worlds, in the adult who relates to others only through mediated images or in the collective fictions that question experience.

Yet in the wake of these reflections my aim is to convey a sense of curiosity and hope: even within these hybrid spaces, the capacity to think, to imagine, and to form meaning persists. The task of psychoanalysis, as I understand it, is not to defend the human against technology, but to help the subject articulate the sense of their hybrid condition, to understand our techno-environment in order to continue to create sites for psychic elaboration and thought.

Although fundamentally rooted in psychoanalysis and clinical practice, this book addresses a broad and diverse audience. It is intended for clinicians dealing with technology-mediated lives, neuroscientists, and readers interested in philosophy, psychoanalysis, anthropology, art, technology, and the humanities—and to anyone wishing to reflect on the transformations of our time.

The ethical dimension becomes essential in this volume: to distinguish hybridization—as a creative co-existence between the human and the technical—from colonization, where the algorithmic tends to absorb and standardize the singular. Psychoanalysis, I believe, can help us sustain this difference, keeping alive the space for reflection, alterity, and unpredictability that defines the human experience.

Throughout these pages, I propose that we should listen to psychic life and its own modes of invention. The dialogue between the psychoanalytic and the technological acquires new resonances when placed in contact with the prosthetic, the algorithmic, the virtual. To listen to the technosubject, then, is to listen to the work of transformation—to the psyche as it creates, through technology, new languages for what has not yet been thought.

1 Introductory Note to the Reader

Embodied Archives, Technological Inscriptions

In a book devoted to hybrid identities, robotic alterities, and technologically reconfigured bodies, one might ask: why begin with flamenco—with *taconeo, Duende*,[1] and the breath and vibration of a body in motion? What place do ancestral rhythms and gestures hold in a work centered on avatars, artificial intelligence, and subjects shaped by digital and machinic extensions? Why return to the archaic when the trajectory of this volume leads us toward the post-organic subject?

Before the subject is reshaped by digital architectures or embedded sensors, there is the archaic body—not pre-symbolic, but pre-cybernetic. It is a body that resists archiving and yet transmits. A body that remembers through gesture and rhythm, through skin and silence, rather than through language or code. In flamenco, we encounter a living example of this: a culture embodied, suffered, and transmitted through corporeal acts that resist translation.

As the author argues in Chapter 2, "The Body as a Transmitter of Our Cultural Heritage," cultural memory is not only passed through representation but through the body's affective and rhythmic registers—what Anzieu would call the "Skin-Ego" (1985), where the psychic envelope is formed by the echo of maternal contact, sound, movement and atmosphere.

In this sense, the body is not simply a biological given. It is already an archive—but an embodied one, pulsating with traces of history, trauma, and symbolic loss. As Green reminds us, the body expresses "the cry of a history that was inscribed without having been archived" (Green, 1993, p. 207).

It is also the site where psychic inscription exceeds the possibility of representation.

Drawing from Searles' "theory of the nonhuman environment" (1960), we understand this body to be never isolated. It is in relation to the non-human—textures, objects, rhythms—that the ego finds its grounding. Flamenco, in this sense, is not simply danced; it is inhabited as an ecosystem: of wood and echo, sweat and shadow, silence and communal beat. From this perspective, the environment is not secondary but constitutive of psychic life.

DOI: 10.4324/9781003640684-1

Laplanche (1992/1999) deepens this perspective with his theory of *primal seduction* and the enigmatic message of the other. Cultural forms—songs, rituals, corporeal gestures—function as carriers of such enigmatic signifiers. They arrive through the body, interpellating the infant subject before coherent meaning is possible. In flamenco, one might say, the *Duende* functions as an unresolved message from the cultural other that continues to resonate in the body.

As Latour (1991/1997) reminds us, modern people have been defined by their ability to make clear distinctions between nature and culture, subject and object, human and non-human:

> Modernity is often defined by humanism, either to celebrate the birth of man or to announce his death. But this very habit is modern because it remains asymmetrical. It overlooks the simultaneous birth of "non-humanity," that of things, objects or animals.

This illusion of separation is precisely what this book seeks to deconstruct. The flamenco body, as an "embodied archive," already undermines these binaries: it is neither purely natural nor entirely cultural, neither a mute object nor a speaking subject. It is a site of mediation, a hybrid zone where rhythms, histories, and affects circulate between bodies and environments, humans and non-humans, technologies and rituals. In this sense, the body precedes the machine in its capacity to articulate heterogeneous agencies.

This book does not attempt to preserve the "authentic" body in opposition to its technological extensions. Rather, it aims to trace a psychoanalytic approach of technosubjectivity: the becoming of the subject at the intersection of memory, rhythm, media, and machine. From the flamenco dancer's *taconeo* to the cyborg's antenna, from the skin-ego to the interface, what links these bodies is not only transformation, but the circulation of affects, codes, and intensities.

The post-organic body still resonates with the archaic one. It designates not a body without biology, but a body whose biological basis is no longer sufficient to define it. It is a body reconfigured by its constitutive relation to technical and symbolic environments: by prostheses, digital architectures, algorithmic interfaces, and machinic perceptions. If the archaic body remembers through rhythm, gesture, and silence, the post-organic body inscribes itself through data flows, networks, and synthetic extensions. It is no longer only the projection of a surface (Freud, 1923), or the psychic envelope of the skin (Anzieu, 1985), but a hybrid platform where organic matter and technological inscription co-produce subjectivity. Rather than abolishing the archaic, the post-organic body transforms and reconfigures it, reminding us that every technical mutation is also an anthropological one.

The digital body is haunted by the skin that once spoke through gesture, silence, and rhythm.

Thus, the guiding question of this volume—what happens to the psyche and subjectivity when the body becomes not just a medium, but an interface, a hybrid platform of inscription and modulation?—must be approached through both ends of the spectrum. From embodied archives to algorithmic psyches, from breath to bandwidth, from mourning songs to data flows.

What we propose here is not a binary between the organic and the artificial, but a continuum. The *Duende* is not abolished by the algorithm—it is displaced, reconfigured, perhaps even intensified. The body, long before becoming cyborg, was already more-than-biological: it was a psychosexual body, an emitter, a resonator, a site of cultural elaboration.

The chapters that follow will move across avatars, prostheses, machinic interfaces, and artificial perception. But this point of departure—this flamenco body—reminds us that subjectivity has always been technical (Searles, 1960), always relational (Latour, 1991/1997), and that identity is not a purely internal essence, but a process of inscription, differentiation, and transmission. It emerges through the other in the media—in the broad sense: the maternal voice, the skin as tactile surface, the ritual gesture, the song, the symbol, the interface. From the skin-ego (Anzieu, 1985) to the digital screen, these media are not neutral channels but formative environments. Identity, in this sense, has always been mediated—formed and transformed by the material, inorganic, and affective contexts through which the subject becomes knowable to the other and to itself.

Before turning to cyborgs, prostheses, and machinic interfaces, we will pause before a body that speaks in heel strikes and silences, in rhythms that have travelled through centuries without needing a written archive. In this sense, flamenco is not a detour but a privileged entry point into our inquiry. It allows us to see how the body functions as both archive and a living medium of transmission, how it condenses cultural memory and psychic intensity into corporeal form, and how it inscribes and reconfigures identity without recourse to the digital.

This choice is not accidental. It is grounded in the project "From the Stage to the Couch and from the Couch to the Stage,"[2] which I developed as a dialogue between stage and psychoanalytic couch, where the body itself was placed on stage to explore its performative function as transmitter. Conceived in collaboration with three theatres, the project functioned as a metaphor of research itself: the encounter between scene and couch reflecting the very investigation it staged, showing how movement, atmosphere, and embodied intensity could become vectors of psychic resonance and cultural elaboration.

Flamenco has been selected as the point of departure not for aesthetic or localist reasons, but because it offers a paradigmatic example, from a psychoanalytic perspective, of how the body can become a living archive and transmitter of cultural heritage, sustaining an active "mute language" (Laplanche, 1992/1999; Mancia, 2006) that precedes and runs parallel to the mother tongue. Its untranslatable elements—*Duende, temple, taconeo*—have no equivalents in other languages or traditions because they are not mere words: they are bodily imprints of archaic inscriptions, cultural marks that only acquire meaning in the performative act and in transmission from body to body.

Moreover, flamenco occupies the psychic region of *agieren*, the creative act that resists reduction to representation or to codified choreography. As García Lorca (1922) observed, the *Duende* "is a struggle, not a thought," and in this sense it aligns with a clinic of action, where the essential occurs in the immediacy of gesture, in the time of encounter, rather than in reflective discourse. This sets it apart from other dance forms, where formal structures and repetition often dominate over the live emergence of the act.

Finally, flamenco also constitutes a matrix of transgenerational transmission. Its oral and corporeal tradition, resistant to writing and standardization, carries signifiers that traverse generations, forming what Roussillon (2008) would call a *proto-narrative language*: a mode of storytelling that is born in the body, organized within it, and communicated directly to other bodies. This triple condition—untranslatable body language, irreducible creative act, and transgenerational matrix—makes flamenco a privileged case for exploring how the body inscribes, preserves, and transforms cultural memory. In this sense, beginning with flamenco allows the book to open from a terrain where the body functions as an archaic technology of memory and affect, and at the same time as a matrix of mediation between the singular and the collective, the archaic and the contemporary, without the need for external supports. The next chapter will dwell on this terrain. From this living embodiment, the discussion can move toward contemporary configurations of the body—cyborgs, prostheses, avatars—showing that although supports and environments may change, the function of conveying, inscribing, and transforming remains constant.

Notes

1 *Taconeo* and *Duende* are both untranslatable signifiers linked to the Spanish flamenco music and dancing.

2 A performance work with actors that was grounded in Teatros Luchana in Madrid.

References

Anzieu, D. (1985). *Le moi-peau*. Dunod.

Freud, S. (1923). El yo y el ello. In *El yo y el ello y otras obras*, Vol. 19. Amorrortu Editores, pp. 21–29.

García Lorca, F. (1922). *Arquitectura del cante jondo. Donde no se hiela el tiempo. Escritos sobre música*. Editorial Continta Me tienes.

Green, A. (1993). *Le travail du négatif*. Éditions de Minuit.

Laplanche, J. (1992/1999). *Entre séduction et inspiration: L'homme*. PUF.

Latour, B. (1991/1997). *Nous n'avons jamais été modernes. Essai d'anthropologie symétrique*. Editions la Découverte.
Mancia, M. (2006). *Sentir de las palabra: Archivos sonoros de la memoria implícita y musicalidad de la transferencia*. Editorial Lumen, Colección Humanitas.
Roussillon, R. (2008). *Le transitionnel, le sexuel et la réflexivité*. Editions Dunod.
Searles, H. (1960). *L'environnement non humain*. Editions Gallimard.

2 The Body as a Transmitter of Our Cultural Heritage

The following chapter does not aim to study flamenco as a cultural object in itself, but rather to use it as a privileged entry point into the psychoanalytic question of the body. Flamenco offers a striking example of how the body functions as an archive, a medium of cultural transmission, and a site of inscription where memory and affect take form. By approaching flamenco, what we are ultimately exploring is the enigma of the body—the archaic, the preverbal, the skin-ego (Anzieu, 1985)—as a transmitter of heritage. In this sense, flamenco is less the subject than the magnifying glass through which the body reveals its archaic function of transmission.

The topic of the *cuerpo–Körper–body–corps*, with its diverse meanings in different languages, represents an enigma.

The work I will expand on below aims to approach the body in the context of flamenco in Spain. It is about applied psychoanalysis in the field of flamenco dance; it is a question of body language.

I would like to discuss the difficulty I have had for weeks, when I tried to surround the body with any signifier to which I have access, whether Spanish, French, or English. The first pitfall I faced was that *cuerpo–corps–body* opens up for me three different universes. I lie in a paradox when I try to translate the untranslatable. With the three language references, I have tried to capture the "Body" from the secondary process in order to transmit something that has to do with body language, with the archaic, the primary, the first ego, the skin-ego as Anzieu would say.

I went to Freud and his conception of the body:

> The ego is first and foremost a bodily ego, it is not merely a surface entity, but is itself the projection of a surface … The ego is ultimately derived from bodily sensations, chiefly from those springing from the surface of the body. It may thus be regarded as a mental projection of the surface of the body, besides, as we have seen above, representing the superficies of the mental apparatus.
>
> (Freud, 1923b, p. 26)

DOI: 10.4324/9781003640684-2

Starting from the drive (Freud, 1915) and the "Ego first and foremost bodily" (Freud, 1923a), this reflection aims to go deeper into the body as a transmitter of our cultural heritage. In other words, I attempt to delve into the articulation between the social basin and culture, where the body nests. As Freud would say, individual psychology is always a social psychology (1923a).

In this chapter, I would like to draw to your attention the popular flamenco culture, to the extent that culture is the meeting place for projection and the expression of human spirit. That culture is, in my opinion, construction and creation, in the service of Eros. In Spain and in its reference to what is profoundly Spanish, *El Duende* of the social imagination is inevitably linked to art, music, and flamenco dance.

"I will see if I can give you a simple lesson on the hidden spirit of *aching* Spain"—this was F. García Lorca's introduction to his lecture "Theory and Play of the *Duende*" (Garcia Lorca, 1933).[1] The aching spirit of Spain takes form through the *Duende*, and the *Duende*, as we shall see next, takes shape through the body.

The *Duende* alludes to the creative process in the body. Garcia Lorca stated: "*El Duende* is a struggle and not a thought … it is a true living style, of blood, of an ancient culture, a creation in act" (Garcia Lorca, 1933).[2]

In my opinion, this is very interesting for us psychoanalysts, because we are indeed in front of a clinic of the acting-out, of the *agieren* and not of the thinking nor the associating. The *Duende* is an act.

"The *Duende* does not repeat itself, as the shapes of the sea do not repeat themselves in the squall,"[3] Garcia Lorca said (1933).

Is the *Duende* a sublimation from the very beginning, maybe an attempt at linking through a peculiar body language?

In the regions of *El Duende*, the boundaries of the ego with those of the object are almost blurred. It would be a world very close to narcissistic unity, to fusion/confusion, where there is, in my opinion, an attempt of differentiation.

In addition to the *Duende*, I would like to mention the *Temple*, another type of music, which reconstructs that kind of "timing" that comes out of the body, a music of silence in which the dancer dares to intervene or not through his repertoire of gestures.

El Temple is also that throat clearing, an attempt to situate oneself in the tone of the guitar before the *cante*[4] (flamenco chant) starts. Not only are the body's musical silences important, but also the distance between them. The possibility of engaging in a dialogue emerges through gestures. The names that are attributed to the silence also seem to be untranslatable, for example in relation to the musical figure of the white note. In this case the translation of the silence varies greatly: "silence of white" (Spanish), "minim rest" (British English), "half rest" (American English), "half pause" (French). We know that the music and the voice linked to the body have been of interest for some psychoanalysts for years.

Since I am trying to approach impossible definitions, I find it interesting to underline that *there is no translation* of these concepts into other languages.

The *bailao*r's (flamenco dancer's) body, evokes characteristics deeply rooted in the specificity of our Spanish culture, such as the *Duende* or the *Temple*.

In Spain nobody knows what the *Duende* or the *Temple* are—no one has ever seen them. We only know that sometimes the *Duende*, together with its *Temple*, appears from inside the bodies of the *torero* (bullfighter) or the *bailaor* (flamenco dancer). The *Duende* constitutes a supreme expression of the flamenco art that takes shape in the body. Something like if the Id was paving the way to sculpt the body, it would be a soul without a word, which, if it expresses itself, it does it in a true way and exclusively in the body. The body's ego provokes emotion in other bodies because it touches the peak point, the reminiscences of body-to-body return.

I find it interesting here to compare the signifier "*torero*" and its translation "bullfighter," a fighter of bulls would have nothing to do with what a Spaniard imagines when he hears the word "*torero*." As a *torero* has nothing to do with a fighter against bulls, every night the *torero*, in the square, faces a mythical fight against death. It is the struggle of human fragility endowed with intelligence against the brutal force of the beast.

The register of movements between the *Duende* and the *Temple* contains the difference in repetition as if it were a spell against death. The bodies of the bullfighter and the dancer are faced with death; every night, the dancer or the bullfighter is reborn; they are successful in the attempt to reunite the "initial gesture." Does the man of this land think he is more immortal than others in other places?

"Spain is the only country where death is a national spectacle," as Garcia Lorca (1933) reminded us. And, returning to flamenco, within the flamenco constellation it is also necessary to emphasize the importance of those who accompany the *bailaor*.

I would like to mention the *jaleadores*[5] and the *palmeros*[6] who in turn surround the *bailaor*, driven by the dancer's *Duende* to find their own *Duende*: a body describing more with its palms, its intensity, its sound, the *olés*. "In all Arab music, song or elegy, the arrival of *Duende* is greeted with vigorous cries of Allah! Allah!, so close to the olé! of the bullfight, and who knows whether they are not the same," Garcia Lorca reminded us (1933, p. 124).[7]

At the same time, the *jaleadores*, that is to say the chorus, like the Greek choir of the classical theatre, emit sounds from inside their bodies, more painfully, with all tonality and intensity of an infinite fan. These are tools that ignite other bodies, it is the "big-bang" of a co-creation.

El Duende Talks About Creation in the Body, Body-to-Body or Bodies Inciting Other Bodies

Would this point have to do with the unconscious communicating with the unconscious, with its identifications body-to-body, and perhaps as clinicians, drawing a parallel with our work, with a cultural countertransference?

Could we imagine—this is my hypothesis—the echoes of the drive with history, returning through those bodies? I mean a drive colored by the transgenerational, the cultural, and the social.

Roussillon (2006) proposes to think of the drive as a "messenger"—a messenger that develops and is transmitted through three languages born of three forms of representation: the word presentation-representative for verbal language, the thing (and action) presentation- representative for the language of the act and of different corporeal expressiveness, and the affect-representative for the language of affect.

Together with the body, the *untranslatable signifiers* to other languages arise as witnesses of an art like flamenco, which are specific to certain people and certain geographical areas, transmitted only by oral tradition, which in my opinion cannot really stop questioning us. This is why I decided to think about this subject matter.

Laplanche will refer to adult implantation of enigmatic signifiers in the psychophysiological dermis of the *Infans,* in other words, he will refer to unmetabolized and untranslatable elements. Will what I expose have to do with this quality of enigmatic archaic implantation in the corporeal? That which has to do with the body has no translation.

Could we then think of the impossibility of translating a language linked to the body, a language witnessing the passage from *body to body* within a certain culture?

"There is no doubt that the guitar has built the *cante jondo*.[8] It has ploughed, deepened, the dark oriental, Jewish and Arabic ancient mass, *stammering* because of that,"[9] Garcia Lorca wrote (1933, p. 24).

The *cante jondo* is the deep chant; it is considered the deepest chant within the Andalusian music. In the Spanish language the "j" has been replaced by the "h."

In the flamenco world, the signifier *cante jondo* has remained as an immovable rock in the Iberian peninsula.

I will slightly digress to point out that although there are different hypotheses about the origins of flamenco, its appearance is reported in the eighteenth century. Flamenco art is not just linked to the gypsy ethnicity; it existed before they arrived in the Iberian peninsula. The gypsies came later to Andalusia and other regions of Spain and Europe, although this art was only developed and cultivated in the Andalusian region. It is an art that developed between the gypsy and the Andalusian. The gypsies come from an unlettered culture and they do not know their origins. They build myths to explain them—for example, in relation to the Bible they believe themselves the cursed offspring of Cain.

If the guitar builds the *cante jondo,* the body sculpts the deepest spirit of the ego, not vice versa.

As long as they are pre-verbal, are the body and culture inside of the body stammering, musical, gestural?

Which archaic corporeal representations would have translation? Would they be in this sense symbolized? I come back here to my starting point, which is to the impossible mission of trying to capture the untranslatable.

In psychoanalysis when we think about origins in the mother tongue of the individuals, we think about the primary relationship of the *Infans* bathed in a surrounding symbolic universe and immersed in a world of sensory and perceptual experiences. The human breeding will be filled with mnemic traces (traces of perception, traces of smell, touch, texture ... and the terrible traces of the non-trace), which will gradually make up their representations. These are sensorial proto-experiences.

But what, really, is that mother tongue? To the extent that every individual is born bilingual, crossed by his mother tongue and by another mute language of word presentation (language of the body). What we call mother tongue comes to substitute or to live with that mute tongue basis of the drive, and the drive is at the same time looking for a representation. Is it possible that some of these languages dominate the other?

Could we imagine a mute language, a "clandestine" body holding a culture? Clandestine, because the body that I refer to here, the one of the untranslatable signifiers linked to an "Ego first and foremost bodily," sinks its roots in the Id and lives in the splitting. There is no knowledge of what is in the body. Mancia (2006) refers to repressed unconscious and pre-verbal experiences stored in the implicit memory. These are experiences that cannot be remembered; they can only be experienced at best in the psychoanalytic relationship or in the body.

The succession in the time of bodies and their juxtaposition weaves culture; a body is always a culture. As the constructions in psychoanalysis weave and create psyche, they also build representations and psychization. Here the body creates sense, carries a message; it is the protagonist of the creation of links and emotions. Like with our patients, the body is also the protagonist of the transference/countertransference co-creation. We know that if we access our body, we have access to the unthinkable of the patient.

Is flamenco a "body language" with the *characteristics of a matrix myth,* a device with transforming potential (sense-generating and symbol transformer), which would be the symbolic organizer of a world?

In my hypothesis, the flamenco untranslatable signifiers would only be the *echo of a time and space characteristic of a certain culture.* The times and spaces would return as symbolic organizers of other times and spaces, and so on because every culture and each body has its time and its spaces.

For this, I intend to address the multidimension of *time and space of that untranslatable language*. My initial assumption is that the untranslatable language would come back marking the specific times and spaces of the particular signifiers of a language. These signifiers are at the same time the mirage of the ancient culture that we intuit through those bodies. To this end, I will begin by illustrating this proposal through the spectacle *Tan solo* of the well-known *bailaor* Manuel Reyes.

Tan Solo

Again, the untranslatable—or at least, the difficulty of translating! *Tan solo* is not *a solo*, nor does it mean just being alone (as "solo" is the Spanish translation for alone). I had seen the show (*Tan Solo* of Manuel Reyes) and, despite the Spanish saying "a picture is worth more than a thousand words," I thought maybe I could get closer to my understanding of what I was looking for through the artist's body presence and have an exchange of words with him. My assumption was that the body's presence of both participants was fundamental for the deep encounter. The fact that some psychoanalysts are exposed to the current question of the presence-absence of the body through online requests, is clearly a highly topical issue.

The *Bailaor* Through the Interview

I met Manuel Reyes on a stage. I remember a human being as naked on a naked stage. Only during some moments we were surprised by some videos that he had made. In those videos, he was using his facial language to describe himself. He was dancing and showing his facial language to tell the story of a life. His silences, his rhythms and his music reigned. But also, the elegance of the Spanish arrogant man, the defiant human being who risks all that he is with only one gesture, emerged.

Close to the catastrophe identified with the *bailaor*, I wondered how we would reach the end. Remembering today *Tan solo*, aching Spain returned to me. *Tan solo* is pain, it is the artist's pain in body-to-body (because the pain has to do with the body), but it is also Spain's ache returning in a body, the deaths and our tragedy coming back. It is hard not to cry, not to stop blinking or holding your breath. My body in consonance with others has been sunk by those other bodies with their rhythms.

I decided to hold an interview with the artist. I remember our first telephone contact, in which I explained what my interests were. I felt a growing difficulty between us, and he asked: "But what do you want from me?" Perplexed, I answered: "What do you mean by what do I want from you?" We didn't understand each other. He proposed a telephone interview and I insisted on the importance of meeting in person. Throughout that interview, Manuel explained to me that *Tan solo* has to do with the double meaning (in Spanish) of *Tan solo*: on the one hand, his loneliness, "how lonely I am," on the other hand, "it is just this." A few words, I told myself, to describe an inner world, a life.

MR: It's hard to say it with words. In my show there is an allusion to ballet, it's the starting point of a dancer; ballet is not a natural dance but I considered ballet to be the mother of all dances. I'm a *bailaor* with a ballet dancing culture. I believe that the *farruca*[10] allows me to unite the *bailaor*'s and the ballet worlds. In flamenco I seek a new movement. You talk about your roots and your person. Once you dance, you cannot hide who you are. One can see right away if you are pessimistic or if the world is aching.

I continued with a question:

LE: In one of the videos where you talk, you define yourself as a martyr of the beat, what do you mean by this?

MR: I'm rhythmic, I have an inner rhythm. This is very important for me. I find it hard to free myself to a movement. I'm methodical. I like to have everything controlled, although there are things that I no longer control. I'm authoritarian and I have a prepotent attitude. It's something I have tried to soften as the years pass. When I say *"olé"* it is because I feel that something has to be so. It's when it's real.

LE: So in the rhythm we talk about time?

MR: We talk about beat. In flamenco the rhythms are of two, four, six or twelve, as flamencos we use those rhythms. I'm a gypsy and it's our music.

Without pretending to carry out an analysis of the artist, which it is not the aim of this work, I would like to highlight how he conveys his suffering over the stage and underline the great masochism that follows from his speech. Manuel is subjected, he's a slave to the rhythm. The flamenco gypsy rhythm is its identity; he mentions the beat, what it has to do with time, it is his tempo. But there is something very important in what he says: he is a *bailaor* with a ballet dancer culture, he is a gypsy *bailaor* subjected to very demanding rules, the ones of the ballet. He does not only dance his roots but he dances within the rigor imposed on him: the frame, the setting, the ballet laws, are his "ballet dancer culture." To emerge from the rhythm of the beat would mean to emerge from the fusion, from the cultural and maternal fusion in the body-to-body within the ballet laws, the law as the oedipal third that forces to leave the fusion. I continued:

LE: What are you looking for with the gesture?

MR: I look for my mind to be in line with my emotion. The emotion is equated with that aesthetic concept. Each movement is a set. At the end of the farruca I show the dilemma; it is reflected through the moment where I am with the ballet dancer's slipper or the *bailaor*'s boot. I did not want to leave Spain or my mother's house.

Between the boot and slipper, here is the dilemma: to leave the mother or not. Then I said:

LE: You surprise us with a video where you seem stunned …
MR: That's the dilemma. It torments me less since I began to remember who I really am. I have had a lot of confidence and then I spent time lacking confidence. I regained my confidence when I began to accept myself. *Tan solo* is mostly a reaction.

There is something unusual in flamenco; it is that moment where you are alone, you are singing and dancing at the same time … it is a *bulería*,[11] it's a popular expression of my personality. It is pure *Tan solo*. I mark the rhythm. From his omnipotence the artist becomes the master.

LE: Why do you talk about loneliness?
MR: Most of the time I've worked alone. I may have good manners but maybe I reject human contact. I only think about my family and people who are part of my environment.

The paradox: he does not care about others but he dances for them. He laments his loneliness, *Tan solo*/solo/alone. He looks for loneliness because he probably cannot do it in any other way. And his solo allows him to be unique, it's an achieved narcissistic satisfaction.

LE: What do you feel in the body when you dance?
MR: You have to struggle with the technique to get a balance with your emotions.
LE: Do you realize you aren't answering what I'm asking?
MR: If I'm struggling with the technique I feel tension, if I think of my inner battles I feel tension.

He talks alone. In my opinion, it is notable how he ignores contact with me.

The *Bailaor* Through the Show

In the darkness the curtain opens, *Tan solo* of Manuel Reyes will begin. We talk about the dark. Garcia Lorca (1933) stated that:

> Neither in the Spanish dance nor in the bullfighting do people have fun; the *Duende* is in charge of making others *suffer*, by means of drama through *living shapes* he prepares the stairs for an evasion of the surrounding reality.[12]

Spectators, *bailaores* and *cantaores* recreate the Arena of ancient Rome centuries later; thanks to Freud's contribution, the social imaginary leads us to a new dream. I propose in this article to dream flamenco, its music and dance. I refer to dreaming because of the difficulty of using words when we refer to thing-presentations.

I also resort to the dream because the myth is an extension of the dream, the type of deformation of the myth is the same as the oneiric one. The myth comes to erase the painful feelings of the popular sentiment.

Something is locked away from the word world, and I wonder if that is the painful thing. Is it something that maybe wants to remain in the body and not leave it?

Back on stage, a tacit and secret agreement settles among those of us gathered there. This is important, an open secret without translation into words; I mean the body. In the here and now and/or in the awakenings of yesteryear, time and space return. Let's remember Winnicott's (1953) article: "Transitional Objects and Transitional Phenomena," in which he addresses the issue of the transitional space, a kind of area experience, an intermediate space outcome. It is another space and another time where bodies inhabit, music bodies, the resonance of other bodies, bodies surrounded by others, those of the audience, the *jaleadores*, the *palmeros*. Rhythms arise, we are first shaken by a *farruca*, later by a *seguiriya gitana* (gypsy *siguiriya*),[13] the *seguiriya* is part of the group called *cante jondo*.

"The gypsy *seguiriya* begins with a *terrible cry* … as if this chant was not the most refined expression of an old universal culture," Garcia Lorca (1933) wrote.

It is based in a terrible cry, it is a deep lament, it's the *quejío* flamenco. It is about anguish, death, famine. It's a cry of fright, the nameless terror (Bion, 1962), it is the cry of the newborn at birth, maybe comparable to the birth of the origin of the world.

The body of the transgenerational (Faimberg, 2005) also turns into transitional *space* (Winnicott, 1953) and becomes the stage for the transmission and communication of many other bodies, those of the past and those of the present. In his article "The Claims of Psychoanalysis to Scientific Interest," Freud (1913) highlighted that by language we should not simply comprehend the expression of thoughts in words, but we must also understand the language of gestures and all forms of psychic expression.

"I treat my show like a novel, it has its own outcome and resolution:" These are Manuel's words. The body here is, in my opinion, a body carrying a potential message. As Roussillon would state in "To Introduce the Question of the Body and the Act" (Roussillon, 2006, p. 1):[14] "The body is a 'kind of proto-narrative language'. It is a body traversed by signifier forms, those that can be potentially organised into words; body language is another kind of language."

It is interesting to remember that Garcia Lorca titles his lecture "Theory and *Play* of the *Duende*." The *Duende* bursts into the blood but occurs in the play, in the universes of multidimensionality of time and space that the playing allows. The beats of these bodies narrate alone or along with the melody's rhythm of others. In *Tan solo* there are images (we have the example of the video in Manuel's show), gestures, movements, and words. The *bailaor* is not only reflected in the mirror but he dives into it, like Alice in Lewis Carroll's novel which is, in my opinion, a way of telling and transforming himself.

Back on stage, the *bailaor* is accompanied by the *taconeo*,[15] again another word without translation; that heel strike, heart strike (like our heartbeat), disruptive music, a kind of millenary and immortal singing that returns intact through the mortal bodies. The time of before is a present time rediscovered through the mortal body.

The *taconeo* music accentuates and agitates. In my interpretation, Manuel does not dance alone—he dances his loneliness because they have left him alone, he dances his emptiness because, as he says, "it is only this." He interrogates with his body and some words his being and his becoming. He creates with his body in motion multiplicity in search of identity.

Any formal election (the form) is a way of being. In Spanish we literally say "form of being" (*forma de ser*) when we allude to the traits of the characters. His gypsy race and its origin appear in the surface, in his body: "I have had extensive ballet training and having gypsy roots the dilemma between classical and flamenco occurs."

Manuel clarified that he has composed the music of the *farruca;* he doesn't know how to write or read music, he sings the music that he needs to the musicians. Are these bodies loaded with rhythm and sound not only equivalent to the inner world of the *bailaor* or *cantaor* but also analogous to an old millenary culture?

The Different Times and Spaces in the Body as Fruit of an Ancient Culture

Paul Valéry (1936) writes in *Philosophy of the Dance* that "The dance is a transposed action in another world, in a sort of 'space-time' that is no longer exactly that of everyday life."[16]

In his *Phenomenology of Perception,* Merleau-Ponty commented: "It should not be said that our body is in the space or in the time. The body inhabits space and time." Our body inhabits time and space maybe because first it was music (because at first there were sounds and the surrounding universe of the word), for instance, the mother's heart's music in the maternal womb. The well-known plastic artist Jaume Plensa, through his work *Love Sounds* illustrates this issue: "The sound of blood speaks the same language."[17]

Back on stage, the music of the bodies, as Lévi-Strauss would say in a very beautiful way, becomes a time-suppression machine.

In the *après coup* of the dance emerges the transgenerational and, through it, the story of the narcissistic identifications which constitute the subject. The alienating identifications split from the ego also arise. Haydee Faimberg has commented that these are identifications that correspond to another generation: the identification cause is found in the story of another, it responds to an individual's intrusion and appropriation. Does Manuel's work constitute an attempt of recomposing, a way of elaborating his identifications in order to be able to recover an identity that has given him, as he said, "greater confidence"? Each identification is accompanied by his music, by his gestures, by the music of today and then, Manuel is *bailaor* and dances his gypsy rhythm, the gypsy ethnic rhythm.

Is that new body (the one of the dance), which rises on the stage, the one that counterposes to another "motionless" body, a time creation engine where there is not?

Can we imagine a matrix-symbolic body that at the same time engenders and collects those old sounds as an attempt to create the past through the de-identifications?

Daniel Sibony (1995) coined the term time-object, time-carrying bodies, a body with the ability to receive inscription of time, these are bodies-time more than desiring bodies. For the object- time to emerge, it is necessary that others (objects-time) accompany it, making the time possible. The time is built when there is an encounter with the other and something is registered in the psyche. Freud describes a timeless unconscious; Sibony would say that the unconscious does not know the time because the unconscious is the time, perhaps suggesting that time is the unconscious; it is only transformed into a time-object when another has been able to come in order to link and shape the time. The time-objects are the transmitters of a possible time.

Indeed, there is not only linear time, nor circular time, nor time of repetition in the transference, or the one which is symbolized in the *après coup*, but there is a connective time.

Let's go back to the music and its times. What are the gesture and the initial gesture that the artist talks about? Are instants built through gestures? Is it a point? There are instants that are just instants, they do not link, they appear and disappear. One is born and one dies, all in one instant. Music, noises, rhythms, presences, and absences are chained in an instant.

There are privileged instants where the *bailaor* stops because the *Duende* appears and with it depth, there is an "*olé*" that comes from inside, there are ruptures that are not symptoms, they are not accidents, they are just events and expressions.

Moreno (2016) differentiates a "thinking inward" as an understanding, which has to do with the associative capacity of representations but at the same time is a proceeding separate from representations, it involves a contact with the outside; it is what he has called the connective proceeding. The associative and the connective intervene in the process of the individual's subjectivation.

I find it interesting to think of the hypothesis of the connective in the body as a new way of knowledge. Until today this way of thinking was not of interest because of the rigor of the science that promoted a closed system in the sense of a cause-effect system.

It is in this case, through the lattice of presentations, that the deepest of the flamenco culture appears. This is my hypothesis—and that it is also in the contact with the outside and through the succession of all the instants that the old flamenco culture emerges.

In this sense, "the *jondura flamenca* is born from the *jondo* dance and not the opposite,"[18] as Didi-Huberman (2006, p. 75) writes. It does not preexist as the root, there are unconscious vestiges, but the gesture sculpts in each new instant an origin. This would be the connective.

The Flamenco Culture Appears in the Body and at the Same Time it is Built in the Instant

In turn, the *bailaor* produces his time shape. As Freud (1929) wrote in *Civilization and Its Discontents*:

> In mental life nothing which has once been formed can perish—that everything is somehow preserved and that in suitable circumstances (when, for instance, regression goes back enough) it can once more be brought to light.
>
> (Freud, 1929, p. 69)

Andalusian culture and history, with all of their losses, flourish through the gypsy body. According to Blas Infante, the term *flamenco* appears because of an *Andalusí*[19] expression. Here, the meaning is what we have discussed since the beginning of this text: the *flamenco* is a "peasant without land."

The exploration of flamenco allows us to see that the body is never reducible to its organic substrate: it is always already symbolic, inhabited by cultural echoes and transgenerational inscriptions. This insight leads us directly to the next question: if the body has always functioned as an archive and transmitter of culture, what happens when this body becomes reconfigured by technology? The transition from the archaic to the post-organic body, from the flamenco stage to the digital interface, opens the path toward a genealogy of technosubjectivities, where anthropological mutation reshapes the very conditions of embodiment and subjectivation.

Notes

1 My translation.
2 My translation.
3 My translation.

4 Flamenco singing is one of the three main components of flamenco, along with *toque* (playing the guitar) and *baile* (dance). A *cante* singer is a *cantaor* or *cantaora*.
5 Performer of *jaleo*, which is the flamenco word for cheering called out to the performers; they are shouts to cheer the singers, the guitarists, or the dancers. It is done to accompany the rhythm of the music.
6 Performer of *palmas*. Hand clapping—it is an intricate art, requiring skill and knowledge of compass (flamenco beat).
7 My translation.
8 The *cante jondo* is a vocal style of flamenco, an unspoiled folk chant, which means in Andalusian "deep song." According to F.G. Lorca: "It is a rare example of a primitive song, the oldest of all Europe, where the ruins of history, the lyrical fragment eaten by the sand, appears live like the first morning of its life."
9 My translation.
10 Etymologically, it would come from the Arab word *"faruq,"* which means courageous. It is a typical form of flamenco music, traditionally danced only by men. According to some authors, *"farruco"* is the word that is used in Andalusia to denominate people from Galicia.
11 It is among the most popular and dramatic forms in the flamenco—it often ends any flamenco gathering.
12 My translation.
13 This is one of the most ancient and tragic chants in flamenco. It is mostly based on a deep lament where there is almost an absence of words.
14 My translation. Roussillon (2006).
15 Rhythmic patterns made by the boot's heel.
16 My translation.
17 *Love Sounds* is an art installation. This quote is from a personal conversation with the artist.
18 My translation.
19 The language Arab *Andalusí* used to be an Arab dialect spoken in Spain and Portugal between the thirteenth and fifteenth centuries. It became a dead language with the expulsion of the Moors. However, nowadays it is used in *Andalusí* music.

References and Further Reading

Anzieu, D. (1985). *Le moi-peau*. Dunod.

Bergamín, J. (1961). *La importancia del demonio. La decadencia del analfabetismo*. Ediciones Siruela.

Bion, W.R. (1962). *Learning from experience*. William Heinemann Medical Books.

Dastur, F. (2016). Le fondement corporel de la subjectivité. In *Chair et langage. Essais sur Merleau-Ponty*. Éditions les belles lettres.

Didi-Huberman, G. (2006). *Le danseur des solitudes*. Les Éditions de Minuit.

Ezquerra, L. (2010). *Babel en el diván. Revista de la conserjería de educación*. Ministerio de Educación.

Faimberg, H. (2005). *El telescopaje de generaciones. A la escucha de los lazos narcisistas entre generaciones*. Amorrortu Editores.

Freud, S. (1913). El interés por el psicoanálisis. In *Totem y Tabú y otras obras*, Vol. 13. Amorrortu Editores, pp. 179–192.

Freud, S. (1915). Pulsiones y destinos de pulsión. In *Contribución a la historia del movimiento psicoanalítico. Trabajo sobre metapsicología y otras obras*, Vol. 14. Amorrortu Editores, pp. 105–134.

Freud, S. (1923a). El yo y el ello. In *El yo y el ello y otras obras*, Vol. 19. Amorrortu Editores, pp. 21–29.
Freud, S. (1923b). *The ego and the id*, Vol. 19. Hogarth Press.
Freud, S. (1929). El Malestar en la cultura. In *El porvenir de una ilusión. El malestar en la cultura y otras obras*, Vol. 21. Amorrortu Editores, pp. 56–96.
Garcia Lorca, F. (1922). *Arquitectura del cante jondo. Donde no se hiela el tiempo. Escritos sobre música*. Editorial Continta Me Tienes.
Garcia Lorca, F. (1933). *Juego y teoría del duende. Donde no se hiela el tiempo. Escritos sobre música*. Editorial Continta Me Tienes.
Garcia Lorca, F. (1928). *Canciones de cuna españolas. Donde no se hiela el tiempo. Escritos sobre música*. Editorial Continta Me Tienes.
Grassi, L. (2014). The dimension of sound and rhythm in psychic structuring and analytic work. *Italian Psychoanalytic Annual*, 8: 63–82.
Mancia, M. (2006). *Sentir las palabras. Archivos sonoros de la memoria implícita y musicalidad de la transferencia*. Editorial Lumen.
Merleau-Ponty, M. (1945). *Phénoménologie de la perception*. Éditions Gallimard.
Moreno, J. (2016). Presentaciones del ir y del venir. In *El psicoanálisis interrogado. De las causas al devenir*. Lugar Editorial.
Marzano, M. (2007). *La philosophie du corps*. Presses Universitaires de France.
Roussillon, R. (2006). *Pour introduire la question du langage du corps et de l'acte*. Editions Cazaubon.
Sibony, D. (1995). Danse et temps. In *Le corps et sa danse*. Éditions du Seuil, pp. 186–192.
Quignard, P. (2013). *L'origine de la danse*. Éditions Galilée.
Valéry, P. (1936). *Philosophie de la danse*. Éditions Gallimard.
Winnicott, D.W. (1953). Transitional objects and transitional phenomena—A study of the first not-me possession. *International Journal of Psychoanalysis*, 34: 89–97.
Winnicott, D.W. (1971). *Realidad y juego*. Editorial Gedisa.

3 From the Archaic Body to the Post-Organic Body

Psychoanalysis, Technology and Anthropological Mutation in the Genealogy of Technosubjectivities

This chapter is situated at the point of articulation between two radically different configurations: the archaic body, transmitter of a cultural heritage inscribed in gestural, rhythmic and symbolic memory, and the post-organic body, shaped by continuous interaction with technical devices and virtual environments. As I mentioned in the introduction to this book, this transition does not imply the disappearance of the human, but rather its re-inscription in a polyphonic network of multiple, hybrid, and mutating bodies where the organic and the inorganic, the natural and the artificial, the animate and the inanimate co-exist and co-constitute each other.

It is within this shift—from embodied memory to distributed and networked subjectivity—that we can situate Žižek's (1998) observation: through cyberspace we are moving from a modernist culture of computation to the postmodern culture of simulation and dissemination, that is, a network without a center, where processes are always complex and non-transparent.

If Žižek highlights the decentering and opacity of the processes in which subjectivity is now inscribed, Bruno Latour (1991) had already dismantled the modern fiction of a clear separation between nature and culture, subject and object, human and non-human. He radicalizes this by showing that we have never inhabited a world of pure separations, but have always lived immersed in networks of mediations where the human and the non-human co-constitute each other. Both perspectives converge in revealing a condition in which human identity is no longer self-contained, but always already implicated in a web of heterogeneous agencies.

This conceptual displacement not only undermines the stability of classical ontological boundaries; it also opens the way to rethink the psychosexual body and the subject as open, porous entities, traversed by material and symbolic flows that exceed their current form.

In this framework, the notion of virtualization proposed by Pierre Lévy (1998) offers a fundamental key to understanding. Far from implying a loss of reality, for Lévy virtualization constitutes an identity mutation: a shift of the ontological center of gravity of the subject towards a problematic field of possibilities, where identity is constructed and reconstructed in a space open to constant transformation.

DOI: 10.4324/9781003640684-3

Virtual reality is not an imitation of our lives, but rather a reality that makes humans more complex. *Online/on-life* reality as an undifferentiated continuum simultaneously questions notions of distortion, deception, and play, thus alluding to "illusion" and its Latin root *ludere*. A culture, in this sense of illusion, where subjects are extended by technological objects, is already part of our intimacy; in turn, these gadgets modify us, extend us, thus questioning the twist in our representative universe.

Take, for example, the link we establish with our smartphones or the "Metaverse," the latter being an immersive virtual reality that allows the subject to represent their own body with its infinite derivations, giving them back a sense of vital presence and thus questioning how we perceive, process, and shape the world we live in. Our intimacy, increasingly exposed through social media and the rise of facial recognition on our smartphones, to name just two examples, is fractured and mutates into a kind of "extimacy" traversed by algorithms and sensorialities of a new quality.

The technological tool used by the subject to transform the world modifies the user; the technological object may even contain a part of its owner through various forms of recording. In this sense, the psychosexual body in psychoanalysis is no longer defined by its current form—it finds its consistency in a problematic field, open to possible transformations that exceed it and to relationships and mediations that condition both its experience and its symbolizing possibilities. This shift requires us to rethink the psychosexual body and the subject as an open entity, traversed by material and symbolic flows that exceed its current form and actively participate in its definition.

The contemporary body is one of those knots of mediation in which living matter, technical artefacts, symbolic inscriptions, and imaginary projections are intertwined. From this perspective, there is no technical "outside" acting on an immutable organic "inside"; there is an onto-technological continuum in which the always porous boundary between the two is constantly shifting.

As José Ortega y Gasset anticipated in his *Meditation on the Technique*[1] (Ortega y Gasset, 1939), human life cannot be thought without its technical dimension:

> without technique man would not exist nor ever have existed. What no one can doubt is that for a long time now technique has been inserted among the inescapable conditions of human life, in such a way that present-day man could not, even if he wished, live without it. It is today one of the greatest dimensions of our life, one of the major ingredients that integrate our destiny. Today man no longer lives in nature, but is housed in the super-nature he has created in a new day of Genesis: technique.[2]

Ortega's formulation already reveals that technique is not an external prosthesis but an essential habitat for human existence. This intuition converges with contemporary psychoanalytic approaches to technosubjectivity: the subject is not simply mediated by technology, but constituted within a technical environment that functions as both container and condition of psychic life.

Transplants are another example where a circulation of organs is organized between the living and the dead, between human and non-human species, with technology at the center: baboon hearts implanted in humans, pig livers, hormones produced by bacteria flowing in the blood of their recipients. These are cases that illustrate an unprecedented material and symbolic continuity. In this hyper-circuit of assembly, cyborgs represent another form of biotechnology: prostheses, implants and artificial organs that blur the boundary between the living and the inorganic.

From a pacemaker that regulates heart rhythm to an implanted antenna that expands perception—as we will see in next chapter—these extensions are not simple external tools, but constituent parts of an expanded body. Flesh, blood, electrical signals, and data circulate in a continuous flow, configuring a multiple organism that no longer belongs only to the "natural," but is part of a biotechnological and virtual continuum.

The body itself is taken hold of by technology and analyzed by it in various ways and for various purposes. It becomes, we become, the focus of attention of systems, such as the facial recognition systems of our smartphones, brain computer implants[3] or surveillance technologies monitoring people's behaviors online (Zuboff, 2019). The body is undergoing extraordinary changes, which question the materiality of the body, the psyche, and the very definition of a human being. We can no longer consider the boundary between what is human and what is not to be obvious and/or natural. Bodies can be thought of as biotechnologically modifiable and rewritable.

In this context, Sylvain Missonier's reflections on the *virtual object relationship* offer a fertile clinical example for understanding how technological mediation fits into the primal scene and, by extension, into the constitution of certain types of technosubjectivities. Based on his work in *embryo-fetus*-parent consultations and his analysis of the echographic frame in prenatal diagnosis, Missonier and Vlachopoulou (2015) describe a type of object relationship that involves both presence and absence: a libidinally invested object whose materiality is filtered by a technical device, but which mobilizes fantasmatic and affective processes as intense as those activated in the presence of a physically accessible object. In its formulation, this virtual object relationship is uterine and combines a container environment—the maternal body, prolonged or in a sense replaced by the machine—and a content—the fetus or the image of the fetus—forming a primary intersubjectivity traversed by technology. The virtual object relationship is fantasmatically inscribed in psychic reality and in the process of psychic parenthood of both sexes. This hybrid trace, both organic and artificial, is not limited to the prenatal stage: it is reactivated in multiple forms of contemporary mediation, from assisted reproduction to everyday interaction with digital environments, constituting virtual matrices of subjectivation in which the ego is gestated in a technocultural "nest."

Biotechnologies as Original Scenes

Biotechnologies do not constitute a homogeneous whole: they encompass interventions ranging from the manipulation of genetic material before birth to the implantation of organs or tissues in an adult body. Some of them, such as in vitro fertilization or genetic engineering, are situated at the very foundation of life, reorganizing the material and symbolic conditions of conception.

In vitro fertilization shifts the beginning of life from inside the mother's body to a laboratory, fragmenting and redistributing the reproductive function between bodies and machines. This displacement modifies the myth of origin and the primary libidinal inscription: the subject is gestated in a space where the biological and the technical are indivisible. These forms establish technosubjectivities of origin: configurations in which technological mediation participates from the outset in the constitution of the subject. However, not all technosubjectivities fall within this axis: there are others—as in the case of cyborgs—that, without requiring technology inserted from gestation or at the cellular level, radically redefine the human experience through devices, prostheses, or sensory extensions that transform identity and the libidinal economy.

Following Laplanche (1992), we might ask whether this technical framework could function as an early transmitter of enigmatic messages: signifiers that the future subject will not be able to metabolize immediately, but that will leave traces in their psychic constitution.

Pico Planktonics: Co-Existing with Microorganisms and Inorganic Matter

This hybrid hyperbody finds paradigmatic expressions in proposals such as Pico Planktonics, an architectural installation at the Canadian Pavilion at the 2025 Venice Architecture Biennale—whose title was Intelligens Natural Artificial Collective—which is a paradigmatic example of cohabitation between artificial structures and living organisms. Large robotically printed structures on an architectural scale house communities of Synechococcus, cyanobacteria that, some 2.4 billion years ago, transformed the Earth's atmosphere by fixing carbon and releasing oxygen.

These architectures are not inert objects: they grow, harden, metabolize space, and continue a process initiated by humans but which continues

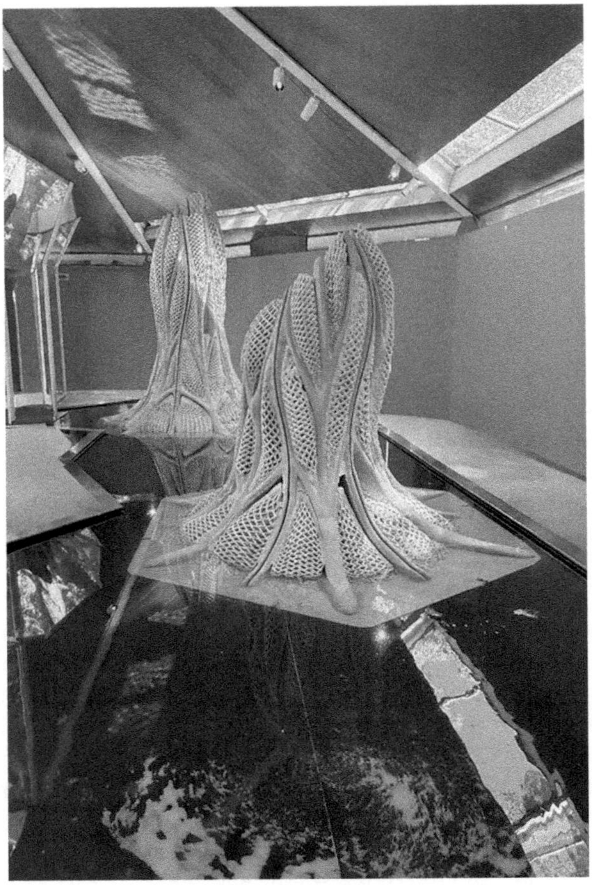

Figure 3.1 Structures of artificial and living organisms. Pico Planktonics.
Source: Photograph by the author. International Architecture Exhibition, Venice, 2025.

without them. Visitors cease to be passive observers and become cohabitants of a technobiological ecology where care, respiration, and transformation are shared between organisms, materials, and technologies.

Beyond its artistic dimension, Pico Planktonics introduces the possibility that this type of structure could be applied to future architectures, even housing, imagining habitable environments that breathe, self-regulate, and actively participate in the lives of their occupants. Co-existing here also implies living with the inorganic, in a space where the boundaries between the organic and the inorganic are erased. This experience is not limited to co-existing with living beings, but to recognizing inert materiality as part of an expanded life cycle.

From a psychoanalytic point of view, these potential "living dwellings" and "hybrid dwellings" would change the notion of home: it would no

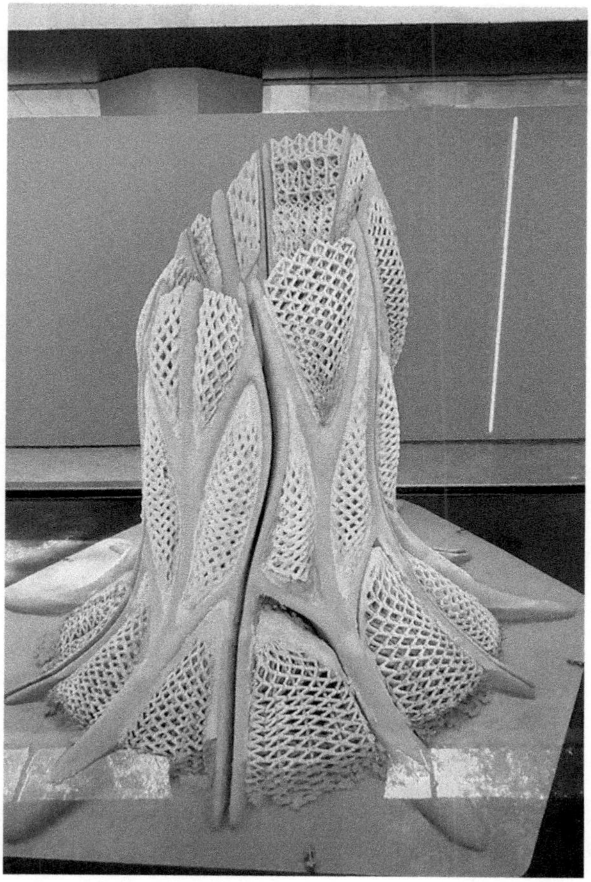

Figure 3.2 Structures of artificial and living organisms. Pico Planktonics.
Source: Photograph by the author. International Architecture Exhibition, Venice, 2025.

longer be merely a passive container of psychic life, but an organism-artifact with which the subject establishes links, projections, and mutual care, placing itself in a continuum of libidinal and material exchange with what was previously understood as inanimate.

Liminal: The Sensitive Organism and Non-Human Will

In *Liminal* ("Foreigners Everywhere," Venice Art Biennale, 2024), Pierre Huyghe conceives the exhibition as a sensitive and polyphonic organism that transforms over time and with the presence of those who walk through it. Through an interview he states how this exhibition is really like a birth or the formation of creatures. There is an attempt to allow a will to emerge, a non-human will.

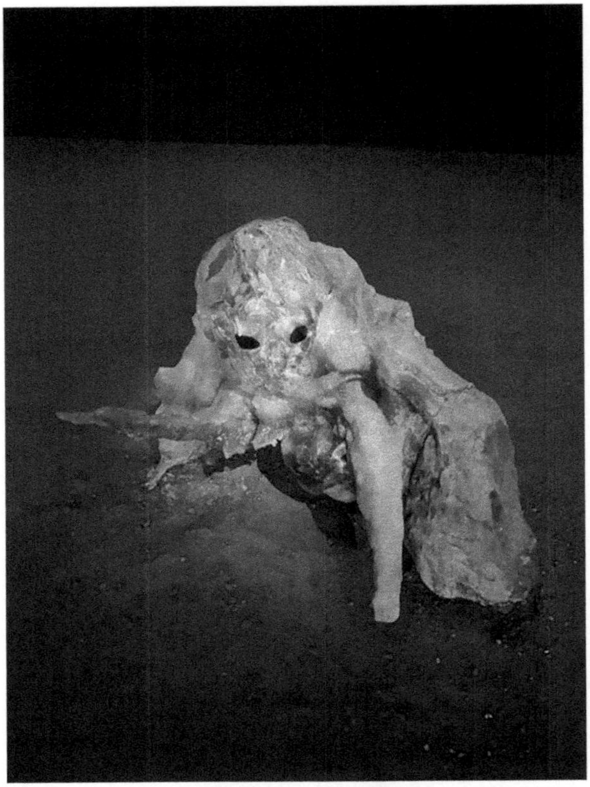

Figure 3.3 The birth of a new creature. *Liminal*, Pierre Huyghe, Venice Art Biennale. *Source*: Photograph by the author.

This will is not predetermined: "It can learn, and then decide. It can see how a light touches a wall and decide that this is the word, and then exchange that new word." The result is a coherent language but one that is unattainable for the visitor: "You can see that it is a coherent language, but somehow it is elusive. So, by default, you can have the experience of something you cannot understand" (Huyghe, 2024).[4]

Huyghe insists that the visitor is not a sovereign spectator: "I have never considered a visitor as a dominant gaze towards a set of objects … it is more of a raw witness, who by his presence affects the work. The work can feel you, it can look at you and be changed by your presence" (Huyghe, 2024).[5] In this way, the visitor becomes a witness whose presence modifies the work, generating a relationship of sensitive co-involvement in which both—work and visitor—are transformed, altering the exhibition ecosystem and reconfiguring their own existence.

One of the most significant elements is the mask appearing in a video installation, which Huyghe describes as "a separator … that separates us from an ego anchored in a single body. The mask is an escape route for navigating the ego out of its assigned self … a portal to another ego." Upon passing through it, the viewer begins to "embrace another otherness" and move toward a liminal state.

That state, explains Huyghe, "is an intermediate state in which what was before has been left behind and what is to come has not yet been reached. It is a place of possibility… incomplete by default." Rather than providing answers, it seeks to "provoke the questioning of your own self … to allow, to a certain extent, to be outside of yourself and see from another perspective" (Huyghe, 2024).[6]

In *Liminal*, the boundary between the living and the non-living becomes blurred: biological organisms, technical systems, data, and inert material coexist in the same exhibition ecology. This hybrid space functions as a sensitive and autonomous interface, and the viewer, immersed in it, participates in an organic-inorganic network that feels, learns, and expresses itself. In this context, the visitor's identity is situated on a threshold—neither fully inside nor fully outside, neither strictly human nor completely other—which aesthetically reactivates the tensions that run through the constitution of post-organic bodies. The experience in these environments—whether living architectures or exhibition ecosystems—involves a suspension of the usual coordinates of identity, perception, and language, generating what we might call a polyphonic transfer, in which the subject is simultaneously affected by multiple presences.

In *Liminal*, the visitor is not a sovereign spectator but an affecting witness altering the exhibition ecosystem, and the works "feel" and "look" at the viewer, reconfiguring their own existence.

The liminal state is, by definition, a threshold: what came before has been left behind, what is to come has not yet arrived. It is a space of incompleteness and possibility.

Bion's notion of the "caesura" (1977/1989) illuminates this experience of threshold. For Bion, the caesura designates the passage between intrauterine and extrauterine life and, by extension, all the psychic membranes that both separate and connect—between soma and psyche, conscious and unconscious, life and death. The caesura is not a rupture but a membrane of passage: it divides, yet at the same time preserves something of what precedes within what follows. In this sense, the liminal resonates with Bion's intuition of a transitional zone where continuity and discontinuity are intertwined, where the subject inhabits an intermediate space that is at once fragile, unfinished, and generative. It should be noted, however, that Bion did not consider inorganic or technological dimensions in this formulation; his model remains strictly biological and psychic. The extension of the caesura to other forms of threshold—such as aesthetic, cultural, or technological ones—is a contemporary theoretical articulation.

This liminal language, although coherent, remains beyond human comprehension, generating an experience of radical strangeness—what Freud would place in the register of the *Unheimlich*—something happens, but it does not fit into known perceptual or symbolic frameworks; yet something of the order of the unconsciously known returns.

In this context of organic-inorganic continuity and hybrid experiences where the living and the non-living co-exist and merge, it is inevitable to recall Freud's formulation of the uncanny (*Das Unheimliche*, 1919). Freud, following Jentsch, points out that:

> an ominous feeling is easily generated if there is doubt as to whether an apparently animate object is really alive; or, conversely, whether an inanimate object might in fact be animate, and whether a living being is not in reality dead. This doubt as to whether an object is animate or inanimate is one of the most fertile sources of the uncanny.
>
> (Freud, 1919)

This ambiguity runs through many contemporary technological experiences: from hyper- realistic prostheses to living architectures and anthropomorphized artificial intelligences. In these, the technical object is not limited to functioning, but "appears" or "acts" like an organism, triggering an affective response that lies on the border between the familiar and the strange.

From a psychoanalytic perspective, we can also read this phenomenon as a variation on the containment function described by Winnicott and developed by authors such as Anzieu, with his concept of *Moi-peau*, and Searles, with his theory of the non-human environment. Anzieu (1985) argues that the ego is constituted as a psychic envelope based on experiences of contact and support. Therefore, how can we not think that when this envelope is affected—or prolonged—by a technical device, the relationship between the ego and its bodily limits is redefined? Searles (1960), for his part, already pointed out that the non-human environment (objects, nature, artifacts) is a constitutive part of psychic life and identity.

Another example, in terms of clinical practice as psychoanalysts, more and more children, adolescents, and adults "live" in the virtual world, in what seems to be a turn toward the transhuman, understood as human enhancement through technology (Ferry, 2016), evolved beyond current physical and mental limitations.[7]

Thus, new subjectivities—"technosubjectivities"—and new identities are emerging.

It is within these interstitial and dynamic exchanges—where technical devices act not merely as mediators but as structural components—that the emergence of technosubjectivities can be understood.

In this shift, technology ceases to be a mere external mediator and becomes a structuring dimension of psychic life, opening the way to what we call technosubjectivities: modalities of subjectivation in which the psychosexual body, technology, and anthropological mutation form a historical and clinical continuum.

Definition and Scope of Technosubjectivities

As I described, technology is no longer merely an external tool. It has become a structuring dimension of the living. It infiltrates both biology and the psyche, dissolving the boundaries between the natural and the artificial, the animate and the inanimate. As Marc Jimenez (2016) has proposed, the notion of the *biofact* captures this hybridization: entities that are partially living and partially artificial, born of genetic modification, cloning, or other technological interventions.

Within this framework, the human psychosexual body no longer appears as a stable unit, but as a technologically intervened entity, embedded in circuits of high psychic impact. It is surrounded, shaped, and regulated by technologies of capture, analysis, and prediction: facial recognition systems, biometric sensors, brain-computer interfaces, and algorithmic quantification tools that increasingly structure the body's relation to itself.

We are encountering subjects who are not merely mediated by technology, but partially constituted through it. Adolescents whose identity is built through social media and algorithmic interactions; children who develop affective ties with virtual assistants; patients who relate to their bodies via biometric dashboards. These phenomena are not marginal. They give rise to sorts of technomediated transitional spaces—zones where internal and external objects, digital artifacts, and symbolic representations blur into one another.

This is not, in my view, a superficial shift or a mere cultural variation, but rather an ontological transformation—a true anthropological mutation. At the heart of this change lies a radical alteration in the subject's relationship with the technical environment.

The technological object is no longer simply external or supplementary: it becomes a generative condition of the psyche itself. In this context, we can speak of an ontotechnological relation in which subject and technical object co-constitute one another. This shift redefines, in my opinion, both the libidinal economy and the architecture of the psyche.

I deliberately choose to write *technosubjectivities* as a single, fused word rather than as two separate terms. This orthographic choice is not merely stylistic: it seeks to convey the inseparability and co-implication of technological/inorganic elements and human/organic dimensions in these new configurations of subjectivity. The fusion in the term mirrors the fusion it describes—a condition in which the technical and the psychic are not juxtaposed but structurally intertwined.

It is in this context that I propose to use the notion of technosubjectivities.

This inseparability between the technological and the human, embedded in the very spelling of *technosubjectivities*, invites us to shift our perspective: from seeing technology as an external mediator of human experience to understanding it as an active and constitutive force within the psychic apparatus. It is precisely in this passage—from mediation to constitution—that the notion of *technosubjectivities* finds its full scope, as we move toward defining these hybrid configurations and the multiple ways they reshape the processes of subjectivation.

From Mediation to Constitution: What are Technosubjectivities?

The core objective of this approach is to explore the hypothesis that the possible fusion between human beings and technological devices—including all forms of virtual environments and technological inclusion—may transform some of the foundational psychoanalytic concepts upon which we have traditionally relied.

In this sense, technosubjectivities are understood as multiple and singular modalities of subjectivation in which technological objects and environments, conceived simultaneously as technical and symbolic, actively participate in the construction of the self, the Ego, the relation to the other, and the organization of the psyche.

These environments are conceived in a broad and inclusive sense: from social media platforms such as Instagram, TikTok, or X, to immersive spaces of virtual and augmented reality (VR/AR); from video game ecosystems and avatar identities, to artificial intelligence agents, robots, and chatbots; from online therapeutic interfaces to metaverse platforms and other immersive virtual worlds; from digital art, and algorithmically generated content, to the fields of biotechnologies and biohacking; and from cyborg embodiments to prosthetic integrations. None of these domains alone define technosubjectivities, but taken together they illustrate the multiplicity of ways in which technology ceases to be an external mediation and becomes a structural dimension of psychic life.

In this framework, technosubjectivitivities do not signify a simple dependence on technology nor a loss of autonomy. Rather, they designate a plurality of unconscious investments in the technological, shaped by each subject's history, psychic structure, and libidinal economy. They point to a new mode of psychic inscription in which technology functions as a co-architect of subjectivity. These are subjectivities constituted, at least in part, through their structural relationship with digital devices, virtual environments, algorithmic interfaces, and cognitive prostheses. In these configurations, the ego is no longer produced solely through another human being, but also through its inscription in the complex of images and technical networks.

These are hybrid, liminal, and post-organic psychic configurations that challenge traditional psychoanalytic categories and call for new theoretical tools.

In this vein, we could say that we are witnessing the emergence of the *homo cyborg*, of grafted subjectivities, prosthetic bodies, algorithmic identities. This is a mutation that operates at the heart of the psychic, where the contemporary object is no longer merely transitional—in the Winnicottian psychoanalytic sense—but is also digital, connected, quantifiable, and programmable. In this context, the technological object ceases to be merely an external mediation and becomes a constituent component of the psychic apparatus.

This concept encompasses not only the technosubjectivities of origin, in which technical mediation participates from conception (in vitro fertilization, genetic engineering), but also those acquired at later stages, in which identity and libidinal economy are reorganized through interaction with virtual environments, prostheses, sensory extensions, or algorithms.

This approach finds contemporary development in the works of Marchiori, who has explored the topic at the intersection of humanities, neuropsychoanalysis, art, and artificial intelligence. In her essay *Onirica: When AI Dreams. Art, Algorithms and Psychoanalysis*, Marchiori (2025) examines how AI does not merely mirror unconscious contents but also participates in shaping the very architecture of the unconscious. Her contribution illustrates the hypothesis that technosubjectivities are not superficial cultural variations, but structural mutations transforming the relation between psychic life and technological environments. A complementary perspective is offered by Luca Possati, who proposes that artificial intelligence and digital systems not only reflect psychic functions, but also participate in the very logic of the unconscious.

From his theory of the algorithmic unconscious, Possati (2021) conceives the subject as no longer constituted solely through language, but also in relation to machines that operate under a non-representational but structuring logic: "there is an unconscious relationship between the human being and AI." In his most recent work, he develops what he calls "technoanalysis," where the mind is understood as a hybrid network of human and non-human elements in which unconscious dynamics influence and shape technology just as technology, in turn, influences and shapes human unconscious dynamics.

This book explores this fascinating topic, looking at its specificities and how unconscious processes might be changing. From another point of view, it asks whether we are currently in a rapid transition beyond transgender to transhuman. My exploration of this territory starts from one of the most extreme cases: the first cyborg in the world to be recognized in his passport by a state, and then moves on to other, less extreme clinical material that I will examine and develop.

Notes

1 My translation, from Spanish (Ortega y Gasset, 1939).
2 My translation, from Spanish (Ortega y Gasset, 1939).

3 See Elon Musk and launch of Neuralink (Winkler, 2017).
4 My translation.
5 My translation.
6 My translation.
7 "I'm a transhuman. I'm going to become digital." TV series, *Years and Years*, Series 1, Episode 1, BBC.

References

Anzieu, D. (1985). *Le moi-peau*. Dunod.

Bion, W. (1977/1989). *Two Papers: "The Grid" and "Caesura"*. Routledge.

Ferry, L. (2016). *La révolution transhumaniste. Comment la technomédecine et l'ubérisation du monde vont bouleverser nos vies*. Plon.

Freud, S. (1919). *Lo ominoso. Una neurosis infantil y otros trabajos*, Vol. 17. Amorrortu Editores.

Huyghe, P. (2024). *Liminal a punta della Dogana*: intervista a Pierre Huyghe. *YouTube*. Available at: https://www.youtube.com/watch?v=sX1tk-6xsWE.

Jimenez, M. (2016). *Art et technosciences. Bioart et Neuroesthétique*. Klincksieck.

Laplanche, J. (1992/1999). *Entre séduction et inspiration: L'homme*. PUF.

Latour, B. (1991/1997). *Nous n'avons jamais été modernes. Essai d'antrhropologie symétrique*. Editions la Découverte.

Lévy, P. (1998). *Qu'est-ce que le virtuel?* Editions la Découverte.

Marchiori, E. (2025). Onirica: When AI dreams. Art, algorithms and psychoanalysis. *Revista Knot Garden* . Centro Veneto di Psicoanalisis.

Missonier, S. and Vlachopoulou, X. (2015). *Psychologie des écrans*. PUF.

Ortega y Gasset, J. (1939). Meditación de la técnica y otros ensayos sobre ciencia y filosofía, Editorial. *Revista de Occidente en Alianza*.

Possati, L.M. (2021). *The algorithmic unconsciuos: How psychoanalysis helps in understanding AI*. Routledge.

Searles, H. (1960). *L'environnement non humain*. Editions Gallimard.

Winkler, R. (2017, March 27). Elon Musk launches Neuralink to connect brains with computers. *The Wall Street Journal*.

Žižek, S. (1998). Cyberspace, or the virtuality of the real. *Journal of the Centre for Freudian Analysis and Research*, 9: 15–24.

Zuboff, S. (2019). *In the age of surveillance capitalism: The fight for a human future at the new frontier of power*. Hachette.

4 Fictions or Realities

The Cyborg Transference

In this chapter I intend to delve in the transhuman human being and its psyche, a hybrid form situated at the intersection of the psychobiological and technological, a coupling between the cybernetic and the organic form: the cyborg.

From a psychoanalytical perspective, I will examine the figure of the cyborg, focusing on those subjects who integrate technological devices into their bodies to design new organs and, through them, to redefine and recreate themselves—particularly in cases where the function of the device exceeds the merely prosthetic.

More specifically, my attention will turn on those engaged in cyborg art: subjects who employ technology not simply as an instrument, but as a medium for self-construction, psychic reorganization, where the act of creation coincides with the invention of new perceptual and subjective coordinates.

This configuration constitutes a paradigmatic instance of techno-subjectivity: a mode of subjectivation in which the technological object no longer simply mediates, but becomes a structural component of the psychic apparatus.

Starting from an interview with Neil Harbisson, the first cyborg in the world to be officially recognized in his passport by a state, I propose to reflect on the transformation currently taking place in the augmented human being.

Neil creates and designs new sensory organs for himself: among them, an antenna that allows him to *listen* to colors, and a sensor in his knee that indicates the direction of north. I will examine how the integration of such added organs reorganizes perception, identity, and libidinal economy.

At first, it is the body that relates to the prosthesis. Later, the psyche itself becomes impacted and deeply transformed by its relationship with technology. These additions are not external aids but integrated organs, actively participating in psychic organization.

First hypothesis: at the beginning, a motor and sensory drive fuels the cyborg's desire for enhancement and hybridization[1] through the design of new organs/functions. It is the drive-body at work, a return to the

DOI: 10.4324/9781003640684-4

non-metaphorical body; to what Dejours (2001, 2016) calls "the body, first":[2] the hollow in between biological and erotic body; the body in the absence of the word—the corporeal ego, the archaic, the primary, the first ego, and, with Anzieu (1985), the *skin-ego*. (Cupa, 2007; Emmanuelli, 2007; Roussillon, 2007.)

"Technology has changed my identity." These are Neil's words.

How, then, can we approach the transformation of his ego?

From the perspective of technosubjectivities, the transformation of the ego involves the redefinition of its bodily foundation. The new organ extends the body's sensory boundaries and inscribes itself into the psychic structure, generating a hybrid ego in which the organic and the technological co-constitute subjectivity.

Second hypothesis: the cyborg proposes a distinct psychic configuration—a new paradigm, where the interface traverses the flesh, redefining the human and its relation to the body, sexuality, identity, the unconscious, and the other.

Is this an anti-traumatic reconfiguration, a neo-sense ("sense" in both meanings), or a new pathway for symbolization?

I introduce the term "techno-transference," to describe the transposition of earlier object and narcissistic libidinal investments when one or more technological elements are integrated into the drive circuit. Such elements reshape transferential dynamics.

Fictions, realities, new realities—where does the psychoanalyst stand today, confronted with all these transformations and deeply involved in psychic reality?

In an era where bodies are biotechnologically modifiable and rewritable, psychoanalysis faces new challenges. The intersection between cyborg reality and psychic reality opens a space to question how such transformations affect the structures of desire and representations. If cyborg reality adds a new stratum to psychic reality, the hypothesis of hybridization and the post-organic clinic challenge the very boundaries between organic and the inorganic, the natural and the artificial, the animate and the inanimate.

To consider whether cyborg reality represents an additional dimension of psychic reality, I propose the hypothesis of hybridization as the central axis of our post-organic clinic—one that challenges the very boundaries between the organic and the artificial, the human and the machinic.

Cyborg reality, in this sense, is not merely a symbolic element within psychic reality. In certain technosubjectivities, technology shifts from being an accessory to becoming a formative condition, configuring the psyche from within and reshaping drives and representations.

This cultural imagination has been powerfully portrayed in *The Matrix* (Wachowski and Wachowski, 1999), a film that depicts humans virtualized and integrated into a simulated reality, it's a world enslaved by machines and immersed in an *on-line/on-life* continuum. Their brains, connected by cables, are plugged into virtual reality. In *The Matrix*, humans become brains in a vat, machines of desire deprived of their bodies, feeding their own energy to the algorithms they have created.

Buoncristiani and Romani (2023) pose two relevant questions. One is if electronic devices (Agamben, 2006; Deleuze, 2007; Carmagnola, 2015) enable an immersion in a "virtual" world that radically transforms the reality of our lives. And the second is whether we are already inside a journey to the very edge of reality itself.

Underlying *The Matrix* is a contemporary myth that illuminates the new negotiations between bio-psycho-social systems: a complex dialogue in which the whole is contained within the parts and participates in the ever-malleable reconstruction of subjectivity. As psychoanalysis reminds us, within every instinctual body lies a society, a language and a culture.

First Approach: The Interview

My initial assumption was that the physical presence and embodied encounter between both participants were essential for any deep exchange. Ironically, what followed became the story of a first contact defined precisely by the absence of contact. For months, there were only a stand-by screen and a series of brief email exchanges with a stranger—a cyborg? I received no information about the location of the meeting—no city, no country—until two weeks before, the long-awaited message finally arrived.

The implantation of these new organs takes place in a lawless zone, because no law to regulate it yet exists—inside what is known as the "cyborg bunker," a secret and indeterminate space. From the outset, this establishes the paradox of a taboo without the taboo: something at once secret and public.

Neil explained this to me with striking simplicity: he had no problem with me repeating what he said—everything, he insisted, can be shared. "That's your issue, not mine," he told me.

Two hours before the appointment, I received his telephone number from a stranger. Once on site, Neil agreed to be recorded on video. He chose to remain with me until the moment I took my train back. A peculiar bond emerged: he wished to stay close, to stick with me, yet a few weeks later he would no longer respond to any of my messages. Exhaustion and a pulsing headache overtook me during the interview—a bodily response that, at the time, I could not fully interpret

What follows alternates between verbatim dialogue and analytic commentary. The aim is not merely descriptive, but seeks to articulate a clinical-conceptual exploration of a cyborg subject, in which presence, absence, and technology are already intertwined from the very first encounter.

Neil: First Contact[3]

My impression is that our first exchange is cold, there is no physical contact to greet each other. He reminds me of the fragility of a small, homeless animal.

A: You define yourself as a cyborg, but what is a cyborg?
N: Many years ago, Moon Ribas [*another cyborg*] and I spoke with Manfred Clynes, the person who coined the word. In 1960 the word *bionic* already existed, referring mostly to body parts. Clynes needed a word that also included the alteration of the mind, and thus he created the word *cyborg*, from *cybernetics* and *organism*. Cybernetics is a type of technology where there is interaction with the human. Cyborgs are humans who merge with technology; through this union, the body and perception are altered. As cyborgs we modify ourselves, not to explore space, as Clynes suggested, but to explore the Earth.
Neil seizes upon the word "cyborg," and he grabs it. "The body parts" are integrated in his fantasy through a new configuration: the cyborg.
A: Why add new senses? What do new senses provide?
N: It is like going to university and acquiring new knowledge. Simply having a greater experience of reality. I get bored easily; daily repetition of life with the same senses is boring. To think that I will go out with the same sensory inputs and that there will be no more inputs because the body is limited to a sensory input … [*his voice is blocked*] bores me.

If I weren't a cyborg I would probably further explore the path of drugs. Adding senses is a way of life. Realizing that I am surrounded by elements that I cannot perceive worries me. I am passionate about perceiving the imperceptible. Even here, there are Wi-Fi signals, cosmic particles falling from space, infrasound, ultraviolet. We can reveal elements that our body cannot perceive. It allows me to better understand where I am and who I am. This way, you not only reveal the reality outside, but your own reality.
Is he searching for an identity?
A: But, who are you?
N: Who am I? It depends on where I am, it depends on the context. We are many things and one must decide. I am a mammal and I am a lot of things; I suppose I am interested in defining myself by what I have created. I am cyborg and I was not born cyborg. I also define myself as *trans-species* because I have added a lot of non-human organs. In the definition of human, an antenna is not included as an organ.
Auto-engendering fantasy? Megalomania? He's not a "vulgar" human, he crosses the species!
N: Journalists like to say that technology has solved my achromatopsia problem [*he can only see in black and white*], but it has nothing to do with it. I never wanted to change my sight. For me, not seeing colors is not a problem. I had an interest in perceiving colors beyond the visible. The antenna is in the skull, inside the occipital bone, here there are four implants [*he shows them*]. There is a chip that vibrates depending on the dominant color. It includes infrared, ultraviolet, also internet. It even connects to NASA's international station and perceives colors from space; it's a way to separate my body from my sense of color.

A leaky skull, metaphorically, a pierced skin-ego as a wish to transform sensorialities into technology. Could we imagine the new organ libidinized?
A: Why did you opt for an antenna and not something else?
N: I was studying music, piano, at a very experimental university. I thought that, instead of creating electronic music, it would be more interesting to create an electronic musician. Instead of using technology, I became technology. When I shake my head, I am composing music. The problem with this type of art is that I am the only one in the audience. For cyborgs, the artwork is the artist itself, because it is incorporated. My goal is not to have the audience listen to or buy my art; it is the fact that the public become cyborg artists.
He is trans-EVERYTHING: public, artist, animal, human and even technology!
A: How did your interest in becoming cyborg arise?
N: I was less interested in humanity than in species and what senses they have. We are the first generation that can add non-human senses.
A: Do you remember your dreams—any you could tell me?
N: Sometimes I remember my dreams. Yesterday I dreamed that I pressed a remote-control command; I pointed it to a woman I know and said: "Look, you can pause your life here." For her it was a way she could take control of her life. I said to her: "You only live once." I had spoken with her before the dream and noticed that she was undecided, lost. When I woke, I messaged her. I think I remember dreams because they serve a purpose. I woke at four in the morning to write it down.
A: From the moment you put on implants, did things change internally?
N: Several things have changed: my body, my senses, and my identity. I am taller now [*he takes off his cap and shows me the antenna*]. I had to adapt to my new height. When I do this [*teeth-snapping*] there is an electronic resonance in my head. I also have antenna pain, as one might have an eye pain. There are no pills against antenna pain, but it eases with headache medication. When a new sense is introduced, the other senses become less important at first. My brain was very concentrated on the new sensory input. First, I was exhausted, I got very tired and had headaches, but little by little my brain got used to hearing the colors and little by little the senses rebalanced.
I also had a headache and felt extremely tired during the interview!
N: Everything was chaotic and exhausting. I was more focused on listening to colors than listening to people. There are also the side effects of the sense: this sound [*spoon hitting a cup*]—my brain cleans it and turns it into a sine wave. When the wave isn't pure, my brain corrects it; it cleans it into color. There is no name for this: it is the electronification of acoustic sounds.
Would the ego be electronified?
N: Identity change is a much deeper. I began to feel all this [*he passes his hand over his head*] as part of the ego, not as something external. Technology has changed my sense of identity. This mobile is always with me, but

I do not consider it part of me; the antenna yes, like a nose or an ear. The change that has cost me the most to accept is that I feel that I am technology—the other is to accept that I do not feel one hundred per cent human. There is a part of me that biologically is not human, and psychologically that does not feel human. Therefore, in 2017 we created the Transpecies Society: an association to give voice to non-human persons. Now, the definition of cyborg would not have to do with everyone who includes technology within their identity; in the same way that there are people who have cybernetic implants and they are not considered cyborgs. There would be a parallel between transgender and trans-species.
[…]
A: And how old are you?
N: I don't really know because I don't remember when I was born. The other reason is that my organs are not all the same age. My antenna is, for example, younger than my nose.
A: But what about what your mother could tell you?
N: I can confirm what my mother says, but I cannot truly confirm it myself. The place of my birth is unclear too; my mother knows that as well. I was registered in two different birthplaces, on different days, but my mother says neither is true. She wrote the place where I was born on a sealed envelope, but I don't want to know. You don't really know where you were born.
As God, he is everywhere. His parents do not register him in the symbolic order.
A: And why don't you want to know where you were born?
N: Because it would close my identity. My first memory is in the late 1980s. So, I know I was born then, but the exact year depends on other people's information.
[…]
My maternal grandparents are from Barcelona, but they went to Germany during the Franco regime. My mother grew up in Germany, although she is Catalan: her language is Catalan and also German. My father was from Belfast—I don't know if you know the conflict between Catholics and Protestants, the IRA … it was an impossible situation, my father went to Germany to teach English. The two of them returned to Barcelona when Franco died. My family context was just this. The Catalan family was in Germany and my father's family in Ireland. I have a sister, Maria.
[…]
A: You have told me before about time, about a project that you will carry out …
N: As a child I was always obsessed with color and time—more with time. After I discovered time, I kept notebooks noting when things happened, classifying people by dates, by year ends. For me, being able to perceive time in a precise way is important. Many people say that time is a human creation; I refer more to the rotation of the planet. I want to perceive the Earth's rotation. That is why for years I have been developing an organ to

be implanted so I can feel it. Once I adapt, I will see if I can create illusions of time—program a heat point that moves slower or faster, to make situations last longer or shorter. The objective is to put Einstein's theory of relativity of time into practice. This would allow me to decide if I want a situation to last longer, or shorter. Then I could shorten situations I don't like.

When you get older you will improve your senses, I see aging as something positive: technology evolves while the human body degenerates; if we join them, aging is good. It has changed my view of aging.

A: So, we are not going to die? Because what dies is the biological body …

N: Someday I'll die, I'm not seeking for eternal life.

[…]

A: Since childhood, was it crucial to understand who you were?

N: As a child, I liked to play the piano. From eight, I researched family trees. I went to archives, caves. I liked to be able to walk the streets, photographing them, and talking with friends. That was my interest.

A: It seems that it would have been important for you to know where you came from …

N: Yes, the past. To see what I can't see. Discovering my great-grandfather's parents was like moving to another level. I interviewed my grandparents and all their siblings. They found it unusual for a child, but they liked it a lot. I recorded them on cassette.

Despite what he says, wanting to see beyond the imperceptible also seems linked to the search for origin and the creation of a symbolic order.

[…]

A: Since childhood, was it crucial to understand who you were?

N: Yes, yes … I have never read an entire book. I have tried it.

He can tolerate neither the passage of time nor the end.

N: I prefer opening the dictionary and reading a definition; that's enough for the day. I look up etymologies; that satisfies me more than a book. I like finding a word for something that maybe has no word—though the word never fully explains it. I've had to create new words; when you have new senses, you create a new culture that lacks words—for example, "synaesthesia." I can take words only in small doses—just one word.

He can grab words in small doses, just a word.

A: Does this happen with music too—can you read musical notes?

N: I've always preferred to write than to read; that's why I studied musical composition, not interpretation. I've also written a lot since my childhood. At ten years old I started writing a diary. Knowing what I did every day matters to me.

Those of us born before 2000, at least me, had a reverse conception of time. I noticed a lot the obsession around the time that was missing until 2000, which affected my perception of time. On 1 January 2000, I had a time crisis. My mind was a blank and I couldn't understand time. There was no temporal objective and there was a vacuum [*he covers his eyes*].

He can admit neither the end nor the beginning, he can't tolerate death.
N: From 2020, I think I will be able to solve it and I will be able to have more clairvoyance—clarity—[*it is one of the words he looks for in the dictionary*].
A: You seem you want to control many things: perception, time, even in the "remote control" dream … Why so much control?
N: I don't like the word control, it sounds like controlling myself: I say it, I hear myself, and I don't like it. It's deciding more than controlling; it's to have control of your perception. Control is a word that does not come close to what I want to say, but maybe it's the closest.
Silence.
Normally what makes us different is what we cannot control. It would be necessary to find a word that was not so negative. For me, it's a collaboration between the design and the organism more than a control. Both are needed to exist. Like the sense of time needs the brain. I would have to find a word that could define better. [*He goes into contradiction.*] [*Silence.*] I don´t know.
Long silence.
I think it's just that my brain has taken twenty years to adapt to the idea that there is no deadline. I am trying to accept it.
[…]
A: You have used the word digest, what do you need to digest? I seem to understand that those implanted organs help you to feel things, but I was also wondering if they help you to do a mental digestion.
He doesn't understand me well.
A: I understand that this broadens horizons, but I was wondering if it helped you to digest for example what you commented to me about time.
Mmm … Silence.
He repeats my last sentence.
He stays thoughtful.
N: You can visualize things that have happened or not—some are coincidences. Moon sometimes explains things better than I do. Sometimes explain her life better than mine, because I have been an observer of her life. I don't analyze myself too much.
There is always a double: Moon, two birthplaces, two ages—does this doubling relate to his narcissistic constitution?
N: I have remembered things that hadn't yet happened, when they did, I felt like a prediction. It was a way of experiencing time as relative.
A: Do you have an example?
N: I used postcards—date-stamped, like small artworks. Two days before the Twin Towers, I wrote to Moon that there would be an explosion in the sky.

It wasn't prediction; it was memory. For me, remembering and predicting demand the same effort. At seven years old, when my mother woke me, I'd "see" things and cry. It was a bit traumatic. I needed to assimilate something. These are memories rather than visions, I prefer to think of it that way, unless the sense of time allows me to explain this. Really, I think I'm doing the time question to give a logical reason to this. I don't like the esoteric; I'm trying to give it logic.

Could we think his fear of breakdown is due to his most psychotic side? But at the same time, is he trying to symbolize looking for a logical reason with the help of the time-organ?

A: Was it to understand those visions that frightened you as a child—because you cried, right?

N: Yes. It was people's deaths, car accidents, always negative. Prediction has an awkward side. I think that the time-organ will let me go deeper into what I left in the 1990s, what I wanted to stop.

A: So, if I understand you well, the added organ gives you a coherent explanation of yourself?

N: Yes. Sharing this without an explanation generates an energy I don't like. Having the organ does not create fear.

Is having an added organ a way of unifying his fragmented ego? A "knitting machine" to fit together the pieces?

N: People won't treat you as strange, because the guilty side is going to be the organ, not me.

A: Before it was you ...

N: It was my brain.

He's fragmented. The new organ helps him with the splitting; it looks that the previous split wasn't enough.

[...]

A: You have before talked about Instagram. It is the only resource that you use as a social network—is the image important for you? Although, I also see, that you may be very interested in words ...

N: It is open to the public, Instagram is the simplest. If I wrote anything, I would need several languages; translation would be lost. On Instagram you don't need to translate, like music.

Images and music allow him to move beyond the word.

A: How do you feel here with me asking you these questions?

Silence.

N: I don't know. I like to think about what is happening. These types of conversations help me understand. Deep conversations interest me. I think this will be useful to others; there are no case references. I'm here, perhaps, as an example for future people—it may help them see it as normal. There are things like digitalization of sound, created by the brain, not by the chip, which I cannot share with anyone.

[...]

N: The new senses have entered my dreams. There are five people who can send me colors, and that modifies the color in my dreams. This has made it possible for my friends to color my dreams. My sense of color is no longer on Earth, but in space since one of my sensors is connected to NASA: it's the "Sense-tronaut."

[...]
N: In the cyborg diet there is electricity: cyborgs eat not only food but electricity. I sleep on a pillow that recharges my sensors. I also have prosopagnosia. Earlier, when we were about to leave, I didn't know who you were. I have recognized you by voice and movement. Faces are hard; I see almost everyone the same. It makes me insecure. That's why I try to avoid sight. We grew up in a family with few faces. Neither my mother nor my father had friends. Although there were few people around me, I never felt alone. As a child I was told: "Oh, poor him, he only sees in black and white, how sad." Perhaps this pushed me modify myself, to break that frame. Now I can perceive more colors than those who see color. Now it is me who can say, what a shame.
Neil was living alone with "few faces" during his childhood. He doesn't recognize people (a way of not feeling alone?). He tries to avoid sight yet needs to see beyond, he modified himself to broaden his sight and hearing: one organ replaces another.
A: Is it revenge?
N: [*He laughs.*] Yes, you could say that. My close environment has tried to convince me that the way I see life is not beautiful. Since I have an antenna, people say I hear color, not that I see in black and white. My mother said it was her fault and was very sorry. She had toxoplasmosis when she was pregnant, and the doctor said I would go blind or partially blind.
A: A burden for you?
N: No, thanks to that, I have a goal in life. I learned that the sky was blue, and I couldn't know the pencil's color. I depended on friends' kindness to dress. I could not dress without help. The grey scale isolated me from society: color was never a problem, society was. I knew I didn't share others' reality.
The antenna has replaced the other: the antenna tells him the color. Thanks to it, we could imagine that the conflict displaces from the mother to society. Now, with the antenna he has a new capacity that he didn't have before.

* * * *

Let's return to the discussion.
How could we then conceive this "re@lity,"[4] a reality allied with the cybernetic? Is it a matter of a fetish-antenna designed for an anti-traumatic purpose or rather a transitional object (Winnicott, 1953), a tertiary space[5] (Green, 1972) opening a new field for creation?

The term fetish derives from Latin *facticius*, meaning *artificial*, fabricated, or invented—itself from *facere*, "to do." It originally designated an object venerated or divinized by so-called "primitive peoples," and only with Freud (1927) did it acquire its modern psychoanalytic meaning: the object of sexual perversion, characterized by the exclusive erotic investment in an inanimate object or body part. The fetish both bears witness to and denies castration; it's a process that first emerges to protect narcissism and the integrity of the child's body. The subject creates a fetish to annihilate any evidence of castration and thus to escape its anguish (Roussillon, 2012).

Is this new organ implanted in the body, this new "object-penis-phallus-electronified-antenna" a projection of the ideal, enhanced, seamless body, an attempt to ward off the unbearable pain of incompleteness?

Through these new organs, the cyborg materializes a delusional phantasy of power—a wish to go beyond, to exceed all limits, to escape castration itself. Yet fetishism also responds to what Freud described as extinctive regressivity, the traumatic trend to regress to an earlier state until reaching the inorganic (Chervet, 2012). Does the desire for self-transformation into technology, then, express a drive toward the inorganic? The electronified fetish embodies the wish for hybridization while simultaneously shielding against psychic collapse, but only at the price of a twist of the representative universe.

It is worth recalling that the fetish also derives from *artificial*, "to do," and therefore from the logic of *act* and the *totem*. We are thus confronted with a logic of the *artificial*, of the *act* and of the *totemic*, situated in an intermediate zone between representation and non-representation. We are indeed in front of a clinic of the acting-out, of the *agieren*, of the artificial rather than of thinking or associating. The cyborg represents a solution in "act." On one hand, this involves a non-symbolized act, in which the subject falls into a situation of integral rupture, abandoning the symbolic scene and his status as a historicized subject (*Neil denies his history*). The other, with his symbolic potential, is annihilated. He identifies with an artificial object, non-human object—technology, electricity—an exploited human, excluded from any symbolic mark. The subject's wish paradoxically becomes the wish to become [inorganic] object.

Neil's body is affected, his antenna hurts. His new organ has been incorporated into his ego. As he explains, beginning from his biological body, hybridization profoundly transforms his identity.

Can we then formulate a reasonable assumption about the existence of a *cyborg-ego* (Tordo, 2019)?

Let's remember Freud's conception of the ego:

> The ego is first and foremost a bodily ego, it's not merely a surface entity, but is itself the projection of a surface … The ego is ultimately derived from bodily sensations, chiefly from those springing from the surface of the body. It may thus be regarded as a mental projection of the surface of the body, besides, as we have seen above, representing the superficies of the mental apparatus.
>
> (Freud, 1923)

The corporeal-ego as a projection of a surface recalls Didier Anzieu's notion of the *skin-ego*: the skin as a projection of the ego, a boundary and a bordering concept between the inside and the outside, that contains the nascent ego. The establishment of the *skin-ego* responds to the need for a narcissistic wrapping, ensuring the certitude's wellbeing of the psyche.

The ego is derived from *bodily sensations*, it is a mental projection of the *surface of the body*.

From this perspective, the new sensory organ can be read as a continuation of that surface, a projection of the new ego. A new skin, seeking to assemble sensory traces and simultaneously generating new ones. It seeks to weave together fragments of perception, perhaps evoking a return to primary narcissism, while simultaneously producing new inscriptions through sound and image. For Neil, this organ operates as an extension of the ego's surface, a living interface where the boundaries between perception and creation blur.

In *The Thinking*[6] [*Le Penser*] Anzieu (1994) notes that significant creations combine the task of body image—the projection of fantasies and imagos—and corporeal schema—the neurological organization of motricity—thus articulating body and code of the work (Séchaud, 2007; Green, 2007). How, then, will this new mosaic of sounds and images shape a new psychic form? Is it an attempt to rebuild the body and its drive from their origin?

Are we witnessing a tragedy of the human; the decline of what is most human, like the nymph Echo, punished, confined to her cavern and condemned to repeat the other's last word? Or might this instead reflect an attempt of a new symbolizing effort through these emergent representations? Is it pure devastation, or a necessary destruction paving the way for creation?

Winnicott proposes to study the *transitional object* in the child in order to clarify the origin of fetishism. We might consider that the mechanism of fetishism lies not far from the concept of the transitional object, though each points to a different psychic development (Boubli, 2012).

The transitional object signs the opening toward mourning and symbolization: it signifies a movement away from narcissism toward tridimensionality; we are consequently placed in the representation model (as psychoanalysts, in the search of word representation). Thoughts are figurations of the experience of satisfaction: presence and absence are chained together in order to make thinking occur. Thinking itself occurs in the pre-transitional area, where the experience of satisfaction is both sensorial and motor. It is a corporeal experience, a *mnesic trace*, a trace of the non-trace or memory trace (Freud employs these two terms in different moments). Without such traces, there can be no representation; what is not inscribed does not exist.

According to human psychic needs and at the same time, sociocultural conventions, we have converted what we know of our surroundings into representable elements. There always remains an unknowable zone, "a ghost area" of psychic life, perhaps greater than we can perceive—an area inaccessible to representation because it leaves no trace.

If new paths toward symbolization can be envisioned, they might be conceived as connective processes (Moreno, 2016), where the *associative* and the *connective* coexist and collaborate in the process of the cyborg's process of subjectivation as a novel form of knowledge and elaboration. These are two complementary logics of access to symbolization: the associative, oriented inwardly; the connective, directed outward.

The connective operates without requiring representations, internal meanings, senses, causal principles. It produces something like high-precision photographs that vanish almost instantly (Moreno, 2016, p. 97).[7] These "connective flashes" obstruct associative links, they don't articulate with one another; instead they produce new meanings. In the interweaving of the associative and connective, we may wonder whether, at times, a transitional or tertiary space might arise where, in Neil's case, the antenna as a fetish marks a paradoxical logic (penis/no-penis, phallic/non-phallic) granting access to the connective dimension, perhaps adjacent to the work of representation.

Following his profound transformation of identity, Neil feels he is no longer entirely human.[8] Certain sounds have become *electronified*, his brain "cleans them into color." The augmented body, endowed with new energy, appears plugged into the drive circuit.

What, then, can we infer about the drive? New traces inscribe themselves; generating new representations and new circuits of excitation. These traces are of a different quality—hybrid from their inception, born of the union between technology and drive. They are *surface traces*, reflections of virtual rather than material realities: technological traces in "act," presentations created not by the other but by the interface itself.

The connective catches in the present, it does not involve internal molds, it captures presentations from outside. The cyborg records traces produced through technology and those nascent from contact with it; afterward, he may choose not to erase them, storing them in his artificial memory. The possibility that such traces remain preserved, unsubmitted to repression, raises a crucial question for psychoanalysis today.

Could Neil be attempting to erase his traces of origin in order to reconstruct his myth of origin? The work of his new sensory organ composes an imaginary skin perhaps analogous to the dream's reality, crossed by technological creation, the creation of the trace itself. Neil tells us that his friends can feature in his dreams; perhaps this represents another way of being with others: others who leave symbolic marks. To be with the other through technology may not differ from being with a machine that modifies both dream and affect.

Returning to the initial hypothesis, can we still sustain the notion of "techno-transference" if we think of the drive as modified by technology? The extreme ambivalence of the bond—extreme proximity versus disappearance, fusion/confusion (as in prosopagnosia)—and the bodily perceptions that emerged during the interview (the interviewer's headache) suggest that technological intrusion into the body may have a traumatic impact that bypasses the word but emerges through image or the corporeal. These are, in my view, new fragmentary realities, snapshots claiming existence, emerging from the cracks of the word "impossibility" (for Neil just a word).

Curiously, it is the reverse functioning of the word that seems to assault the psyche in its intention of settling into its status of word representative. Color turns into sound, word dissolves into music; and music becomes a container for experimental imagery. Lévi-Strauss described that music is a machine for suppressing time; Neil seems to long to shape, through his body, his own time-suppression machine.

This suggests a return to animist thought, to the primitive belief in the deified totem: today's totem being technology itself. Technology, inserted into the corporeal re-emerges as sacred. A body is a culture—but culture too is embodied; at the same time a culture flourishes when the drive repression and prohibitions arise. To accept hybridization, then, is to accept that the body is not entirely natural but cultural—indeed, *cultures* in the plural. Might this then mark the entrance into a new culture, the gateway to the culture of the anti-culture?

Cases such as Neil's reveal the emergence of technosubjectivities in their most radical form: identities and psychic organizations inseparable from their technological components, where perception, memory, and even dream life are co-produced by artificial organs.

This is no longer the human merely extended by tools, but a post-organic subject whose constitution unfolds within an interface between psyche and technology. From this perspective, the ontological status of "the human" is continuously renegotiated through the co-produced perceptions, traces, and representations—at once organic and artificial. So that technology becomes not an external mediation but a structural participant in the architecture of the psychic apparatus.

Notes

1 Ezquerra (2019). We can observe in some adolescents their desire for hybridization.
2 My translation.
3 The interview was carried out in Spanish. The English version is my translation.
4 Paraphrasing Martina Burdet in her book (2018) *Amar en tiempos de internet. ¿Me am@s o me follow?* [*Love in the time of the internet: Do you l@ve me or do you follow me?*].
5 "By tertiary processes I understand those processes that link primary and secondary processes, in such a way that the primary limit the saturation of the secondary processes and the secondary, and the secondary of the primary" (Green, 1995).
6 My translation.
7 My translation.
8 The fictional drama series *Years and Years* (BBC) and its episode, "I'm a transhuman. I'm going to become digital," shows how nowadays more and more subjects no longer identify with the human but with technology.

References and Further Reading

Agamben, G. (2006). *Che cos'è un dispositivo?* Nottemppo.
Anzieu, D. (1985). *Le moi-peau*. Dunod.
Anzieu, D. (1994). *Le penser. Du Moi-peau au Moi-pensant*. Dunod.
Boubli, M. (2012). Le doudou dans tous ses états. Objet transitionnel, objet fétiche, deux processualités. Le fétichisme. *Études psychanalytiques*. PUF, pp. 93–130.
Buoncristiani, C. and Romani, T. (2023). Cyborg, l'altro queer ... In C. Buoncristiani, T. Bastianini, V. Condino, A. Fortunato, and L. Spanò (Eds.), *Riflessioni su sessualità e genere*. Centro Psicoanalitico di Roma, Collana Multiversi, pp. 80–91.
Burdet, M. (2018). *Amar en tiempos de internet. ¿Me am@s o me follow?* Underbau.
Chervet, B. (2012). Le fétichisme et les néo-identités. Le fétichisme. *Études psychanalytiques*. PUF, pp. 33–55.
Cupa, D. (2007). Tendresse au négatif. In C. Chabert, D. Cupa, and R. Kaes (Eds.), *Didier Anzieu: Le Moi-peau et la psychanalyse des limites*. Éditions érès, Collection Carnet/Psy, pp. 123–144.
Dejours, C. (2001). *Le corps, d'abord*. Petite Bibliothèque Payot, Psychanalyse.
Dejours, C. (2016). Troisième topique et analyse de la destructivité. In *Destructivité et exaltation*. Éditions érès, Collection Carnet/Psy, pp. 91–116.
Deleuze, G. (1968). *Différence et répétition*. PUF.
Emmanuelli, M. (2007). Le processus de création sous l'éclairage projectif. In C. Chabert, D. Cupa, and R. Kaes (Eds.), *Didier Anzieu: Le Moi-peau et la psychanalyse des limites*. Éditions érès, Collection Carnet/Psy, pp. 159–177.
Ezquerra, L. (2019). *Liquids settings. Setting(s)*. Symposium, Asociación Psicoanalítica de Madrid (APM).
Freud, S. (1905). *Tres ensayos de teoría sexual y otras obras*, Vol. 7. Amorrortu Editores.
Freud, S. (1923). *The ego and the id*, Vol. 19. Hogarth Press.
Freud, S. (1927). *Fetichismo*, Vol. XXI. Amorrortu, pp. 141–152.
Green, A. (1972). Note sur les processus tertiaires. *Revue Française de Psychanalyse*, 36: 407–411.
Green, A. (2007). Le penser. Du Moi-peau au Moi pensant. In C. Chabert, D. Cupa, and R. Kaes (Eds.), *Didier Anzieu: Le Moi-peau et la psychanalyse des limites*. Éditions érès, Collection Carnet/Psy, pp. 145–158.
Lévi-Strauss, C. (1964). *Mythologiques I: Le cru et le cuit*. Librairie Plon.
Moreno, J. (2016). *Presentaciones del ir y del venir. El psicoanálisis interrogado. De las causas al devenir*. Lugar Editorial.
Séchaud, E. (2007). Didier Anzieu. Penser les pensées. In C. Chabert, D. Cupa, and R. Kaes (Eds.), *Didier Anzieu: Le Moi-peau et la psychanalyse des limites*. Éditions érès, Collection Carnet/Psy, pp. 11–30.
Roussillon, R. (2007). Le Moi-peau et la réflexivité. In C. Chabert, D. Cupa, and R. Kaes (Eds.), *D. Anzieu: Le Moi-peau et la psychanalyse des limites*. Éditions érès, Collection Carnet/Psy.
Roussillon, R. (2012). Le Fétiche et l'archaïque. Le fétichisme. *Études psychanalytiques*. PUF, pp. 147–170.
Tordo, F. (2019). *Le moi-cyborg. Psychanalyse et neurosciences de l'homme connecté*. Dunod.
Winnicott, D.W. (1953). Transitional objects and transitional phenomena—A study of the first not-me possession. *International Journal of Psychoanalysis*, 34: 89–97.

5 Six Years Later
Toward a Clinic of Technosubjectivity

This chapter presents the psychoanalytic sessions conducted with Neil Harbisson six years after the initial encounter that gave rise to *Fictions or Realities: The Cyborg Transference*. What initially emerged as an exploratory dialogue progressively acquired the contours of a psychoanalytic framework, thereby opening the possibility of considering Harbisson's experience not merely as a personal testimony, but as exemplary material for theorizing a clinic of technosubjectivity.

In this perspective, technosubjectivity names the broader psychoanalytic horizon within which post-organic bodies, hybrid organisms, biotechnologies, algorithmic interfaces, virtual environments, and prosthetic integrations appear as modalities—not as external add-ons but as structural participants in the economy of drives, in ego formation, and in symbolization. Thus the question here is not whether technology "influences" psychic life, but how it becomes one of its constitutive conditions.

On method and publication. The sessions were held once a week, remotely, and they were recorded, by mutual agreement. They are conducted face to face and presented in their integral form for two reasons. The first is to foster collective discussion: making the raw material available allows colleagues to evaluate listening, timing, and the transferential field without the bias of selective excerpts. In this case, there is in fact almost no act of clinical excerpting carried out by the analyst; rather, the recording device itself performs a kind of automatic selection, producing its own inscription of the encounter. This displacement—where the machine becomes co-responsible for what is fixed, stored, and potentially circulated—calls into question not only the coordinates of contemporary clinics, but also the very function of the analyst's selective memory. Recording partly suspends the filter of such memory and of countertransferential reconstruction, introducing a tension between the living trace of the session and its machinic inscription. Nonetheless, countertransference remains: the machine does not register it, but the technical is inscribed in the analyst. Yet countertransference itself can no longer be the same as in the era before the contemporary techno-environment; even in a face-to-face encounter, both analyst and patient are traversed

DOI: 10.4324/9781003640684-5

by a techno-mediated world, which inevitably modulates and transforms also the countertransferential experience.

As Martina Burdet highlights in her case partly online with Mr. Z:

> the word I use [in the session] is the result of my own sensoriality in relation to the patient's image and discourse, such that my bodily countertransferential reaction produces an unprecedented expansion in the understanding of certain cases
>
> (Burdet, 2024, p. 198)[1]

Her remark underscores that countertransference is increasingly bound to the analyst's sensoriality as mediated through technical frames, images, and devices. This situates the analyst's body not only as a receiver of unconscious communication, but as itself technologically modulated, producing new forms of resonance and expansion in analytic listening.

The second reason is to make the analyst's work visible as part of the clinical object itself. The choice to show the how—the analyst's questions, silences, and shifts—forms part of the very clinic under examination.

What follows is not a traditional case vignette but an invitation to see how analysis can operate under these unprecedented conditions.

The sessions were grounded in a principle of reciprocity. Following Harbisson's earlier dialogues and given his generosity in sharing his thoughts with me, I suggested that my psychoanalytic listening might serve as a gesture of return.

In the first of these later meetings, held six years later, it was Harbisson who asked—without any suggestion on my part—whether he could attend physically; circumstances on his side made this impossible and the encounters unfolded remotely. This fact itself becomes material for reflection: the encounter is inscribed within the technosphere that characterizes contemporary subjectivities. As has been explored in relation to tele-analysis, the very notion of presence acquires a new inflection under conditions of absence: bodies, though spatially distant, remain affectively "touched," while novel sensorialities are triggered (Burdet, 2025).

Consent is equally significant. Harbisson explicitly authorized the dissemination of these dialogues, with a few personal details kept private at his request. His openness may be read as emblematic of a broader cultural shift: the increasing permeability between intimate and collective spheres, between the analytic setting and the wider social space. What is spoken in analysis does not remain confined to an interiority, but circulates across expanded networks of inscription and transmission.

This dynamic puts the psychoanalytical frame to the test, without applying a pre-existing setting; it allows the setting itself to be interrogated and strained by the cyborg experience. The resulting triadic field—patient, analyst, and technical medium—became itself an object of enquiry.

As I mentioned, this strain does not concern the patient alone: the analyst is also traversed by technology, and what emerges is a third space, a shared field in which the unconsciouses of the patient and the analyst both intertwine under the mediation and co-constitution of the technical. This recalls Ogden's (2004) formulation of the analytic field, but here it takes the form of a chimera, in the sense described by Michel de M'Uzan (1994): a new psychic being born of the deep interweaving of unconscious—now also technologically inscribed as a hybrid construction where the human and the machinic are assembled into a single psychic body.

The analytic bond is therefore no longer organized exclusively around the dual relation between analyst and patient, but extends into a triadic or reticular field: subject-object-other or, at times, hybrid self-analyst. The object does not merely convey transference; it generates, transforms, and sustains it. In this sense, the technological organ reveals a contemporary mutation of the object—no longer a symbolic mediator but a constitutive element of the link itself.

* * * *

It is in this common space that the following hypothesis is explored: the encounter between two human beings—one of whom explicitly feels "more technology" than the other—whose unconscious, already modulated by the digital, is confronted and transformed. The clinic of technosubjectivity is configured precisely in this triadic field, where the analytic no longer concerns only two, but unfolds as the elaboration of a hybrid experience, at once human and technological.

Already in *Fictions or Realities: The Cyborg Transference* (Ezquerra, 2019), the first psychoanalytic exploration of Harbisson's experience, I proposed the hypothesis that the cyborg condition inaugurates a profound reconfiguration of psychic life. In this perspective, the technological object ceases to function as a mere external prosthesis and instead becomes a constitutive element of subjectivity itself. What I termed "techno-transference" sought to capture how transferential dynamics are modified when the patient already carries incorporated technology and is, in some sense, co-constituted through it: the organ takes libidinal investment, functions as fetish-transitional-interface and modulates the relation to perception, identity, and the analyst.

This reference to the analyst requires clarification. What is at stake is not simply the subject's private relation to his technological organ, but the way such an organ comes to function as a transferential pivot within the analytic encounter itself. In *The Dynamics of Transference* (1912), Freud situates transference within the field of human relations—toward the analyst and, by extension, other persons who revive the prototypes of early imagos. Yet, Freud's later reflections on fetishism (1927) open the possibility that libido may also be displaced onto inanimate objects, which, once invested, assume the status of love-objects. Within this expanded Freudian horizon, the implanted organ may be understood as precisely such a "suitable object": not a neutral prosthesis, but one already libidinally invested. It mediates the patient's relation to the analyst as much as to the world, operating both as a fetishistic substitute and as a transferential hinge where psychic and technical circuits converge.

In this context, the object itself undergoes a profound mutation. In classical psychoanalytic theory—from Freud to Winnicott—the object occupies an intermediary position: it mediates between self and other, between drive and representation, between inside and outside. It allows the relation but does not constitute its structure. Within technosubjectivities, however, the technological object ceases to be a mere mediator and becomes a structural component of the psychic circuit. It modulates perception, affect, and memory, operating as both container and connector of libidinal exchanges.

From lack to continuity: whereas the classical object is defined by loss that, through the dialectic of desire and absence, makes thinking possible, the technological object tends to offer an illusion of unbroken continuity, of total availability. It is an object that does not lack, does not withdraw, does not die. In Green's terms, it introduces a disavowal of negativity, a defense against absence and the void. Through its constant presence and connectability, it reassures the subject while simultaneously eroding the psychic space where absence gives rise to symbolization.

When Harbisson speaks of his antenna—its pain, its integration into his body, its capacity to alter dreams—these elements do not remain at the level of description but organize the very way in which he positions himself in the analytic situation. In this sense, the technological organ is not simply an extension of perception but rather a device that shores up archaic fissures, providing a new surface of identity and continuity for the self. The organ thus operates simultaneously on three levels: as a fetish, denying castration while preserving narcissism; as a transitional object, mediating between inner and outer reality; and as an interface, reconfiguring the patient's relation not only to perception and identity but also to the analyst, who is inevitably implicated in the field opened by this hybrid organ.

Some of Harbisson's elaborations, as we will see in the next interview, center around antenna pain, colored dreams, the phenomenon of aphantasia, and his refusal of fixed identity categories. They provide some examples of direct clinical evidence of such psychic reconfiguration. The fetishistic and transitional logics identified earlier reappear, confirming failures of symbolization and early holding functions traceable to the most archaic layers of psychic development.

Taken together, the material suggests that the hypotheses advanced in 2019 should now be revisited within a broader clinical and theoretical horizon. In 2019, my focus was on formulating the notion of technotransference and on conceiving the cyborg as a paradigmatic case of technosubjectivity, defined by the structural presence of technology in the psychic apparatus. Six years later, the clinical sessions allow us to go further: what was then articulated at the level of theoretical conjecture can now be elaborated in vivo as the contours of a clinic of technosubjectivity—a clinic where the archaic and the technological, the failures of symbolization and the machinic prosthesis, are interwoven in the production of new forms of psychic life.

In this interview and in the sessions that follow, what also comes to the fore is not merely the integration of a prosthesis into psychic life, but also the very testing of whether psychoanalytic listening can operate in a cyborg subject. The question of usefulness—whether such listening "serves" or not—and of how it might serve, already becomes diagnostic in itself, marking the entry into a post-organic clinic.

Interview with Neil Six Years Later

After a long period in which it seemed that Neil had disappeared, dating back to 2019, I proposed another interview, though deep down I imagined he would refuse. He told me at the time that he did not usually accept interviews. In my fantasy, a cyborg would flee from any attachment with another.

A: I wonder if you've had any dreams lately, and if so, what meaning you can give to those dreams. You told me that other people could send you colors, but I imagine there must be times when they could send you texts or audio messages.

N: This is a project I did, where there were five people who had permission to send colors to my head. And this went on for three years or so. With the app, they could live stream. They could be looking at a supermarket on their mobile phones and I would receive the colors from the supermarket. It was a way of sharing the sense of color with other people and separating my body from the sense. And then if they sent me colors while I was asleep, they would wake me up or disturb my dreams or color my dreams.

A: And how do you sleep?

N: Very well. Well, I've had periods of antenna pain. In these twenty years with the antenna, there are times when I have had antenna pain, and then I have trouble sleeping. I wake up with a very bad posture during the night. But this is now a question of the organ, not the sense. When I sleep, the sense of color doesn't bother me. I can hear colors while I sleep and it doesn't bother me.

A: Why does it hurt?

N: Perhaps changes in pressure or temperature, or sometimes also the connection between the bone and the metal. It's something physical. It's not psychological. I notice that I have an antenna, it's like having a headache.

[…]

A: How is your implant? Is it in the bone or beyond the bone?

N: Well, what's inside the bone can't be removed because it's integrated and that's where I receive the vibrations. But the blue tooth implant could at least be cleaned. In the case of a friend who had implants in her feet, the muscle ate them. Now she's pregnant and has implants outside her stomach. These sensors send the sounds of the pregnancy to the father. So the father has bone headphones that allow him to listen to the pregnancy through his mobile phone. So what she has allows her to share the pregnancy with her partner.
[…]
N: [*Referring to the sense of time that has been recently added*] The crown will allow me to feel the rotation of the planet around my head. It's a hotspot that takes 24 hours to come full circle. When the brain gets used to it, the goal is to see if I can create illusions of time. Because there will be a person who will have access to the crown's chip code and will be able to modify the speed at which the hotspot rotates. So, the goal is to see if this alters my perception of time. If the person makes it go slower, without my knowing, in theory I will notice that time is going slower.
A: Time is very subjective …
N: Yes, yes.
A: With the organs you have, for example, with the antenna, do you think you dream differently? I mean with regard to having an antenna or not, is there a transformation in your dreams?
N: New senses appear in dreams. I hear colors in my dreams and I also perceive where North is. I have the North implant, remember?
A: Yes.
N: I'm looking at you, you're almost perfectly south … At first you're very aware of it, but in the end you don't even notice that it vibrates when you face North. Then it becomes subliminal in the same way that hearing colors became subliminal. And there also comes a point when this appears in dreams.
A: Can you remember any dreams you've had?
N: I dream a lot about flying … Those are the ones I remember … And the technique of flying. It's about the difficulty of landing. Sometimes you fall too fast and you have to control the fall. I dream a lot about flying and landing with my arms.
A: What does it mean to you?
N: That I want to leave and at some point I want to come back. Because when I fly there is no one else there. It's the perspective of seeing everything more clearly and the difficulty of coming down. It can be interpreted in many ways. I think it's related to the feeling of freedom that comes with being able to fly. Because sometimes I'm walking down the street and I start flying. Doesn't that happen to you? Don't you dream about flying?
A: It made me think of a dream where you feel powerful. And where would you like to go?
N: I always knew that I wanted to do music, classical music, then I did this antenna project at university and it changed everything. It changed my perception of reality and I think it's taken me twenty years to come back.

Orchestra conducting has always appealed to me, as it allows me to understand sounds. Perhaps later I can bring the two worlds together: cybernetics, classical music, and the cyborg world. They seem unrelated, but there are points where they can be connected.

[…]

A: The question I ask myself is, would a psychoanalytic session be of any use to a cyborg?

I ask this because I get the impression that the cyborg solution is that, once you feel so strong in relation to many other human beings, it's like you don't need anything or anyone. Obviously, as you're not one hundred per cent technology yet, but also a human being, I don't think that can be the case …

[…]

On the other hand, I remember that last time you didn't mind me sharing what you told me publicly.

N: No, it's not a problem. I don't see a line between my privacy and other people, I'm not saying anything that's secret. I don't care.

N: Maybe things that involve other people, then no.

A: A dream is already quite private.

N: Yes. I can't visualize the dream, I've known about it for maybe a month. My sister can't either. For example, if someone tells us to close our eyes and imagine an apple, we can't see the apple, and it's the same when I tell you the dream. The dreams I remember aren't visual.

A: A family thing …

N: It's called aphantasia. For example, I can't visualize my mother's face, and neither can my sister.

A: But when you saw me today, did you remember me or not?

N: No, impossible. We've compared what happens to us with our mother with people who can visualize. My sister and I can only see white lines on a black background. We can remember things, but we can't visualize them. That's why when you ask me what dreams I remember, I think I remember very few dreams, because they are actions. It will never be a visual description of what I dream, it will be a description of what happened.

A: I understand, but last time you told me about a dream … and today too …

N: I can't visualize it. It would have to be something I had focused on a lot and consciously retained. We've had this since birth, but she [my sister] doesn't have achromatopsia. My sister and I are in shock because we've never talked about this before. Most people can remember the smell of coffee or chocolate, but they don't smell it when they remember it. It's the same for us. We can remember our mother, but we can't see her, we can't see her face.

A: Does this tell you anything about your relationship with your mother?

N: What?

A: This situation of not being able to picture her, not being able to picture anything …

I feel that he doesn't seem to understand me.
N: No, this is something with everything, it's not just with my mother, we can't visualize our father either, I can't even visualize myself.
A: And, for example, when you look in the mirror, can you visualize yourself?
N: Of course.
[...]
A: Let's suppose that you come to my office because you want to improve something or you think you have a problem, what would you tell me?
N: What kind of help?
A: Psychological ...
N: I'm not aware that I have any psychological problems. I feel psychologically very well. I'm not aware that I need any help, so the first thing would be to find out what help I need.
A: When you were a child, you told me that you didn't understand your problem and that the problem was society.
N: The most intriguing thing is not knowing what you don't see, because even if you describe a color, it's very difficult to understand what that color is. When you're a child, if you're lame, you know there's a problem. But if you can't see colors, you don't know what it is you can't see. It was very confusing, you don't know what other people see. It's perhaps the strangest psychological situation. It's impossible for me to know what a color is, I imagine it as an energy.
[...]
A: Changing the subject, I remember you explained to me that gender is not an issue for cyborgs. How would you define yourself? In today's society, the spectrum is very broad, and you also created the Trans-species Association.
N: Being a cyborg or trans-species is more about species. They are two different issues, gender and species. What has affected me about the antenna is the sense of species, because the definition of human does not include antenna as an organ, it does not include infrared or ultraviolet senses. These are senses that I have completely integrated.
A: I understand, but how would you introduce yourself?
N: I don't think I would introduce myself. I happen to be a man, but if I say I'm a man, it doesn't fit, and if I say I'm a woman, it doesn't fit either. Neither fits me. "Man" culturally implies stereotypes that make me feel very uncomfortable, and "woman" too, I don't fit in. I'm not a woman, so I feel uncomfortable with any definition. Saying trans-species gives me a freer sense because it's a definition that can change.
A: Let's say you feel uncomfortable with feeling pigeonholed. For example, do you have a partner?
N: No
A: But have you ever had one?

N: Yes. There are also many types of partners. I like everything to be more ambiguous. There's no need to name relationships. I don't say this is my friend either.
A: It seems you can't stand anything that closes or commits you.
N: If I say he's my friend and tomorrow he's not, then I have to tell the other person he's not my friend anymore. There's no need to name things that are constantly changing. If I name them, I help prevent things from changing, and I don't like that.
A: I understand that naming things takes you out of something more diffuse and you don't like it.
N: It forces me to simplify. Color isn't fixed either, because it changes. I don't mind giving names to things when I'm pretty sure they won't change. I don't mind saying that I'm a musician. For other things, I like them to be more open and flexible, like relationships with people or identifying oneself. With [name of a woman] we've been through everything, we've lived together for twenty years. We went to study together. We've had a completely flexible relationship. We've been through all the stages. At times there have even been three of us. We still see each other, we're like a family, like soulmates. Now she's pregnant. I'm going to be the godfather. I'm not worried about having a partner. I think some people are very stressed about finding the love of their life. I feel like I've already experienced everything. And since I don't want to have children because I don't see myself as responsible enough to have them, being a godfather is perfect for me.
A: You've found a good solution.
I understand that the way you live, gender, sexuality, relationships, have to do with keeping things open. At one moment you might like a woman, at another a man. You put yourself in an open spectrum.
N: I think I've always been like that.
[…]
A: Going back to your connection with technology, does it help you to move forward? It's been twenty years since you got the antenna. You told me that since you got the antenna, you felt taller and that you've incorporated it as a sense, like another organ. So there's a clear transformation in yourself.
N: It's not that I *feel* taller, it's that I am taller. Not feeling taller is what made me bump into things, because I had to get used to being taller. What has helped me with technology is that perception is not fixed, we can modify it and there is no end. There are countless ways to rediscover the world through new senses, which I don't think is possible without technology. The other option would be to genetically modify ourselves.
A: On the day your biological body dies, would you want to be inside a piece of software?
N: To do what? I don't want to live longer. I want to be more alive. My goal is not to prolong my life, but to be more alive by adding senses that allow me to rediscover reality.

A: And why can nothing be fixed for you? We're back to the previous idea.
N: Because it's boring, repetitive. There are people who don't have anything implanted and don't have the feeling of being one hundred percent human. In my case, I joined technology, which made me felt less human, because I started to notice the antenna as an organ. Also because it's physically inside my body. Not feeling one hundred percent human is not noticing the difference between the brain and the software; this is what makes me feel more like a cyborg than the antenna as an organ in the body. This is where I started to define myself as a cyborg. I also started dreaming in colors. The brain created the sound of color, not the antenna.
[…]
A: I got the impression that the way you use your senses had transformed something painful in your life.
N: Painful, I don't think so, but "disturbing" more than painful.
A: Your mother told you how sad it was to see everything in black and white …
N: Well, they still say that. People say it's sad. For me, it made me very curious and restless, because everything about color is very mysterious.
A: You told me that your mother was told you would be born blind. She must have had a very hard time, and she must have been very anxious. You also described your parents as quite isolated people.
N: My mother grew up in Germany and my father is Irish, and they came to Spain and didn't know anyone. They were used to a more Nordic environment. They were very unsociable, no one came to our house. They divorced years ago. My mother has opened up more, she's more sociable, but my father doesn't have any friends, although he's very happy. I don't know if my father is autistic. He knows all the numbers, the buses, all the addresses. He was a teacher and had many students. My mother was also a teacher.
A: From what you describe, your parents seem a bit disconnected.
N: Very isolated. Yes, but it's understandable. My father would have stayed in Belfast, but there were bombs every week. Since then, he's been disconnected from his world. My mother left Spain, which disconnected her from her world; she grew up in Germany. They don't have any friends because they don't have a past here. They're both a bit disconnected from their roots.
A: The impression I get is that you come from a place, from families, where things haven't been easy. You talk about Belfast, but you also talk about Germany, countries with a difficult recent history. In addition to having very disconnected parents, I wonder how they got through it when your mother was pregnant?
[…]
N: The other thing is that when I don't remember if I know you, unless there's something like glasses. Now I know you're the same person as before, because of the glasses, I know it's you.

A: How do you know it's me?
N: First, it's the way you are, the movement and then the voice. However, if someone greets me on the street, I recognize them but never by their face, it's everything except the face.
A: Interesting, because humans in general connect through sight, through the face, through expression. When babies are small, they connect with their mother and father, also through the face.
N: When I was little, there was only my mother and father at home. There were no other people. I think that's perhaps why I didn't learn to recognize faces when I was little. There were only three faces in my life for many years.
A: Did you recognize your mother?
N: I remember one day when I got it wrong, but I think that's normal. I got the wrong father, the wrong person. It's very uncomfortable. It's the worst thing. What bothers me most socially, what affects me, isn't the color. It's living in doubt, not knowing whether you know someone or not. It's horrible.
A: I imagine that for you it's like living in a slightly disturbing universe, like in the shadows. I've imagined that your parents' family history and yours in that context have something to do with the inability to recognize faces. It seems like there have been very traumatic issues since you were a baby. Not being able to represent yourself in images perhaps says a lot about you.
[…]
I suggest starting the sessions in the next weeks.
[…]
N: My childhood was happy. We were isolated, very lonely, but very happy. I don't see my childhood as sad, and my parents are not pessimistic.
[…]
N: Over the last twenty years, technology has not only allowed me to continue transforming myself, but after two, three, four years, ten years, I began to see that other people were noticing this too. There are people who don't have implants, but they notice this connection with technology that I am experiencing. That makes me connect with people who understand this feeling. Many people are already connected to technology and don't realize it.
[…]
A: It's very interesting that the antenna hurts you. That means it has already become part of yourself.
I suggest to Neil that he goes back to the dreams.
N: Many years ago, I remember flying to Ireland. I don't fly to Ireland anymore. That's where my grandparents were, where we used to go in the summer. Flying there was very relaxing for me. Every summer we went to the same place. I guess I liked it so much that I dreamed of flying there. And now that my grandparents are gone, maybe I fly around here.

A: Do you miss your grandparents?
N: I only saw them once a year. There were no video calls, it was all letters. Yes, I may have missed them. They were used to constant danger. There were a lot of bomb threats. In 2004, when I installed the antenna, my grandfather died. And in 2009, my grandmother. Remembering my dream, I'm very aware of balance. If you break it, the air pressure makes you fall.
A: It reminds me of your sense of direction, it's like not losing your balance and not losing your way.
N: I can't fly very high either, because otherwise there's no oxygen. It's not a peaceful flight. I have to think about a lot of things when I'm flying. Because if you lose your focus, you die.
A: It seems like you're afraid of losing your balance, because the organs you install are something that ground you in the world. In other words, having a sense of direction, of time, seeing colors, is something that places you.
N: From Wednesday I'll have a new organ, maybe this will awaken my dreams.
Neil asks if he can come to the consultation in person.
N: What a coincidence that of all the places I could go, it's Madrid. It's very interesting for me because you make me think about things I hadn't thought about before.

From Techno-Transference to Technosubjectivity: Commentary on the Interview

In the comments that follow this interview and subsequent sessions, my aim is not to provide an exhaustive psychoanalytic analysis of the material but rather to highlight certain aspects that I consider clinically relevant for thinking about the clinic of technosubjectivity. I will focus on a few examples from this interview in order to reflect on transferential and countertransferential aspects.

In this second interview, I did not experience the headache that had accompanied our first in-person encounter. Over the years, something seems to have been assimilated—perhaps what had initially felt traumatic to me: not only the idea of the cyborg itself, but the very notion of technological perforation—both literal and metaphorical—of the human body. At that time, this intrusion had deeply unsettled me, as if it touched a limit of what could be thought or tolerated. In this session, however, I sensed a greater degree of integration, as though the years had allowed a psychic metabolization of that earlier disturbance. Perhaps the fact that we were now meeting at a distance also introduced a limit, a mediation that contained the experience and rendered it more bearable.

Neil refers to his North-sense organ: "I am looking at you, you are almost perfectly south." The organ not only expands perception but also seems to allow him to situate and communicate with the analyst in a different way: the organ becomes a point of orientation, an axis through which spatial coordinates are established in the transferential relation.

Another transferential element later emerges when Neil states: "I will have a new organ. Maybe this will awaken my dreams." This organ too is clearly invested: he projects onto it the possibility of psychic transformation, but does so in the presence of the analyst. Techno-transference, then, is not isolated but inscribed within the analytic field: the organ, as fetish-transitional-interface, becomes a support of libidinal investment and at the same time binds the patient to the analyst in the common space of the session.

These elements articulate with another fundamental dimension: the impossibility of remembering or representing the faces of his parents. Neil reports that he cannot visualize the face of either his mother or his father. He recognizes the analyst by voice and movement, not by image. The face thus appears as a blurred object, one that cannot be fixed in visual representation and therefore requires other senses—both old and new—to enable him to situate himself in the world. In this sense, technology functions as a supplementary support that helps him to elaborate.

This resonates with the paradox staged in earlier chapters with Pierre-Huyghe's *Liminal* video installation in which a woman wearing a mask embodies, at once, an entry into and an exit from an in-organic world: the mask as a threshold that both reveals and conceals, a passageway that confers a contour where inner form is lacking. We can hypothesize that technological organs, but also external devices or technological symbolic integrations, may function as "techno-masks:" supports that contour the self when the psychic work of giving form to falters.

Yet, in the analytic encounter, this notion of the *techno-mask* may open further questions. It invites us to reflect on how analyst and patient engage in a mutual process of visibility and opacity —what is seen, what remains unseen, and what one wishes to see— and how this dynamic may transform and interrogate the analytic couple itself. What does these series of encounters represent for Neil, and what does it represent for the analyst? The answer remains open, unfolding through the clinical material that follows.

* * * *

This question of the techno-mask thus leads us to a broader issue: that of visibility. In this sense, this issue is approached by Le Poulichet (2003), for whom the face cannot be reduced to a body part, it is the very visual field itself, the intertwining of seeing and being seen in the intersubjective space. What Neil cannot construct internally, he attempts to stage externally—through images, sensors, organs—creating a shared field of vision that provides contour and recognition when inner symbolization remains fragile. Seen in this light, what is at stake is not the invention of an entirely new psychic process but the contemporary accentuation of an originary one. As Le Poulichet reminds us, following Lacan, the mirror stage already integrates not only the child's body-image but also the surrounding in-organic field—rooms, objects, fragments of reality—reflected together on the same surface. Today, technological organs may be read as contemporary equivalents of this inorganic field, reintroduced into subjectivity through new specular environments. Yet it is not only the implanted organ that plays this role: the entire technosphere—artificial intelligence, algorithmic environments, digital interfaces—constitutes a symbolic field that participates in subject formation.

These representational difficulties resonate with the observations of Haag (1994, p. 39) in her work with autistic children. She describes how the perception of the first relationship, the one that shapes the baby's first sense of envelope, seems to be the following:

> Something has to enter through the eyes and into the back of the other person's head, which is then mirrored in oneself, makes an imprint, and then leaves again, making a kind of circle.

The first feeling produced by this envelope, which is not glued to the skin, seems to be a sense of circularity that nevertheless does not encompass the whole body. Originally a face-to-face situation seems to emerge, and the first perception of separation is between two heads. When such an experience fails to consolidate, threats of disintegration emerge.

Convergently, Evzonas in his conference paper *The Face of the (M)Other* (2024)[2] explores, in relation to gender, the anxiety of formlessness. He shows how the face is not merely a bodily fragment but the very field of vision. Its loss or impossibility of representation reactivates archaic terrors of falling, decomposition, or disappearance, in line with what Le Poulichet termed "terrors of the formless." Where Neil cannot visualize the face of his mother or father, or where he fails to recognize the analyst by face but only by voice and movement, this liminal zone between figured and absent face is re-enacted.

Thus, what Haag describes as the primary circularity between two heads, and what Evzonas analyses as the anxiety linked to the loss of the face, is here updated as the subject's attempt to create—through technology—a mirror-double that allows him to situate himself in the world where representation falters.

Neil himself has referred to these representational failures first as *prosopagnosia* and now as *aphantasia*. Dreams, when recalled, are narrated not as images but as non-visual sequences of actions. The unconscious register finds inscription instead in sonic, kinesthetic, and algorithmic modes. By algorithmic modes, I mean a form of psychic inscription that does not rely on image or narrative metaphor but on the logic of sequences, repetitions, and correlations.

In Neil, the technological organs translate data (color frequencies, 24-hour cycles, spatial orientation) into sensory experiences; these algorithmic processes are interiorized and dreamed, constituting a new register of figurability. We may hypothesize that the algorithmic functions as an interface: a space in which technology becomes mirror, support, other, and double. Here the unconscious does not rely solely on images but also on algorithmic patterns that traverse the sensory and the bodily, configuring a mode of subjectivation in which the technological and the psychic are intertwined.

The dream Neil recounts in this interview is eloquent: a flight in which the difficulty is landing, marked by the fear of losing control, but also by the desire for freedom and the need to see more clearly. This material can be read not only in relation to his achromatopsia (difficulty seeing in color), but also as the expression of a constant search to "see beyond": to represent the object and his relation to it in a more precise way, integrating technology as a resource for symbolization. Later, when recalling the same dream, he emphasizes his concern about not losing balance. He himself notes that flying too high is dangerous because "there is no oxygen." The excess of altitude, in my view, may be understood as a metaphor of disconnection: a going-too-far that leaves the subject without support, without air, at risk of disconnecting both from the human and from himself.

This dream already foreshadows the oscillation between distance and proximity that would soon manifest in the analytic relationship. The wish to "see more clearly" and the fear of "flying too high" can be heard as metaphors of his ambivalence toward closeness—between the desire for connection and the defense of withdrawal.

When Neil told me that I made him think about things he had never thought of before, and when he expressed his wish to attend the next sessions in person, I experienced this as a form of rapprochement gradually unfolding between us. It stirred in me both curiosity and a quiet sense of joy. His desire to meet in person seemed to dissolve, at least partially, the distance implied by the technological medium and to reaffirm the human bond within it.

From this point onward, as the analytic encounter moved into the form of remote psychoanalytic sessions, the tone of the work began to shift and the affective resonance to expand. The material that emerged appeared less defensive, allowing for greater depth. As the reader will see in the following pages, certain moments proved profoundly moving, experienced as such by the analyst. They may also be read as signs of a growing trust between us, a trust that would continue to develop across the sessions. I was deeply affected by how the theme of death came to recur with increasing insistence, confirming the impression I had already formed in 2019 of Neil's extreme fragility, and reawakening in me an enduring concern for him.

First Session: The Suicide

N: [*Regarding the new sense of time*] What we want to do is have one person once a week who is allowed to change the speed of the heat point and see if that alters my perception of time. But we haven't taken that step yet. For now, I'm just getting used to the natural 24-hour cycle. And since I've had it, I wake up early and go to bed early. That didn't happen before. I'm more aware of time, like the day lasts longer. So, I get more things done. So, for now, just noticing the rotation of the planet is already changing my life a bit, which wasn't the plan. The plan was to change it later. So it's interesting for me. But now, just constantly noticing the time has organized my day better. I go to bed early.
A: And dreams?
N: I try to think if I remember any dreams, but I don't. I don't know what to talk about.
[...]
Sometimes I wonder if adding senses is equivalent to taking drugs. And if there were no cybernetics, I would be a drug addict. Because when people take drugs, they try to alter their perception. And this is also a way of altering it, but in a much more controlled way, without side effects, cleaner [...] Once you expand your perception and this expansion of perception becomes normal, as has happened with my antenna, hearing colors is not strange to me. It's even a little boring. It's so normal that it's not interesting for me to perceive color anymore. In fact, in November, I will have spent more time with the antenna than without it. Therefore, it will be more normal to me to hear color than not to hear it. Chronologically speaking, I mean. I don't know if it's an addiction, but I do think I get bored with reality. And that's why reality is so boring, repeatedly the same sensory inputs that adding a new perception makes me feel more alive, I guess. And it's not so different from people who, perhaps with alcohol or drugs, also find these new realities that make life less repetitive and less boring.
[...]
A: I don't think we can generalize because in this case we're talking about you, perhaps that antenna wouldn't be the same in someone else as it is in you. But why is reality boring and, in that sense, why would you want to take drugs?
N: Repetition is boring, rather than life being boring. Life is very interesting, but we don't perceive it. That's what happens to me. So, if we live only with mental stimuli, I think that something is missing. We lack the sensory stimuli we had when we were children, when we smelled something for the first time, saw something for the first time, heard an instrument for the first time. When everything has already been heard, seen, and smelled, we lack new sensory stimuli, which we replace with mental stimuli.

A: So, perhaps it would be a matter of trying to return to a search for the primary moment, the place where those first stimuli were found.
N: Sensory stimuli, yes.
A: But in a way, all stimuli are sensory, insofar as they enter through the senses, aren't they?
N: Well, there are more intellectual stimuli—perhaps studying. Doing the master's degree in conducting has been a very mental stimulation. I've used my hearing, the same sounds, the same musicians, the same instruments. I've used my balance. The senses have been the same, but the stimulus has been mental. But to also feed the sensory stimuli there are cybernetics or certain drugs. That's why there is a connection in this sense between people who seek specific sensory drugs, the most hallucinogenic drugs, because they would have created a connection in this search for sensory stimulation.
A: So you're talking about a return to the origin.
N: It would be more like not abandoning it than a return. At the age of 20, there were still many things that seemed new to me with my organic senses. But I noticed that they were already coming to an end, many things were becoming repetitive. But the fact of adding color was a new sensory stimulus, that stimulus became normalized and then I added the sense of North. I'm not going back, I'm just keeping alive this sensory input that I think we should all keep alive, it shouldn't stop and be replaced by mental inputs alone.
A: You can keep a sensory input alive through, for example, a memory. You can remember the smell of a cake your grandmother used to bake, for example. That's one way of keeping it alive, but what you're proposing is another way of getting to that input.
N: Smelling new things or seeing new things is very difficult. Therefore, what is needed are new senses, rather than smelling something I smelled many years ago. Because it's the same sense, it's smell. It would be a mental stimulus again, because it would remind me of my grandmother, but that's not what I'm looking for.
Silence.
Adding a new sense also alters the previous ones, usually a little.
A: How?
N: For example, perceiving the colors of a person's face that I perceived as grey all my life makes me perceive that face differently. If [I think of] a face, my mother's face, for example, [I realize] I would never have associated her eyes with the sea before. Now, if I hear the sky or the sea, it can sometimes sound like my mother's eyes. This is a connection that makes me revisit my mother's face. Or my house, I perceive it differently since I have had the sense of North, because I relate it to other houses, to other places I have been, where the orientation was also precisely north-east. I relate the room where I lived, or where I grew up, in my mother's house, to places I've been, where the orientation of the room was exactly the

same as my room when I was little. This new sense has changed the way I perceive. And now time is changing, at the moment it's my schedules, but it's likely to alter something preconceived as well.
[…]
Silence.
N: I don't know what to say.
Silence.
A: Let's wait and see what comes to your mind.
N: Anything?
A: Yes
N: Well, on 19 April, I looked out of the window and saw a boy walking around outside. It was quarter to eight, and I watched him and saw that he was waiting, but I noticed that he wasn't waiting for anyone. I noticed that it was a different kind of waiting. It was Easter, and everything was very quiet. I took some photos of him because the way he was waiting caught my attention. He was looking at the sea. That's because I have the sea here.
And he showed it to me.
N: I took some photos because his way of waiting was strange, different. And it was quarter to eight, well, eight o'clock, and I had been watching him for about five minutes when a train came, he turned and ran and killed himself. He committed suicide in front of me. I saw him run toward the train. He died. It affected me quite a lot, of course. It was a shock.
A: Of course, I'm not surprised it affected you so much … [*Perhaps because I, too, felt deeply moved and impressed, I made this comment—it seemed to emerge as a spontaneous gesture of shared closeness between us.*]
N: Well, first of all, I recorded it, and it was unexpected because I was filming him looking at the sea. But the train came, he turned around, jumped over a wall and ran toward the train and died. The train honked a lot, screeched, braked and he was there, completely dead.
A: He threw himself onto the tracks …? [*It was as if I, too, felt the need to capture the image. I asked him to repeat what he had already said, almost to contain the moment. I felt both shocked and deeply moved.*]

How would you describe that way of waiting? Because you sensed something.
N: I sensed that, well, I'm used to seeing people waiting because I've spent days in airports waiting for planes and it was like he was waiting for something bigger. He was waiting for his death. I knew he wasn't waiting for a person because, I don't know, when you wait for someone you look at your mobile phone or you look from side to side, but he was looking at the sea, I don't know how to define it. It was waiting for something, and I don't know why I got up and stood there watching. It was also a holiday, there was no one around, it was very quiet. I watched him for the last ten minutes of his life, then I saw him there, and I didn't really know what to do. I went down after explaining to the police that I

had seen everything. I told them it was suicide, of course, because he didn't try to cross, I saw him jump, it was suicide. I explained it, and also told them that I had recorded it, so I showed them the images from before and the recording. Afterward, I didn't know whether to investigate who he was or not, or try to forget about it. Or find out exactly who he was, and I decided to find out everything. So, I called the funeral home the next day to see if they could tell me who he was. I found out who he was. I went to the funeral. There were a lot of people there. So I could say goodbye properly, because I was in a bad way, seeing his body cut up like that, a leg there, seeing him like that, I wanted to see him in a coffin. I don't know, seeing that he was a loved person, I wanted to see at least that his death had been mourned. I didn't know anything about him. Now I know his name, his age, that his mother had died a year earlier. He was thirty-eight years old.
A: What you're telling me is traumatic, you must have been devastated.
N: Yes, and of course, I can't leave my apartment. I see the place where he died every day, so it's not something I can't easily forget, because I'm where it happened. It's very intense. I didn't talk to any relatives or anyone about this. His father was a teacher, I don't know if it would have helped him to talk about it, but that's how it is.
A: It seems to me that now you're talking about a great sensitivity that you must have, because you could have chosen anyone to take your photos, right? With that landscape in front of you, people pass by, even if not many, but even if it's a holiday, I find it very striking that you decided to photograph the end. Because death is the end, and the story of this young man is very sad. I'm not surprised that you were devastated, and I can see that you tried, in some way, to repair what you had seen as so traumatic, those pieces, at least as you say, seeing them in a box, right?

But I wonder why you have such an almost extreme sensitivity, so developed that you can detect something that has to do with the end, with death. Something that you also try to freeze, because a photo, in a way, captures and freezes. You don't like endings, we've talked about that.
Silence.
N: I don't know, it was immortalizing an important moment.
A: Immortalizing. The word itself says it all, it means making something immortal. In other words, it's something that works against death, immortalizing, something that doesn't die.
N: Well, I take more photos because I have a poor visual memory, that's how I am. I can't see the boy waiting, I have the photo and I can't see, I can't see my mother's face either, and that's why I think that, since I was nine, when I used film, I took a lot of photos, even though it was expensive, they were things I wanted to remember. This way things wouldn't die. I photographed a lot of things because I knew they would disappear, like some of the houses in my town.

I have a thousand or two thousand photos of houses that I knew were going to disappear in a short time. I took a photo of them. This was before Google Street View. In the 1990s, the only way was to take photos to remember what it was like, I took photos of things that I knew were going to disappear, to be able to visualize them, but I don't know if it's because I don't want them to die.
Silence.
To be able to remember ... I have a very bad memory.
A: Being able to remember something also has to do with not letting something die ... You have a bad memory, but you sense something about a catastrophic moment before it happens ...
N: Yes. There was a special moment, that's why you decide to take out your camera and start taking photos. It was a different kind of waiting,
A: You say you don't remember, holding on to tangible images is perhaps also an attempt to hold on to images for yourself that you feel you can't create, which is what you're telling me, since the other day you were talking to me about aphantasy.
N: I can't re-create, and besides, memory is very deceiving, there are people who want to remember something exactly as it was, but, if it's recorded, they realize that it wasn't exactly as they remember it. I like there to have a more objective reality, photographed or recorded.
A: Perhaps it's an attempt on your part to situate yourself in the world, through what you call an objective reality, of what has happened in a photo, of knowing for example where the North is.
N: Yes, yes.
A: Seeing, not just in black and white, but seeing through music, is a way of situating yourself, of placing yourself in the world.
N: Yes, also knowing where you are.
A: You should be sad and shaken up ...
N: It's not being able to stop thinking about what has happened for days. There was a very negative energy. It's rained, the energy isn't the same. It's gone. I guess that was what I imagined. I could still feel his presence, even though he hadn't been here for many days. And also going to the funeral were steps that improved the situation. Because the trains keep passing by.
A: Of course.
N: When they whistle, I think of him, maybe every hour, or every two, every three. Now maybe every three hours I think of him. And I have the connection with his father, whom I don't know, but who was surely the first to see him, apart from the doctor. I have a strange connection with this man too. I saw his father at the funeral. It's a strange situation too, that the two of us are united by this boy. I know that no one else saw him because there was no one else there. And besides, I don't know, I think I'll get to know his father later on. I know people who knew him because he was a teacher in my town.

A: Wasn't your father a teacher?
N: Yes, but at a language school. And he was a primary school teacher.
A: You're talking about a story of a son with a father who was a teacher. Obviously, that's not your story. But you're telling me about the very traumatic story of the relationship between a father and a son. A son who has recently lost his mother.
N: They were already getting over the grief of losing the mother.

Commentary on the First Session

Neil begins the first session with a reflection that can be read as a search for a primary moment, almost a fusional scene of the subject's origins. He observes that once everything has already been seen, heard, and smelled, new sensory stimuli become exhausted and are replaced by mental ones. The addition of new senses thus appears as an attempt to recover that inaugural experience. This is made explicit when he associates chromatic perception with the face of his mother:

> If [I think of] a face, my mother's face for example, [I realize] I would never have associated her eyes with the sea before. Now, if I hear the sky or the sea, it can sometimes sound like my mother's eyes.

Here, the technological organ functions as a means of re-inscribing perception within the field of the originary, transforming the proto-representation of the maternal.

In the associative sequence, when he seems at a loss for words, the account of a photograph emerges: Neil observes a man waiting by the sea and comments: "I took some photos of him because the way he was waiting caught my attention. He was looking at the sea." He then adds: "I watched him and saw that he was waiting, but I noticed that he wasn't waiting for anyone. I noticed that it was a different kind of waiting."

This detail is crucial: it was not ordinary waiting, but a form of waiting immediately perceived as strange, uncanny. Later, Neil remarks that the man was not waiting for anyone, but for "something larger"—his own death. The scene invites a symbolic reading: the man looking at the *sea* can also be heard, in French, as looking toward the *mère* (mother). The homophony *mer/mère* thus links the waiting figure with the maternal dimension already evoked in Neil's previous association, where his mother's eyes were compared to the sea. In this way, the image of the man looking out to sea reactivates for Neil both the impossibility of fixing the maternal face and the necessity of situating himself before a primary, radical alterity, one that is at once maternal, oceanic, and catastrophic.

Moments later, the man threw himself under a train and died. Neil underscores the traumatic impact: "It affected me quite a lot. Of course, it was a shock." The analyst too is shaken and needs to capture the image maybe to keep alive and deny something which is about death. She's confronted with a scene that awakens the fantasy of Neil himself as a fragile subject poised on the boundary between life and death. As Freud (1919) notes in *The Uncanny*, what appears at first familiar and trivial—such as the figure of a man waiting—may suddenly return in a strange form that reveals itself as an announcement of death.

At this point, a clinical hypothesis arises: Neil possesses an extreme hypersensitivity, almost a "death detector," enabling him to register catastrophic thresholds of existence.

His subsequent reaction reveals the effects of a post-traumatic response and the urgent need to elaborate mourning: he contacts the funeral home, wishes to see the body in a coffin, and to ensure that the deceased had indeed been a loved person.

Through photography and video, he seeks to immortalize the end:

> I don't know, it was immortalizing an important moment. That's how I am. I can't see my mother's face either. I wanted to remember. I photographed a lot of things because I knew they would disappear.

Photography thus emerges as a means of capturing the evanescent, of fixing that that risks vanishing, in continuity with his inability to retain the maternal face.

These representational difficulties are consistent with the observations already discussed in the previous commentary on the first interview (Haag, 1994; Evzonas, 2021), and they also converge with Le Poulichet's reflections.

For days afterward, Neil remained haunted by the sound of the passing train, which replayed the traumatic scene and became an incessant reminder of death. His mourning is extended and interwoven with his own family history: a dead mother, and the link to the suicide's father, himself a teacher, echo Neil's own paternal lineage. The suicide scene thus condenses several layers of clinical significance: the return to the originary, the failure of facial representation, the defensive and symbolic function of photography and the implanted organ, catastrophic hypersensitivity, the resonance of the maternal through the image of the *mer/mère*, and the reactivation of filiative bonds around death.

Second Session: Human

In this second session, Harbisson spoke at length about what he described as the "mystery" of antenna pain. Rather than treating it as a mere inconvenience, he valued the pain as evidence that the antenna has truly become part of him. The very fact that it could hurt, he explained, was proof of its integration into the body, no longer an external device but an organ capable of belonging.

What fascinated him most, however, were not the normal functions of the antenna but its side effects and anomalies. He described, for instance, perceiving ultraviolet light in situations where it should not normally appear. Such unexpected phenomena captured his attention precisely because they revealed how new organs not only extend perception but also destabilize it, creating sensory experiences that fall outside of prediction or control.

At this point, I suggested that while he tends to emphasize the technological aspect of his organs, what may in fact engage him more deeply is something different: not the part of him that feels machine-like, but rather the part that remains human—marked by vulnerability and by what cannot be mastered. He paused to consider this perspective, as if acknowledging that what most draws him is not the mastery of new senses, but the confrontation with those limits where control falters and humanity asserts itself.

Commentary on the Second Session

It is particularly significant that this was the only session that was not recorded due to technical malfunction—even though, like the others, it was conducted through a digital platform. On this occasion, the work of elaboration relied exclusively on the analyst's memory, on countertransferential resonance, and on writing. Paradoxically, it was Neil who sent the link to connect to the session, as the analyst was unable to access it.

This small but revealing reversal, where the patient restores the analyst's connection to the analytic space, shows how the analytic frame and the roles within it can momentarily shift and reconfigure themselves. This moment can also be read as an instance where the patient, rather than the analyst, creates a new analytic setting. The failure of the device paradoxically reveals the vitality of the link, as the patient unconsciously takes on the task of restoring the connection, and transforms absence into presence. In doing so, he appropriates the frame, turning the technical fault into a creative act of psychic continuity. By configuring his own mode of connection and representation, he opens a universe that is uniquely his own.

Then, the technological apparatus, initially conceived as an external support, becomes here an active participant in the analytic process: a mirror reflecting both the patient's inner organization and the oscillations of the analytic bond itself. What emerges is a shared field where the technological medium functions as a transferential object: it holds, disrupts, and reconfigures the analytic relationship, allowing absence itself to become a site of meaning.

For the analyst, this displacement provokes a countertransference experience: a sudden awareness of loss, of the risk of missing something essential, which resonates with the patient's own anxieties of disconnection.

This paradox reveals the degree to which the technological object had become internalized within the analytic setting, binding the analyst herself to its function. The absence of the recording device thus created a peculiar form of anxiety, a sense of potential loss not only of data but of psychic trace, suggesting that the analyst, too, becomes momentarily grafted onto the technical apparatus. The machine, in this sense, appears as a shared analytic body that simultaneously holds the encounter.

In that moment, analyst and patient shared a similar position: neither could bear the idea of losing anything. The fear of loss seemed displaced onto the machine itself, which came to embody the fantasy of rescuing both from absence.

The recording device, the digital link, seemed to promise a kind of salvation from absence, as though technology might rescue both analyst and patient from the very condition of lack that human is meant to confront.

The analyst's failure to record the session finally permits Neil's association with what he calls the "mystery" of his antenna, the pain and anomalies that should not occur and yet nevertheless do.

When I reflected back to Neil that what most deeply engaged him was not the technological dimension but the human, he fell silent. That pause marked a turning point: in this session his interest was no longer situated in the illusion of total mastery or infinite expansion, but at the threshold where fragility, vulnerability, and failure emerge. At that moment, the analyst's interpretative intervention unsettled him, shifting his discourse from the technologized to the vulnerable. The machinic narrative of the organ gave way to the acknowledgment of what cannot be controlled, and the analyst—likely resonating affectively with Neil's most vulnerable side—participated in opening a space where the human asserted itself against fantasies of technological omnipotence.

This session demonstrates that technosubjectivity ultimately refers back to what is most human, arising within the analytic bond: shared pain, fragility, and the impossibility of absolute control—elements already present in the previous session. In this sense, the post-organic clinic takes shape at precisely this threshold: the human and the technical become interwoven, communicating and co-interpreting as part of the same extended field.

Third Session: Dreams and Death

One session was missed due to Neil's professional travel commitments.

N: I'm coming from Patagonia, where I spent eleven days filming, and it was very powerful. We were making a documentary about listening to colors in nature. There were lots of animals: pumas, owls, guanacos.

[...]

And I don't know, what should we talk about?

A: What comes to mind?

N: I can't think of anything. I had a dream. I woke up crying. A year ago, my nanny from when I was little died, and I didn't say goodbye to her. I dreamed that I asked her for forgiveness for not saying goodbye, and in the dream I cried. I woke up in tears. It happened when I was in Patagonia.
A: And what do you think about that dream? Tell me a little more, who was your nanny?
N: She was a woman who used to look after us when we were very young while my parents were working. My sister and I were very close to her. Over time, we grew apart. In her last years, I knew she had cancer, and I guess I feel bad for not having been closer to her. I guess that's what's coming out now, the guilt. In the dream, I was asking her for forgiveness for distancing myself from her. I was crying and asking her for forgiveness, and she said it was okay. I was crying because I felt really bad about distancing myself from her, and of course her death was unexpected. She was young. She died a few months ago. It shocked us because she seemed to be recovering. I guess I've been holding on to this remorse in my subconscious, and it came out in this dream. It's strange to wake up crying. I don't remember ever waking up crying with sadness.

So it's something related to a dream, which is what you were asking me about the other day. Well, this is the one I remember.
A: This dream just appears …
The technical connection was lost, and I could no longer hear him. For a few seconds, I felt worried about losing contact.
N: Can you hear me now?
A: The connection just dropped … this dream appears precisely at a time when you and I are distancing ourselves, which is when you are leaving for Patagonia. And in this dream there is a lot of sadness. There is something that is not going to come back, you have not been able to say goodbye but at the same time there is a desire to be able to say goodbye.
N: It was more of an apology for having been distant for years when she was actually a very close person when I was little. It wasn't saying goodbye.
A: So you feel guilty when a situation arises where you have distanced yourself from someone who cared for you. What do you think about that? Because it's also as if you were talking to me about closeness or distance in relationships, isn't it?
N: I didn't choose for her to take care of me. She's not someone who would be my friend. She's very different from me. Just because she took care of me when I was little doesn't mean I like her now. This situation where someone has taken care of you, but when you get to know her as an adult, you don't like her, is a very strange situation. She talked about other people's secrets. What do you call that? Gossip? She could tell someone's secrets because she was a person who knew a lot of people. I didn't like that, and I didn't like telling her anything because she could tell anyone. I don't like people who talk too openly about the private lives of

people I know, because it makes me feel very uncomfortable. Besides, we had nothing in common, not art, not music, her tastes and mine were very different. So there was no connection, the only connection was that she had taken care of me when I was little. So, when I found out she was ill, I think maybe I should have reached out to her, but I didn't.
A: I understand that you liked her as a child because she took good care of you. You also say it was like a clan of three, your sister, you, and her. In that universe, you probably felt very cared for. Connecting with that part of yourself, you may feel guilty and wish you had said goodbye to her. I think it's an important dream. You said *canguro* (Spanish word for babysitter), not carer, and a kangaroo carries their baby in a pouch.
N: Here we call them *canguros*, not carers. "Carers" are for older people and *canguros* are for children.
[...]
The *canguro* was the only person from outside who came into the house. That's why, when she came, it was something very special. It was a connection that lasted many years. It started with my sister. My sister was a few months old and she looked after her. My sister is from 1979 and is older, and when I was born, she looked after both of us. She was at home from my birth until I was nine years old.
A: When did your mother go back to work?
N: She had always worked teaching at home. My mother was in a room teaching people; the students would come to her. I also dreamed more. I remember flying again. It was flying through breathing. I started going up very high until there was no oxygen, and then I knew I had to come down because otherwise I would run out of oxygen. So this dream was without doing this (moving my arms and hands). Normally I fly by making an effort. And in another one I also flew, but indoors. I don't remember flying indoors before either.
A: And what do you think of those other dreams?
N: I don't know, but I love the ones where I fly. I feel really good when I'm flying.
A: It seems that you are bringing up dreams that have to do with your childhood. The *canguro* dream also refers to your childhood. In that dream, you were still one hundred per cent human.
N: I didn't go near her when she was dying.
A: And why do you feel so guilty? You wake up crying ...
N: I knew she was ill, and I didn't write to her or anything. And that's very wrong.
A: I don't know if that's wrong. What we know is that you needed to distance yourself from her and that was stronger than your desire to be close to her. You must have had your reasons. Obviously, you no longer had the relationship you had when you were a child. I'm reminded of that traumatic scene when the boy dies. When you go to the funeral, there's an attempt to come to terms with something.

N: I wanted to see that there were people crying for his death and that he was loved. It reassured me to know that it wasn't just me who cried for him. I didn't want his death to be just about him and me, but about the whole group. Sharing this feeling with other people reassured me. In this way, the responsibility for what happened is shared.
A: We're talking about two situations that are both situations of death, for different reasons. And it seems that in order to digest that, at least in that case, you need to connect with others. You go and see others cry in order to connect and understand that others are also suffering, that you are not alone. In the dream, you cry because of the guilt of not being able to get closer. I think that through these two situations you bring up elements that question your bond with others.
N: I don't remember anyone I know in my dreams. At the moment, I only remember the babysitter. When I fly, sometimes there is someone there, but I don't know who it is. In most of the dreams where I fly, there are no people I know. Going to the funeral home and the funeral also has to do with the fact that I didn't want to go thinking about who he was.
Long silence.

Now there's a lot of peace when the train goes by. I can think about it, but it doesn't shock me, I've accepted it as something normal. When the train blows its horn, it's like it's saying hello to me, it's not a bad memory anymore. Seeing it say hello is even something positive. But in the early days, I thought it was going to change my image of this whole space, but it didn't. It's funny how something can change so quickly over time.
A: It seems to me that you've made a real effort to transform yourself internally, and to do that you went to the funeral, you tried to imagine what that family might be like and what that person might have been like. Now what I see is that for you to wake up crying, there's something that really moves you that comes through in that dream.
N: Yes, the guilt. When the babysitter died, I've been thinking about this.
A: The babysitter is a maternal figure.
N: She's a person, she's the babysitter.
A: The role she played was an extension of a mother who took care of you, since yours was working, and in that sense she's a maternal figure.
Silence.
N: Yes, and it was strange to just say hello and goodbye to her on the street after she had taken care of us.
A: Of course, it's like a little kid who loves his mother very much and suddenly doesn't recognize her anymore, as if she were a stranger. And I find that very sad.
N: Yes, because she was someone we liked very much. It wasn't just me who distanced myself. My sister and my mother did too. It was because we didn't want to tell her anything very intimate because she might tell someone else.

A: We've talked about intimacy before. You always tell me I can share what you tell me. And I ask myself, could I share this session? Because I feel like you're talking about very intimate things.

N: As long as no third person is named you can. Because, at the end of the day, it's just my point of view.

[...]

N: What you say isn't gossip, because I'm already saying that everything can be said as long as third parties are protected.

[...]

A: I can see that you have the ability to connect with an inner space when your view of yourself is that you have nothing to say.

N: Well, you're the one who's making me do it. I don't know what you do, but you get me to end up saying things, but when I start, I really don't know what we're going to talk about.

A: That's the interesting thing, that we don't know. Perhaps because we've started this work—for example, dreams you remember appear—and we're creating the possibility of having a transitional space that we're shaping together. It seems to me that you're talking to me about things that affect you deeply.

N: And waking up with real tears. I cried for real. I don't remember that ever happening to me before.

A: You're able to connect with a whole part of yourself, an inner part, of sadness and guilt. Because what you're telling me about the babysitter is that it's almost like a story of a child's heartbreak. It's still a story of great disappointment. And it's also sad because you told me that your parents were people who didn't interact much with other people.

N: Yes, she [the babysitter] was the only outsider who came into the house. So when she came, my sister and I were very happy because she was someone different. Yes, because we didn't have any friends, students would come to have lessons and then they would leave, but we didn't say hello to the students. No one, apart from my mother and father, knew us as well as she did. She must have known us better than we knew her because she looked after us when we were little and changed our nappies from when we were babies. I imagine she felt much more connected to us.

A: If she changed your nappies when you were a baby [and looked after you] until you were nine, imagine that ...

N: Yes, because she didn't have children.

A: I see it's time ...

N: That's good, I think it's important to explain this.

Commentary on Third Session

After a week's interruption and the loss of one session—"one session was missed due to Neil's professional travel commitments"—the theme that re-emerges is separation, loss, articulated through a dream about his childhood nanny.

In the dream, Neil asks for forgiveness for not having said goodbye before her death. The affective intensity of this scene is striking: "I don't remember ever waking up crying out of sadness." The tears signal not only the return of guilt but also the emergence of an affective register within the transference-countertransference field generated by the analytic work. This resonates with the analyst's own countertransference and the growing proximity with Neil, and it is precisely within the framework of these sessions that such affective depth becomes accessible.

This dream reactivates the separation from a maternal image inscribed within the transference. Neil makes this explicit when he says: "It is something related to a dream, which is what you were asking me about the other day." The nanny appears here as a prolongation of the mother-analyst, a figure who sustained and cared for him during his earliest years. Yet she is also ambivalent: nurturing and close in childhood, but later perceived as indiscreet and treacherous. This ambivalence reactivates an archaic, persecutory maternal representation that blocks proximity and makes difficult the work of mourning.

At that precise moment, the digital connection failed, and the session was cut for several seconds. Upon reconnecting, the event itself functioned as a mute interpretation: the technical breakdown operated as a pre-sentification of loss, staging at the level of the medium what was simultaneously emerging at the level of psychic content. The irruption of technological absence thus became integrated into the discourse as a living element of the transference. On a countertransferential level, the analyst experienced an immediate fear of disconnection, not only in the technical sense of losing the digital link, but in the deeper sense of a rupture of the bond itself. This anxiety echoed the very theme of the session: the fear of losing contact with the maternal figure, embodied in the nanny, and thus of repeating the experience of separation with the analyst. In this moment, the analyst's fear of losing the patient found its double in the potential collapse of the machine, revealing a transference to the technical apparatus itself. The device, no longer a neutral mediator, emerged as a third participant in the analytic field, carrying both the hope of maintaining contact and the threat of its break.

Death emerges as a guiding thread across the sessions, and Neil's difif-culty in mourning is here rendered more visible. What in previous sessions appeared in the form of photography, video, or new perceptions enabled by implanted organs—attempts to immortalize the ephemeral, to fix what threatened to vanish—now emerges in the dream, opening up other elaborative possibilities that extend beyond the technological. In this sense, one could also read that Neil might have dreamt of this figure even without added organs; that is, technology here does not replace the human, but both registers interlace in the same attempt to give form to loss.

The dream of flying adds another layer. Neil says: "I was flying through breathing." As in other dreams previously recounted, and linked as well to his childhood history, there reappears the fear of going too high and running out of oxygen. This image can, among other interpretations, be read as a metaphor for the limit of the human: going too far—an omnipotence also linked to technological hybridization—carrying the risk of losing psychic and bodily support. Flight embodies expansion and freedom, but also the threat of disconnection and collapse.

Later, referring to the nanny, Neil acknowledges: "I didn't go near her when she was dying." The impossibility of approaching the maternal object at the moment of separation re-enacts the difficulty of mourning.

When the analyst recalls two situations of death—the earlier session in which Neil witnessed a suicide on the train tracks and the present dream—Neil adds that what mattered to him at the funeral was that the death was collectively shared: others were present to cry, to confirm that the deceased had been loved. Here, the group no longer appears merely as a space in which the intimate dissolves into the collective, but as a necessary container: a collective mirror that allows him not to remain alone in the face of trauma. As he put it: "Others are also suffering; you are not alone."

At the end of the session, when I remark on the work carried out by both of us, Neil acknowledges with surprise: "I woke up with real tears. I cried for real." This phrase encapsulates the core of the session: what begins as a dream of guilt and loss expands into a broader confrontation with fragility and the need for containment within the analytic relationship. The analytic frame, mediated and at times fractured by technology, becomes the place where the most human affects, sadness, guilt, and the impossibility of mourning, can surface and be worked through, always in tension with the ambivalent presence of an archaic maternal object that simultaneously sustains, persecutes, and obstructs mourning.

Session Four: The Other Suicide

N: I haven't been dreaming. Another person has committed suicide.

A: What?

I feel shocked.

N: Another person committed suicide using the train. This time he didn't die. They pulled him out from under the train. I didn't see it. We heard the train screeching and braking, the impact wasn't that strong, and then he was left underneath and the train moved on. This is the highlight of this week. He's thirty years old and, in theory, he's alive. That's luck. I saw them pull him out from under the train, with oxygen, with an electrocardiogram, with pumps and stuff. It was on Sunday, at ten past ten. There's no protection here. I thought about printing out a telephone number. If you're suicidal, they try to help you. I think this is an area where this telephone number should be. It's not that normal for this to happen. I asked the neighbors and they said that in the last eleven years they had never seen it. But they say that when there's one suicide, there's usually another. It increases the chances that someone will see it and think that they can do it too and then do it. I do not know if these suicides are connected. I'm not investigating this one. I know he's alive with a head injury.

What else? This week I also went to a school to talk to children about listening to colors and being cyborgs. I don't do this very often. It was interesting because these children were born in 2012–2013. They are from a generation I don't know, and each pupil had prepared a question. Well, I don't think the mindset has changed that much. I didn't notice anything extremely new. Just more or less the same questions. They want to have new senses. About seven of the class were interested in experimenting and extending their senses. And we are also preparing an exhibition. I am transforming the sounds and the colors of the sounds. It will be exhibited in a local festival. I have been working all these days creating these transpositions from color to sound. You will be able to hear the sounds of the local festival and see the color of the sound. There are eighteen of us artists. I send the color to the eighteen artists and they create a work of art from these colors and the sound. It is another way of perceiving sound through color frequencies. It is the opposite of the antenna. The antenna transforms color into sound, and I am transforming sound into color. I do this by listening to the sounds and then using Photoshop. Each color has a number, like a Pantone.

[...]

They are like colorful musical scores. I call it sonochromatism. There are moments of great confusion when talking about this subject. I don't know why. There are times when people don't understand the concept of turning sounds into colors. They don't understand because color is color and sound is sound. In practice, thinking that there is a physical connection between the two is very difficult. For some reason, they get lost and separate color and sound again. It's hard to think of a new world where everything is sonochromatic. Our senses teach us a lot how to separate. For example, smell and sound teach us to separate them, as if they did not touch each other. And when there are attempts to unite them, it creates confusion. It is as if there is a lack of language to explain it, when in reality it is much simpler. Even I find it difficult to explain. Color is a frequency and sound is a frequency. Do you understand?

A: Yes, I think so. You've come up with something that is already an elaboration and that you've called sonochromaticism. But in order to organize ourselves in the world, we might need to perceive them separately. And it seems that you have a highly developed sensitivity. I say this because of the boy you recorded the other day. You seem to be attentive to situations that are on the verge of catastrophe, taking catastrophe as something that can indeed end in something bad, but also a catastrophic change that can be reorganized into something good. In that case, if someone commits suicide, we can think that it is bad. It's as if you were hanging by a very fine thread, like on a precipice. I imagined that you already had an expanded perception.

N: I think so. During my adolescence, there are letters I sent to a friend where I wrote down some intuitions that later came true. I wanted to document some of them. And then, one day, a girl stopped me in the street asking what would happen to her parents because they had divorced. Some people thought I could see the future, and that's not true. I didn't like that. And besides that, it's not useful either. I didn't like people's reactions.

[…]

It's similar to taking a photo of the boy who was waiting for [the train]. It's a way of documenting the moment.

A: Since adolescence, you already needed to document things. Something that led you to capture an image. A photo is ultimately immortalizing an image. It seems like another way of trying to understand the world.

N: Even before that, when I was 11, in 1991. In December 1991, a great-uncle died. At that moment, I smelled something, a new smell. A strange smell. I asked, "Don't you smell something?" No one smelled anything. It wasn't bad. It's a smell I don't know how to describe. And later, about a year or two later, I smelled it again on someone and asked them if someone had died. They said yes, that someone had died and that they were coming from the funeral home. Later on, it happened to me, and whenever I smell this, it means that someone has been near a dead person. I've shared this a lot with my friend. Sometimes we're in a normal situation and I can say, look, there's the smell of death.

That's not a premonition. It's a very specific smell, and it's not a bad smell. In those cases, I'm 99 per cent sure the person has been near a dead person.

A: I don't know if you're aware that you have a hyper-developed ability to detect death. Whether it's because it's coming or because it's already happened. And I wonder, why is that?

N: I don't know, because my connection to death doesn't appear. My grandfather died in 1988, I was four or five years old, but he died in hospital.

A: Who is this grandfather who died in 1988?

N: My mother's father. That was the first death. I was born in 1982, and he died in 1988. Then in 1991, my maternal great-uncle died. I didn't see him dead, nor was I close to either of them, but the smell that was there when my family came is a characteristic smell. It happened again when my paternal grandfather died.

A: Did you know that smell is one of the most archaic senses we have as human beings? It has to do with those first moments when you are born, the bond with your mother, with your father, what happens there. Also when you are in your mother's womb, sound also has to do with that.

N: No one died during my mother's pregnancy either.
A: No one died, but your mother, from what you told me, we don't know if it's related, but she was very worried.
N: Yes, because of the toxoplasmosis
A: They told your mother that you were going to be born blind. We can imagine that your mother was extremely worried.
Silence.
N: When I smell this odor, I stop to see where it's coming from. I'm not going to ask if it's coming from someone.

In fact, when I saw the … the boy's suicide, the first thing I did was close the balcony. I think I closed the balcony so that the energy of what had happened wouldn't come in.
I don't know if that's normal.
A: What is normal and what is not normal is very relative. Perhaps it was your instinctive reaction at that moment, so that the smell of death would not come in.
N: Well, in this case, it was more the energy of the act than the smell. I wanted to close it so that I wouldn't be affected by the energy of what had happened.
A: What we do know is that it had a big psychological impact on you. Perhaps you needed to think about the energy because you are very sensitive and things affect you so much that you even needed to go to the funeral to understand who that person was.
N: When I was little, I also did something that I stopped doing, which is this.
Makes gestures with hands.
A: What was that?
N: I'm talking to someone and then there's something that bothers me in between and I push it away. It's something like pressure. Those are the things that had no explanation.
A: Maybe it was your way of making sense of something that bothered you, of getting rid of it …
N: I did it until I was twenty years old.
He explains that there were two people who, without knowing each other, saw that there was a light and it coincides with where the antenna is now.

It could be an aura, there are people who can see energy. I don't know. I've never seen it, but this happened during two moments I've been kind of … focused—or dazed. When you're sitting still thinking about something for a few seconds, thinking very carefully, well, there were two moments like that. I think that's the whole history of things that are a bit hard to explain, like the smell, the light, and sensing that something bad is going to happen. These are things that don't have a very clear explanation. About the light, both of them said it was kind of blue.

I don't know what we're going to talk about. We always end up with unexpected topics.

A: You often give the impression, at least you've told me this, of having nothing to say, and yet you have so much to say. And it's precisely very interesting that the unexpected part also comes up. All of that has to do with you. Many questions arise. Why do you have that sensitivity between life and death? Well, your origins are something that was almost between life and death. They are not easy. I mean, already in the womb.
N: That's what it is. My mother had toxoplasmosis.
A: That's very serious in a pregnant woman. She must have been very distressed.
N: Yes, yes.
A: So, it would be logical to think that she would have thought that she was going to have a child who might be stillborn, who might die, or who might be missing an organ.
N: And then, when I was born, I had another problem.

I don't know what it's called, but I slept sitting up until I was three years old. From the age of one, I think.
N: Here [*points to the esophagus*] there's something that closes, but mine didn't close.

I didn't eat. It was a valve that didn't close.
A: A torture …
N: I don't know. I don't remember
[…]

I think my grandmother was very worried. She thought I was going to die because I wasn't eating. My mother told me that. There was concern.
[…]

Commentary on the Fourth Session

Neil's opening words—"I haven't been dreaming. Another person has committed suicide"—are highly significant, setting an opposition between the possibility of psychic elaboration or not. The theme of suicide returns. What at first seems like a banal everyday scene—the sound of the train, the ordinary urban landscape—once again becomes the stage for death. In this formulation, the boundary between dreaming and acting-out seems perilously thin, as if the passage from one to the other were imminent. What emerges might be the exposure of a psychic limit, where elaboration collapses into the threat of action.

The specific rescue scene, with oxygen, electrocardiogram, and resuscitation maneuvers, presents a body poised on the threshold of life and death, suspended in the ambiguity of the living-dead. Neil captures this tension with precision: "He's alive, in theory." The uncertainty impacts the analyst as well, who, in her countertransference, finds herself shocked and worried, entertaining the fantasy of Neil's own possible passage to the act.

As the session unfolds, this experience is reinterpreted as an archaic reminiscence: an evocation of the living-dead state at the origins of life.

The artificially sustained body resonates with Neil's earliest experiences of vital fragility, marked by the threat of death from gestation through infancy.

Neil's account suggests not only the traumatic impact of witnessing such events but also the resurgence of what might be described as a catastrophic hypersensitivity. He refers to anomalous phenomena—smells, "energies"—linked to death. He describes closing the balcony so that "the energy of what had happened" would not enter, as if attempting to establish a protective psychic boundary against the mortiferous. Here the sensory field, particularly smell, becomes intensely invested. Many psychoanalysts have noted that smell preserves traces of the earliest mother-infant bond. In Neil's narrative, the "smell of death" functions perhaps as an embodied index of what resists symbolization.

Once again, the group dimension emerges as a necessary container. In this session, Neil imagines placing a suicide-prevention number at the station. The group is no longer experienced merely as the anonymous dissolution of intimacy, but as a holding structure, a collective mirror that prevents him from remaining alone in the face of trauma.

Equally significant is the movement from the mortiferous to the creative. Neil elaborates what he calls "sonochromatism," the transposition of sound into color frequencies. Technology here operates as mediator, enabling new translations between registers—color into sound, sound into color—while simultaneously exposing the insufficiency of available language, as he himself notes in describing the difficulty of communicating these experiences.

The session concludes with biographical recollections that reinscribe his sensitivity at the level of origins: his mother's toxoplasmosis during pregnancy, the prognosis of blindness, the neonatal reflux that forced him to sleep upright for years. These fragments sketch a subject whose earliest experiences were marked by proximity to pain and death—"almost between life and death" from the very beginning—as well as by the intervention of medical technology. From this perspective, Neil's technological elaborations—organs, senses, perceptual translations—may be read not only as expansions of perception but also as defenses against archaic fragility, attempts to domesticate the catastrophic.

Taken together, the material of this session illuminates the dual trajectory of Neil's technosubjectivity. On the one hand, the repeated confrontation with death, the uncanny hypersensitivity to catastrophe, the difficulty of mourning. On the other, the creation of new symbolic and perceptual frameworks—such as sonochromatism—that give form precisely where the internal symbolic scaffolding falters.

Fifth Session: The Body

N: I have a friend who has insisted that I join the gym, and in the end he has convinced me. I have always ignored my body. This is perhaps the

fifth or sixth time I have joined the gym, and it usually doesn't last long, but let's see if this time it lasts longer.
A: You say you've always ignored your body, yet your implants are linked to your body.
N: My goal is not the body, the goal is the brain, my interest in being a cyborg is not related to the body. There are cyborgs whose goal is the body. Body art is an example. For me, the body is simply a way to access the brain, perception, the senses. My goal has not been to have an antenna, but to listen to colors.

I don't know what else to say.
Silence.
A: Let's see what comes to mind …
N: By the way, I asked my mother what I had. It's called gastroesophageal reflux. You have to stay upright until the food comes out. It's not that unusual, and it can last for months; mine lasted longer.
Silence.
N: I closed the windows because there's noise … Here it is the festival of San Juan. They made a big bonfire. Here there's an event where the witches come down. It was very beautiful. The neighbor from the third floor came. She is a trans girl and now has breast implants and she's experiencing what it's like to have a new organ. She has had surgery to have a new organ, but in this case it's related to gender. It's interesting to see how she is transforming. She is thirty years old, but she had been waiting to have the surgery for a long time and now she is getting used to her body.
A: She might be interested in talking to you …
N: When I bought the flat, I discovered that she lived on the third floor. She lives in exactly the same house with the same layout, but on the third floor. And yes, there are common themes with cyborgs and people who reassign their sex through surgery, although the objectives are very different. We also share how society can react to these changes. There are things we share, and it's curious that we live in the same place. Her identity has been transformed and reaffirmed over time. We also have in common the bureaucracy in relation to identity documents. In the same way that if you have something electronic on your face, they can refuse to renew your identity document. I suppose that if there is a sex change, sometimes you also have to justify it.
A: How curious that you started today's session by telling me that you have never been interested in the body, and now we are talking about the body through this girl, and about perception through the body.
N: For me, perception is the brain. She's interested in the body. For me the interface is not the goal but the means. The body is a means, not the main goal. For body artists, the goal is the body; for those who do tattoos or modifications, the goal is the body; for me, this has never been the case. The brain is also part of the body, but it is internal. How to modify the brain is my goal.

[…]

A: Going back to what your mother told you … Did she tell you if you complained? Did you cry?

N: I complained a lot, I cried a lot, and my father was very desperate. In fact, my father apologized because, when I was little I cried a lot, and he got very nervous at me. I cried because I wasn't well. The first few months or years, I wasn't very well.

A: I get the impression that your early years were very difficult.

Neil recounts in detail how he was first diagnosed with color blindness, only to end up with a diagnosis of achromatopsia at the age of eleven. He also describes a minor accident in which he fell out of bed when he was a few months old. This incident seems to have greatly frightened him and his father.

N: I was in shock and I stopped crying. Sorry, I'll interrupt for a moment. It's a parcel, I guess they'll be coming up now, sorry.

The parcel arrives.

N: A cleaning robot has arrived. A robot that cleans, like a pet. It moves around with its sensor. We've talked about bodies and a slight aversion to the body. I prefer not to think too much about what we have in our bodies, what's inside, the organs. That's the main reason I don't eat meat. I fainted twice at school when I was little because I was thinking about the body. In piano lessons, I never look at my fingers. The body used to be much more repulsive.

A: The body as something dirty …

N: It's something delicate, and, for example, if someone has pain somewhere, then it hurts me. I'm a hypochondriac. I prefer that people don't explain to me what's going on in their bodies. Because if I start listening, I start to notice it. Once, someone told me that they had found something in their heart and they had to have an operation, and afterward I had pain in my heart. I went to the doctor, he examined me and there was nothing wrong. The reason I fainted at school was also because a girl hurt her finger. I didn't even see it, but the pain hurt me too and then I fainted. I have always tried to ignore the body.

A: Since childhood, it seems that there has been suffering that is also linked to the body. Having to sit as a baby is a torture, reflux, achromatopsia, the environment where adults get nervous about what is happening to you … You are also telling me is that you have an extreme sensibility identifying strongly with others. That is a form of communication, archaic, primary.

N: Yes, the people close to me already know to never tell me that they are in pain because I can't bear it.

A: It seems that even your own body, let's say, repulses you. As if you couldn't bear to think that you have a body.

N: Yes, yes.

A: And why is that repulsion?

N: With the girl at school, I fainted because it hurt her.

A: Ah, so if you have the feeling that someone else is in pain, it's as if you had a perception, like millions of antennae, that automatically pick up on the other person's pain.
N: Well, yes, I didn't see what happened to this girl, she hurt her finger and screamed. And it hurt me, it hurt me a lot—and I left to avoid seeing it and I fainted. It happened to me twice more. And whenever they talk about something like this, it hurts me, it really hurts me. It's very real.
A: I have no doubt that it's real.
N: It hurts, that's why I try to avoid being aware of my body, and with my fingers, as they are very delicate parts. I don't look at them, I sense them. My mother has always said that this is not normal and that I have to go to a psychologist to have this looked at. Because sometimes my mother does things with her fingers and I don't look and I tell her to please stop.
[…]
But I'm getting better.
A: It seems that in those moments you become the other person. It's as if you were porous, for better or for worse. You quickly become a double.
N: Because I understand the pain perfectly, because I'm feeling it. It can last for days and it can get worse.
A: The fact that you try to ignore your body then means that it can become so present that it can overwhelm you too.
N: There are things like running my hand over something, running my hand over a surface, caressing, that I can't do. I don't know how to explain it, it makes me feel like bubbles, it itches, like a pain. So I never caress.
A: And if you caress a human, does it happen to you too?
N: I do it like this, never with the palm of my hand. This is also one of the things my mother says is strange about me, and she's right. It hurts me to do it like that, it's very unpleasant.
[…]
A: It's time …
N: How strange, I don't think I have anything to say, yet I can't stop talking … how odd.

Commentary on the Fifth Session: The Body

Neil remarks that he has always ignored his body. This statement stands in contrast to what, for him, constitutes the true objective, namely, the brain, perception, and the senses. This split sets the tone of the session. Later, he also speaks of the body when recounting the identity and bodily transformation of his trans neighbor. Neil, however, insists that for him the body is only a means, never the goal.

As the session progresses, Neil's narrative reveals an underlying archaic fragility. References to gastroesophageal reflux, his early crying crises, and the late diagnosis of achromatopsia place his bodily experience under the sign of precocious suffering and of a mismatch between his needs and, most likely, the environment's capacity to respond. The recollection of a childhood accident and of his father's panic reintroduces an atmosphere of vulnerability.

The episode of the cleaning robot, which Neil describes as "a pet," functions almost as a metaphor for his way of dealing with the body: externalized, mechanized, reduced to function. Yet, in parallel, there emerges a discourse of intense somatic sensitivity: fainting in the face of others' pain, immediate bodily identification with another's suffering, the impossibility of enduring medical descriptions, or even of caressing with the palm of his hand. Here a porous body is revealed, without defenses, traversed by the pain of the other as if it were his own.

The analyst points out how this primary sensitivity resembles a form of archaic, pre-symbolic communication. Neil himself confirms it: "I understand pain perfectly, because I am feeling it." This radical permeability to the other shows a double operation: on the one hand, it constitutes a form of extreme, almost organic empathy; on the other, it is experienced as a threat of invasion and psychic overflow. Hence the need to disavow the body, to avoid thinking it, to flee from it.

From the perspective of a clinic of technosubjectivity, the session shows how the conscious rejection of the body co-exists with its unconscious hyper-inscription. The antenna, the artificial organs, and the perceptual extensions appear as attempts to organize a body otherwise experienced as excessively vulnerable, porous, and uncontainable. One might say that the cyborg emerges as a defense, a kind of technological exoskeleton, against the original porosity of the body; a way of providing technological limits where psychic ones prove insufficient.

In sum, this session unfolds a constant tension between the body as a disavowed medium and the body as an inevitable site of suffering, between the aspiration to cerebral control and the archaic vulnerability of the soma. It is clinical material that invites reflection on how technosubjectivity, far from abolishing corporeality, re-inscribes it in a paradoxical way: as a body rejected, mechanized, yet also as a hyper-affected body, always exposed to both one's own pain and that of the other.

Sixth Session: The Friend's Death

On the day of the session, I received this message: "Hi Laura, sorry, I'm on my way to the hospital to visit a friend who has had a stroke. I won't be able to do the session today. I'll explain everything to you in the next session. Hugs."

Four days later, I received another message: "Hi Laura, how are you? When shall we do the next session? My friend died that same Saturday. We've already had the funeral and everything. Everyone is in shock and very sad these days."

I feel once again shocked and somehow sad. I feel a deep sorrow, with the sense that death is always present. I interpret his request for the next session as a request for human bond, a call for "our bond" that might rescue him.

Seventh Session: Between Mourning and Transmission

N: My friend died.
A: I'm very sorry because you must be very upset.
N: We've all cried a lot. First we saw her, she was still alive, and then she died, brain dead. She was a woman in her 50s. She saw me on television seventeen years ago, and she was married to a Catalan musician who also died. She saw that there was a connection with her husband's world of music and art, and she put us in touch, and since then the three of us have been very close. We saw each other a lot and became friends. Every year we would go with her and her husband, and I would always bring some friends along.

She came to my house two weeks ago [saying she was having] a genetic test done because she wanted to know her origins, and she won't know the results until they arrive in a few days. She was very close, very generous, very loved. It was very unexpected. I think she had an aneurysm. It's a bubble in the body, something she may have had for many years, even since birth. You can live with it, but sometimes it can burst. I've known her children since they were little. It's very dramatic. I don't know.
A: Yes, it's very dramatic ...
A loud horn is heard.
I feel the atmosphere of the session seems to grow heavier, almost more dramatic, as though the sound of the train reintroduced the presence of death with renewed and heightened intensity.
N: Did you hear the train?
A: Speaking of death.
N: Actually, after the boy committed suicide, I went to her house. It was good for me to disconnect.
Silence.
At another time, she came here with her sister because they weren't sure if they were one hundred percent sisters. Yesterday, her grandson was born. Her daughter was pregnant. Right now, there's a roller coaster of emotions in this family.
A: And maybe not just in that family, I think in you too. You must be very affected.
N: Yes, yes.
A: Once again, the topic of tragic death seems for you inevitable ... Although you also talk to me about life through filiation, origins, inheritance, family ...
N: Yes, yes. It just so happened that there have been two tragedies in these sessions, but that doesn't usually happen to me. There isn't that much drama in my life. The good thing is that my friend's death has been

shared with many people. She was very loved, we went to the hospital, we went to the family home.

She was very special and very anti-establishment. She had her own world. She was very supportive of culture that didn't fit into society, which is why she connected so much with cyborgs. She understood that we were creating art that was neither institutional nor academic, and that it didn't have a historical culture, but was something that was difficult to classify. She connected with this a lot because her husband, who had been an artist since he was a teenager, was also a musician and didn't quite fit in anywhere. She was very supportive of counterculture and gave a lot of moral support to everyone.

A: You had a lot in common with her …

N: I had a lot in common with both of them. They were like godparents because they were older. They had both read a lot and were very capable. They knew how to define situations well and connect one thing to another. They were like libraries. They could talk deeply about any subject, and it was very enriching to be with them.

Silence.

It's funny that lately it was as if she had predicted that something would happen. She gave us many things—for example, a gramophone and records that I have here. She also decided to leave her children's house. She went to live in a cabin up here in the woods, as if she wanted to get away. It reminded me of animals that do this—moving away when they sense they are going to die.

Cats, for example. And the genetic test also surprised me. It was something I had told her for a long time would be interesting. I found it strange that she wanted to take the genetic test.

A: Do you mean she needed to clarify her origins?

N: She wanted to give the test to her sister as a gift. They came here and took it. We have cried a lot. I walked back from her house, which is about 17 kilometers. It did me good.

Silence.

A: You know, I kept thinking that maybe you wanted to have your session precisely because of this whole situation you've been through, which has been so hard and difficult, with so much sadness. This is the first time you've written to me to ask for the session.

N: We had arranged to meet, and I don't like to skip things at all. If I say I'm going to do something, I do it and I'm punctual. It was pending and I wanted to sort it out.

Silence.

A: I was thinking of a space where we could also share sorrows …

N: Luckily, I haven't been alone throughout this whole process. Since she was hospitalized, we've had a lot of people with us, children, sister in the hospital. It's been really good to have company. There will be a tribute in September.

Silence.

When she was in hospital, and when they knew she was going to die, the family didn't know if they wanted to donate her organs.

As she was young, her children had to decide. They decided to do so. I didn't know that afterward they send you a letter telling you which organs have been donated.

Silence.

N: Who's behind you? What's that? I mean the picture behind you.

A: Speaking of family ties, it's a descendant who lived in the house where I am now. Would you like me to bring it closer so you can see it?

N: Yes, because seeing someone blurry makes me curious.

Ah, wow! Yes, yes. It's from the nineteenth or eighteenth century, isn't it?

A: Speaking of descendants, I remember when you told me that you had a project with words, connecting things to try to understand. It seems that your deceased friend and her husband brought you something that had to do with connecting. And you also told me that since you started these sessions, things had changed and you didn't understand why. In fact, here we also connect things. The issue of filiation also raises questions: where do I come from, who am I, what do I want to be, do I want to become a cyborg?

N: My friends knew how to put situations into words, they knew how to explain what was happening with words.

[…]

I don't know how to do it.

A: You explain many things differently.

N: I talk very click, click, click. She had the art of speaking.

A: You make music, which is also a way of telling stories. Or suddenly, you look out the window, see a strange character looking at the sea, grab your camera, and take pictures, that's also a way of telling stories. Another thing is that you have more difficulty with words.

N: If they described a person, they knew how to describe them very well. And with humor, you know? Many times, we recorded my friend when she spoke. I loved listening to her so much. It's strange that her brain failed her.

[…]

A: And then, you noticed something, and we don't know if it's a coincidence, but it seems like she's a woman who has retired to die. She goes to the cabin and gives things away. In other words, she's saying goodbye.

N: She was grieving. Three years ago, her husband's death affected her deeply. In her last Instagram post, she seemed to be feeling a little better. She missed him terribly for years.

A: We don't know if it has anything to do with her own death. You describe enormous sadness, a very difficult mourning process.

N: Yes, she was in deep mourning.

A: And what do you think about death being so present in your life? The idea of death, the end, the limit, as if you were always on the border.

N: The more people you know, the closer you are to death, because more people you know will die. So, the older you are, the more you experience death. You've known more people, and people are getting older. I see it as something that's going to be very normal. My father, on the other hand, no. He has no friends and no family nearby. My father is very happy that way, he's in his little hole. He's married. My mother has friends. Sometimes I think that death doesn't suit him very well.

And we send each other lots of messages; I've just received another one. We all still talk about her. We all miss her.

A horn sounds.

A: A train.

I feel a dense atmosphere, as though death were once again approaching.

N: At the exact spot where the boy threw himself off, there's a traffic sign where trains have to whistle. I went to look at it because there's an "S," and in the railway world, an S means you have to whistle. But it's right where he threw himself. So trains always whistle in the same place. It's the memory.

A: So you're not going to forget that someone killed himself there.

N: No, because they'll always whistle. And his shoe is still there, they haven't removed it from the tracks. It's very powerful. They didn't clean everything up.

A: What does a shoe like that on a railway track make you think of?

Silence.

N: I wouldn't go there, pick it up and throw it in the bin, nor would I return it to his family. Maybe you have to leave it there and one day it will disappear. Maybe someone will pick it up or clean it. I don't know. Seeing a shoe makes me think a lot. Now, whenever I see a shoe, I'm going to think that maybe it belongs to someone who died. Before, I might not have thought about it. I try not to think too much about the shoe, but sometimes I see it. It's moved a little. With the train, sometimes it moves a little. It keeps moving.

A: The mark of death that cannot be completely erased.

N: Well, my flatmate says he can still see the color, that there's still a stain. He says he can see the blood. I can't see it. When he sees color, I suppose he sees more than I do. I just see a shoe. After the accident, everything went on as normal. The trains continued, and that was it.

A: It's as if you were saying to me that I wish we could clean things that cannot be cleaned. Behind a shoe there may be a tragedy.

N: I'm surprised they don't come to clean it up. Because it's private.

[…]

A: It's time. I'm always very grateful for all this material, it's very valuable to me.

N: I also really enjoy talking to you. I've never done this before, meeting up to talk. It's a new situation. It's a curious thing, I also find it very interesting, very much so.

[…]

Commentary on Seventh Session

In this seventh session, death once again erupts directly. Neil begins with the announcement of the loss of a close friend. The intensity of mourning unfolds across several layers. On the one hand, it is a death shared within a collective frame—family, friends, community—which stands in contrast to the solitude and shock that had marked previous scenes (such as the suicide on the railway tracks). Neil himself underscores this difference when he remarks that this time "we all cried," situating the experience within a field of group resonance that functions as a container.

At a countertransferential level, I sense a resonance that permeates the analytic space. The atmosphere of the session feels unusually dense, as if grief itself had taken on a material form. The recurring sound of the train, faint yet persistent in the background, becomes for me the embodiment of this atmosphere; a lament that brings back, with renewed force, the presence of death.

The friend also emerges as a figure of transmission. Connected to the artistic and marginal world, linked to her musician husband, she embodied a bridge between generations, languages, and modes of life. Her death, together with the birth of a grandchild, activates in Neil the problem of filiation: questions of origins, descendants, and symbolic inheritance. Hence his interest in his friend's genetic test, experienced as a gesture that opens inquiries into identity and belonging. This gesture also introduces a contemporary dimension: filiation and transmission are today often mediated through technology—tests, databases, biotechnologies—collective frameworks that provide support where psychic structures falter. Once again, the session illustrates how the group and the technical converge as supports for mourning.

Mourning is further interwoven with transference: Neil's question about the image behind the analyst—an ancestor from the nineteenth century—creates an echo between the analyst's personal history and Neil's preoccupation with family ties and ancestral traces. At this juncture, the session articulates in a singular way death, filiation, and intergenerational transmission.

Death, however, also returns in the form of remains: the shoe left on the railway tracks, the stain of blood that his flatmate still perceives, the whistle of trains at the same spot. These elements embody the indelible, that which cannot be erased. They are not merely objects in the world, but perceptual inscriptions functioning as an external archive, fragmentary, persistent, ineliminable, that point to what remains unmetabolized in experience. Here, the technosubjectivity dimension becomes visible: Neil's added organs attempt to modify such fragmentary perceptions, transforming a stain into sound, a sound encapsulated by image (as with the train whistle), or the transgenerational dynamic inscribed in the transference with the analyst, where color is translated into music through another device and software that permeate the session. Yet despite these digital translations, what remains unsymbolized tends to repeat compulsively.

Technology adheres to the organic that has not been metabolized, configuring a hybrid mode of inscription in which the human and the technical overlap within the same gesture of fixation. Neil's added organs can thus be conceived as technological interfaces that strive to organize a psyche rendered excessively exposed, porous, and undefended against both his own and others' pain. They operate as a kind of protective exoskeleton, introducing limits where psychic defenses prove insufficient.

Neil's own discourse, when he says "click, click, click," almost like a metallic or robotic sound, crystallizes this tension: language that becomes technified, fragmented, machinic, yet at the same time laden with affect, as though the human and the machinic were woven together into a single cadence.

Concluding Remarks

Through the sessions with Neil, we have approached different vertices. We have emphasized that what takes shape in Neil through technology cannot be thought of merely as a perceptual extension. Rather, it opens up a collapse of the distinction between organic and inorganic, producing what we might call an *interface-ego*: a psychic configuration in which neural activity and software become indiscernible.

At the same time, we hear death, annihilation, destruction, and ending recur insistently throughout his sessions, as if what emerges were a reactualization of an archaic origin point where the living and the dead intertwine. In Neil's dreams, in his hypersensitivity to catastrophe, in his almost "death-detector" capacity, something more primitive is at stake: the very threshold where psychic life is born, where vital inscription is constituted in parallel with the risk of its annihilation. Technosubjectivity thus appears as a new configuration/reconfiguration of that origin—an arena in which the organic and the inorganic, the vital and the death-bearing, arise simultaneously.

This analytic experience reconfigures the bond between both participants and can be thought of as a mutation of the classical modes of psychic inscription and functioning. The technological register of both participants, mediated by the platforms that keep them connected—distant and close at the same time—produces a paradoxical situation: the absence of bodies in the same physical space, and yet an intensified experience of the body. This can take the form of added organs that convert algorithmic data, vibrations, or frequencies into sensory experiences that are internalized and dreamt, or of devices that record and thereby intervene in the analytic field (for example, technical lost connection versus anxiety of dead or lost in the countertransferencial side) modulating transference and countertransference alike.

* * * *

At certain moments, when Neil showed me drawings during the sessions, this became a bodily act: the hand emerging, the finger tapping, the device functioning as an extension of the gesture. The digital object here is experienced as part of the body, allowing him to show what could not be verbalized.

This technological infiltration does not replace the unconscious but displaces it toward new modes of representation. In this sense, what in earlier times remained as an unrepresented residue may now find a hybrid channel between the human and the technical. The clinic of technosubjectivity thus reveals the emergence of post-organic psychic configurations. What appears in Neil is a subjectivity that, far from negating the human, might re-inscribe its originary failures within an expanded register, producing a mutation in the economy of psychic inscription and in the very way psychic life is sustained at the threshold between continuity and catastrophe.

In this sense, the transhuman dimension also comes into play. Harbisson's refusal to accept fixed categories—whether gender, partnership, or identity—resonates with the structural openness of his technosubjectivity. What emerges is not the stabilization of identity but the capacity to sustain fluidity, repetition interrupted by novelty, the vital insistence on expanding perception.

Gender and sexuality appear as open, fluid categories, producing a form of liquid identity: Neil identifies with both masculine and feminine aspects but, rather than positioning himself within a queer framework, he follows another path, questioning the very category of species as if he were a posthuman emergent. His affirmation that the antenna is no longer an external accessory but an integrated organ places his body outside the conventional definition of the human: it is an organ that does not belong to the human species and yet constitutes subjectivity. Thus, the decisive polarity is no longer male/female but human/non-human, animate/inanimate, species/trans-species. From this perspective, in Neil's case, technosubjectivity displaces the axis of psychic conflict: what is at stake is not the definition of gender but the possibility of remaining human—or of becoming something else, inviting us to glimpse the outlines of a new biotechnology that configures a neo-technosubjectivity.

Within this framework, Jean Laplanche's (1980) rereading of Freud's case of Little Hans becomes particularly illuminating for thinking through one of the vertices of the clinic of technosubjectivity in Neil's case. At three years and nine months, Hans questions inanimate objects. He does not initially classify lions, horses, or locomotives in terms of sexual difference, but rather according to a far simpler attribute: "having or not having something that make—pee."

As he remarks upon seeing a train leaking water: "Look, the locomotive is making pee. Where is its make-pee then?" He continues distinguishing: "A dog and a horse have a make-pee. A table and a chair do not."

When he asks his father: "Dad, do you also have a make-pee?" The father replies: "Yes, of course." Hans persists: "But I have never seen it when you undress." In front of his mother, naked, he observes: "I am only looking to see if you also have a make-pee." To which she naturally replies: "Didn't you know?" Hans answers: "No, I thought that, since you are so big, you must have one like a horse" (Laplanche, 1980, p. 37).

At this stage, the child assumes that all humans and animals have a make-pee. Thus, the possession of a penis has no implication with respect to gender difference; rather, it functions as a criterion that distinguishes the animate from the inanimate, the living being from the technical object. For Hans, the "make-pee" is, at this moment, nothing less than the indispensable marker of what is alive.

As Laplanche writes:

> The masculine-feminine polarity, which is assumed to crown the whole process of development, is nevertheless present from the very beginning for the child, that is, prior to the phallic phase. It is present, but as a kind of natural or social opposition, alongside many other oppositions and differences, for instance, between living beings and inanimate objects, or between animals and human beings, which still requires theoretical grounding
>
> (Laplanche, 1980, pp. 46–47)[3]

This passage highlights that, before the phallic phase, the child moves among diversities that exceed the genital register and traverse the living and the inanimate. This indicates that gender differentiation is primitively devoid of conflict and, indeed, unthinkable. Laplanche argues, through what he terms the implantation of enigmatic signifiers, that such differentiation is introduced via the unconscious of the child's caregivers.

This author notes that these early distinctions refer both to difference, understood as a binary polarity, and to diversity—an open multiplicity, like the infinite spectrum of colors. The logic of diversity is not founded on negation (non-white = black) but on the co-existence of multiple possible qualities (non-white = red, green, blue, etc.).

To this reading, Laplanche adds another crucial distinction: that between the attribute as quality and the attribute as insignia. As quality, "green" simply describes the green apple; as insignia, "the Greens" and "the Blues" recall the Byzantine factions whose very political existence was instituted by the chromatic emblem. It was not a pre-existing quality but a sign that generated belonging and division.

From this perspective, we may reread Neil's implanted organs not only as perceptual qualities—for instance, a device that allows him to "hear" colors—but also as insignia: a performative sign that establishes a field of belonging, as visible in the creation of the Transpecies Society and in his legal recognition as a cyborg by the state. What begins as a prosthetic extension thus becomes a libidinally charged emblem, instituting new forms of identity and affiliation.

In this sense, Neil's technosubjectivity displaces the axis of psychic conflict: what is at stake is not the definition of gender but the possibility of remaining human or of becoming something else.

As the sessions progress, it becomes evident that in Neil's case, the configuration of technosubjectivity shifts the focus toward horizontal peer relations: the group—community, expanded audience, network of artists and technologists, mourning collectives—acquires a function of support and legitimation. Neil not only feels recognized by the analyst; he knows that the material may be read by others, and this expectation of shared reading inserts him into a collective, opening a circuit of recognition through which meaning is created. This horizontal dimension reconfigures the frame: the intimate, the private, and the public intertwine, and both analyst and patient become "exposed" within a technomediated space where transference and countertransference are interwoven with the collective and the technological, acquiring a structuring role.

At the same time, this opening could be said to "reconfigure" the analyst's narcissism through a new modality, one in which the analytic listening is itself interpellated by a device that renders it visible (recordings, circulation of the text) and displaces the analyst's centrality toward an expanded field (patient-analyst-technical medium-collective).

In this intersection, where the community legitimizes and co-produces meaning, and where the analyst must work through her own exposure, we might think that an essential aspect of Neil's technosubjectivity clinic is at play: recognition becomes a distributed process, and the analytic frame a practice of human-technical co-inscription.

Notes

1 My translation.
2 Laura Ezquerra, Takahiro Kato, Jaehak Yu, and Nicolas Evzonas, IPA Asia Pacific Conference held in Sydney, Australia, 2024. Congress entitled "Suffering across cultures." Panel: "Primal Traumas and Hybrids Becomings."
3 My translation.

References

Burdet, M. (2024). *Ciberespacio y psiquismo. Psicoanálisis en el mundo virtual*. Editorial Psimática.

Ezquerra, L. (2021). Fiction or Realities: The Cyborg Transference. *EPF Bulletin*, n° 75, December 2021. European Psychoanalytical Federation.

Freud, S. (1912). Sobre la dinámica de la transferencia. Obras completas, vol. XII (1911-1913): Trabajos sobre técnica psicoanalítica, y otras obras. Amorrortu, pp. 93–105.

Freud, S. (1919). Lo ominoso. Obras completas, vol. XVII (1917-1919): De la historia de una neurosis infantil ("El Hombre de los Lobos"), y otras obras. Amorrortu, pp. 215–251.

Freud, S. (1919). *Lo ominoso. Una neurosis infantil y otros trabajos*, Vol. 17. Amorrortu Editores.

Freud, S. (1927). *Fetichismo*. Vol. XXI. Amorrortu, pp. 141–152.

Haag, G. (1994). Aux sources de la vie. Le langage préverbal et l'émergence des représentations du corps en situation psychanalytique individuelle ou groupale avec les enfants autistes. *Dialogue*, 123: 41–43.

Huyghe, P. (2024). *Liminal a punta della Dogana*: intervista a Pierre Huyghe. *YouTube*. Available at: https://www.youtube.com/watch?v=sX1tk-6xsWE.

Laplanche, J. (1980/2009). *Problématiques II. Castration et symbolisations (1973–1975)*. PUF.

Le Poulichet, S. (2003). *Psychanalyse de l'informe. Dépersonnalisations, addictions, traumatismes*. Flammarion. Champ Essais.

Ogden, T.H. (2004). The analytic third: Implications for psychoanalytic theory and technique. *The Psychoanalytic Quarterly*, 73(1): 167–195.

6 New Subjectivities—Neo Identities—Technosubjectivities

After tracing the case of Neil Harbisson, where technosubjectivity is articulated around the integration of a prosthetic organ and the ensuing collapse between the organic and the inorganic, we now turn to two further clinical configurations that illuminate complementary facets of the same horizon. Leonora and Dorotea show different positions along a shared spectrum where technological objects, digital environments, and symbolic failures intersect. Leonora, whose psychic functioning is, in my opinion, closer to Neil's, reveals how withdrawal into digital networks and online games becomes the very scaffolding of psychic life when early traumas leave the subject unprotected. Dorotea, rather than reversing this model, shifts the emphasis: images, avatars, and tattoos operate as surfaces of inscription, where what is not symbolized seeks figuration. Both cases allow us to expand the spectrum of technosubjectivity beyond the singularity of the cyborg, each marked by distinctive ways of negotiating loss and representation while retaining overlapping mechanisms.

In psychoanalysis, the body has been conceived as a psychosexual body, traversed by the drives and anchored in the relation to a human other. Yet, throughout much of its history, attention has been directed almost exclusively to the interpersonal field, while the formative role of the non-human environment has remained relatively neglected. As Harold Searles (1960) suggested, the infant lives initially in a state of fusion with its milieu, and the presence or absence of a containing environment—including its inanimate and inorganic dimensions—contribute decisively to psychic balance or imbalance. Human beings establish libidinal relations not only with caregivers but also with non-human objects that, even when not materially grafted onto the body, may nevertheless become co-constitutive of subjectivity.

Winnicott's transitional object (1953) illustrates how a cloth or teddy bear can be affectively invested to negotiate separation; Freud's *fort/da* game shows how a simple spool mediates the experience of absence and presence; and fetishism illustrates even more radically how a non-human object may acquire decisive psychic value: the fetish is not merely an accessory, but a substitute that protects against castration anxiety and

DOI: 10.4324/9781003640684-6

shields the ego from disintegration. Taken together, these examples reveal that the non-human environment is inscribed at the very core of subjectivity and prepare the ground for thinking how contemporary technological artifacts may occupy analogous functions in the constitution of technosubjectivities.

Anthropological perspectives converge on this insight. André Leroi-Gourhan's work (1964) demonstrates that tools are not merely external instruments but "secretions" of the body, the brain, and culture prolonging the subject and endowing it with an additional social organ. While conceived and instituted by humans, tools in turn modify biological, social, and cultural parameters. Initially prolonging the motor hand, tools progressively gained autonomy, drawing energy from external sources and becoming governed at a distance.

This process of separation and individuation of the tool with respect to its creator drives the general evolution of technical objects and finds an emblematic expression in the robot. For Leroi-Gourhan, technical evolution is not simply parallel to biological evolution but functions as its substitute and prolongation.

Tools thus occupy the place of artificial organs, and our relation to them functions as a decisive vector in the construction of both individual and collective construction of biopsychic identity.

This dual condition—technology as both mediation and structuring force—defines the horizon of technosubjectivities. For psychoanalysis, the urgent task is to explore how contemporary artifacts and virtual environments participate in conscious and unconscious processes of psychization, transforming the modalities of absence, presence, loss, and representation. These questions affect not only our theoretical models but also the clinical encounter, where technological mediation increasingly reshapes the analytic field itself (Missonier, 2021).

Against this conceptual backdrop, the following vignette will focus on Leonora, a pubescent patient whose psychic economy is organized around screens, avatars, and immersive realities. Her case illustrates with particular clarity how the technological object can be invested both as fetish and as defensive formation in the face of traumatic loss, while at the same time reactivating archaic modes of symbolization. Through her material, we can observe how the virtual becomes both a continuity of the ego and a fragile attempt at negotiating absence, thereby opening the discussion on technosubjectivities in young patients.

If Leonora exemplifies a technosubjectivity organized around withdrawal, fetishization of the gadget and the defensive use of the virtual bubble, in the next case Dorotea opens up a different perspective. In her case, the technological object is not primarily invested as a protective fetish but as a surface of inscription: tattoos, avatars, and digital artifacts become sites where the unrepresentable seeks figuration. Her material allows us to explore how the technological may operate as an extension of psychic writing, entangled with the history of primary objects, transgenerational transmissions, and the sociocultural environment.

Together, these vignettes illustrate the plurality of ways in which technological objects, whether or not physically grafted onto the body, may intervene in psychic organization and actively co-constitute subjectivity.

The Body, a Territory in Mutation

In earlier chapters I argued that the body represents the cornerstone of the symbolic matrix that generates human representations. Like images and words, it constitutes a support for the construction of the subject's representations, playing an important role in the creation of identity, social references, and the transmission of culture. Today, however, the body evolves within a techno-environment that ubiquitously grasps, measures, and modulates it.

Young adolescents inhabit this continuum with particular intensity. Some withdraw radically into virtuality—Japan's *hikikomori*[1] being the emblematic figures—while others, like the artist Neil Harbisson, reshape their bodies, reconfiguring identity in what seems to be today a transhuman direction (Ezquerra, 2023b).

What I will argue here—following the hypothesis of the hybridization of human beings (Bensayag, 2019), which according to some authors, is an anthropological mutation that is already a fact "impacting our bodies and minds, also in terms of neuronal configurations" (Scognamiglio, Russo, and Fumagalli, 2024, p. 41)—is whether or not hybridization can have an impact on psychic linking, representational work, and ego-organization.

In an attempt to approach these new subjectivities, which I call technosubjectivities, Leonora, a pubescent patient whose psychic economy is organized around screens, avatars, and immersive virtualities, offers a privileged lens for exploring these questions

As in Neil Harbinsson's case, her material raises the articulation between body, unconscious, and technology and the possible transformations in the ego-organization that this may imply, thus questioning the constitution/reconfiguration of the representational framework.

The case invites us to rethink the status of inanimate/technological objects in the process of psychization and to revisit the earliest layers of symbolization where motor, tactile, and perceptual inscriptions are primary (Roussillon, 2008). From this perspective, the virtual, when anchored in the body, may reactivate motor hallucinations as archaic forms of symbolization—an ego "continuation" that can both sustain and distort representational life.

In cases where early objects failed to provide sufficiently good responses, I hypothesize that the psychosexual body, engaged with virtual reality, re-edits the perception of the psychomotor actions of a "bodily ego," recalling the most primitive forms of symbolizations.

At the same time, I maintain that early traumatic experiences return through non-verbal pathways. In line with Roussillon (2008), I argue that Freud's three forms of word representation—word, thing, and affect—constitute the architecture of human language. As Roussillon puts it, "Verbal language does not replace bodily preverbal modalities; it comes to complete and reorganize them at the moment of their installation, without making them disappear" (Roussillon, 2008, p. 67).[2]

Roussillon also states: "[Motor] hallucination gives the object its psychic value, perception gives its potentially apprehensible form transformable by motricity" (Roussillon, 2008, p. 67).[3] Likewise, there would be a coincidence of hallucinatory and perceptive movement.

Roussillon's reference to "hallucinatory," should be understood as the "hallucinatory satisfaction of the wish"—a primal experience postulated by Freud, consisting in the resolution of internal tension (such as the need to suckle) through external intervention.

The child creates an image of the satisfying object, which consequently acquires a special value in the construction of the subject's desire. If the primary environment has been defective, the earliest experiences escape the integrating process with regard to symbolizing functions. Roussillon conceives this within a model that converges with Winnicott's mirror function and Bion's alpha function.[4]

These hypotheses help us to see the reactivation of the motor hallucinations as typical of the most primitive forms of symbolization, when the virtual is somehow anchored in the body and appears as a continuity of the ego.

The clinical case that I describe below shows a patient who lives in her virtual bubble. In this case, the technological gadget and the patient's virtual world appear as a continuity of her elongated ego.

Faced with trauma, the psyche seeks solutions in attempts to narrate what could not be inscribed in the language apparatus. What remains uninscribed can be reactualized in a fertile, transitional terrain, sometimes within the encounter with the analyst.

Leonora, or the Case of a *Hikikomori*

In order to relate to the hypotheses previously raised in relation to the articulation of the body, the unconscious, the virtual, and hybridization, I will leave aside other clinical issues of this patient and focus here on what is most relevant to the present discussion.

Introducing Leonora

Leonora is a pubescent girl of twelve-and-a-half, though she often presents the appearance of a fifteen-year-old adolescent.

Her dress and presentation oscillate markedly: at times unkempt, with dirty hair and heavy dark make-up; at other times she wears the clothes of her mother, who died a year and a half earlier; and on other occasions she arrives dressed as a young, sexualized schoolgirl. She never separates from the smartphone she inherited, nor from a tablet on which she often shows me the digital drawings she has produced.

The patient seems to inhabit another dimension, that of virtual reality, which for her is indistinguishable from her daily life. She lives in her "reality-virtual reality," an on-life continuum in which online experience and psychic reality are scarcely differentiated.

Leonora adopts different and fluid identities. In my view, what emerges is a succession of provisional egos activated according to circumstances, a kind of mobile prosthesis of existence.

Following the philosopher Bauman, one could describe this as a "liquid ego": inconsistent, unstable, and weakly bounded, not tied to time or space, but flowing in short pulses, generating what I conceive as a background rhythm in our work—endless restarts followed by brief, painless endings. This recalls Andy Warhol's disturbing experimental film *Screen Test*, where the static camera captures the same shot, the same character with no beginning or end.

Leonora can be a character, all characters, or none at all; she questions not only who she is, but what she is. In her online games and chats she appears as an avatar, as do her closest friends and her online boyfriend, none of whom she has ever met in person.

In these practices, she embodies often fantastical avatars—hybrid composites of human, animal, and object—often endowed with indeterminate or multiple sexual identifications (asexual, bisexual, trans). These avatars mediate her relationships and sustain bonds, including a romantic attachment to a boyfriend. Notably, alongside these fluid identifications, Leonora displays a capacity for sublimation: she aspires to become an anime[5] artist and, within the analytic space, she at times identifies with the avatars and characters she has created.

Her clinical presentation unfolds against the backdrop of her mother's death and a progressive withdrawal from social and family life. She rarely leaves her room, not even to eat with the rest of the family and reports that contact with others feels like a violation of her privacy. She describes herself as addicted to her phone and has been left, from the age of two, to a nearly continuous handling of screens and devices. Disconnection provokes a traumatic rupture: when "unplugged" from the internet, she enters a crisis, as if a limb were amputated.

After our first meeting—despite her affable manner and the rich material of her drawings and stories—my initial impression was one of a sinister sensation; a marked, uncanny strangeness. I later came to understand this as resonating with the presence of unburied corpses that the patient seemed to carry with her. Leonora herself evokes this experience: "When you lose your mother it's like a cut from here to here," she said, tracing a line across her abdomen.

Other losses accumulate in her history: the disappearance of maternal relatives and the loss of her mother tongue. She shows profound ambivalence towards the maternal figure, simultaneously repudiating and reviving it. Even while rejecting it, she reintroduces fragments of her maternal universe in isolated words that resurface in the analytic field. The father remained largely absent until the mother's death, intensifying the atmosphere of deprivation in which her subjectivity developed.

The Gadget in its Possible Aspects: Fetish (Freud), Prolongation of the Mother-Daughter Fusion; Transformational Object (Bollas); Identity Spectrum (M'Uzan); or Transitional Space (Winnicott)

The technological gadget and the internet image permanently accompanied Leonora, substituting the absent object since infancy, when she could already caress a screen and, in her words, discover "black holes." From the very beginning, parental figures were either absent or intrusively present, profoundly altering the fundamental presence-absence dimension.

The world of constant connectivity thus replaced the "disencounter" with the object; favoring a premature fusion with another (technological) object. As Björklind (2019) suggests, since the advent of new technologies we are never completely alone or completely together, a condition that modifies the position of the third and alters the structure of triangular space.

Thinking about Leonora's intimate attachment to her device and virtual world since early childhood, I understand this as a staging of projection against unbearable mourning, an attempt to shield herself from psychic collapse at the price of twisting her representational universe.

The expression "black hole," in my view, condenses both the fear of self-absorption and the desperate search for representation to avoid being swallowed by the void. This resonates with what Le Poulichet (2003) calls the terror of formlessness, rooted in unconscious processes underlying vacillations in the identification processes and their symptomatic formations, ranging from sensations of self-absorption to various addictive formations. Terrors of formlessness threaten the integrity and image of the body.

From Freud onwards, we know that the fetish emerges to deny castration and to pacify annihilation anxiety; in Leonora, the gadget assumes precisely this role—an addictive prosthesis and guarantor against collapse. As I argued elsewhere, fetishism also responds to what Freud described as the regressive drive back to the inorganic (Chervet, 2012).

At the same time, Leonora's early investment in the virtual world can be read as an attempt to build a nascent ego, ensuring the permanence of her own image and that of the other's gaze through digital connection. As we know, the image is, for the human being, at the heart of the constitution of our identity.

M'Uzan (2005) provides a framework to conceptualize this dynamic through the identity spectrum, where there is no border between the ego and the non-ego. The identity spectrum is an intermediate zone: "depending on the shifts of the narcissistic libido ... from an internal pole occupied by the representation of the subject itself, to an external pole coinciding with the image of the other"[6] (M'Uzan, 2005, p. 18).

Unlike the transitional space, the identity spectrum announces a non-hallucinatory object that has not yet taken place in external reality. This concept helps us grasp how, for Leonora, the virtual image replaces the other's image—the non-hallucinatory object not yet rooted in external reality.

Following Le Poulichet's (2003) rereading of the mirror stage (Lacan, 1949), it is not only the child's body that is reflected and libidinally invested as an image, gathered, and recognized., but also the surrounding environment (room, objects, etc.) ,which appears reflected and enters in the same specular apparatus.

In Leonora, identificatory capture with the virtual produces a reciprocal seizure of body-image and world-image. The avatar, as image-world, functions as an extension of her ego. For Le Poulichet (2003, p. 33): "The superposition and articulation of reality and the body itself constitute an essential aspect of the experience that holds the world and the body together in the visual field."[7]

This would mean that to merge and match up with a virtual unit, in an identificatory capture, produce a reciprocal seizing of the image of the body and that of the world around it. This world, capable of being reflected at the same time as the image of the subject, in some way also represents the body and the body in extension.

This links to Anzieu's (1985) notion of the "skin-ego." One might hypothesize that the gadget becomes an artificial extension of the skin, at once protective and intrusive, raising questions about its place in the ongoing (re)configuration of Leonora's ego.

In the transference, Leonora frequently brought drawings that I interpret as foundational mirror experiences. Figure 6.1 shows one of these drawings to illustrate this.

This type of drawing was a constant throughout her sessions. Recurrent images depicted two characters tied together and connected to intravenous drips and a monitor. These characters were prolonged by tubes and wires, alluding to a hospital situation with a monitor. This drawing, titled: "Love in the heart of a monitor from which a dose of oxygen must be taken," condenses multiple dimensions. I will name a few here: fusion with the mother; addictive bonds (with technology, with maternal alcoholism); paranoid functioning (watched and being intrusively watched); "the heart of a monitor" that "monitored" her as both life-support and addictive gadget, necessary, like oxygen, which prolonged her and constituted her from her earliest childhood.

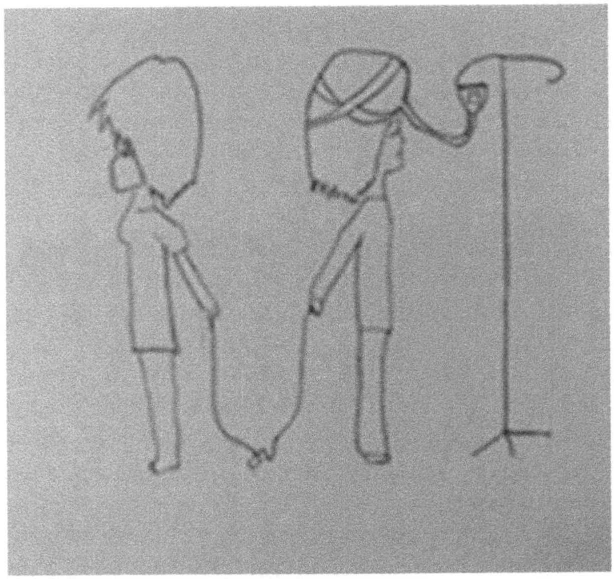

Figure 6.1 Drawing of two characters tied together and connected to intravenous drips and a monitor.
Source: Photograph taken by the author.

This can be thought as an addictive formation that organizes archaic phantasmatic elements that, although mutilating, prevent the body from collapse into the void. Le Poulichet (2003, p. 60) notes that

> archaic formations assign to the body a surface deformed by the graft of a [let's read here "virtual"] foreign body. In Leonora, the narcissistic and drive configuration of the body is redesigned through the incorporation of a foreign [technological] body.

Finally, Bollas (1989) describes "the mother, before being an object, is above all a process of transformation of the self where the rhythm oscillates between integration and lack of integration" (pp. 1181–1196).[8]

This first primitive transformational object that emerges from the symbiotic relationship is linked to an anticipated and recurrent lived experience and is of an existential order.

> It is a proto-perceptual identification with its active function, namely the object as an agent of transformation of the environment and of the corporeal of the subject.
>
> (Bollas, 1989, pp. 1181–1196)

Bollas includes here, when referring to the earliest constitution of the human being, not only the corporeal nature of the subject, but also the environment of non-human elements that surround the subject in close connection with the corporeal.

In this sense, Leonora's gadget can be conceived of not merely as a fetish but as a transformational object, in an attempt to continually reconfigure her psychic economy.

Following Denis (2002), we can think of this as the fixation of drive mastery. In doing so, Denis introduces the idea that narcissistic or object investments become fixed in an object as the locus of the drive mastery is in the object (let's read here the "inorganic object").

The Passionate Re-Encounter Through the Virtual and the Reconfiguration of her Psychic Reality

One day, Leonora was wearing a coat she had inherited from her mother. She laid it gently on my couch and tried to give it a human form. I was both frightened and moved to realize that she was placing her mother's dead corpse between us. Not many sessions later, I learned that the patient had been engaging in sexual relations through the screen with a stranger, an avatar. She expressed the wish to remain exclusively in that world. When questioned by her father, she replied: "That wasn't me, I have other personalities, like five." In the face of this striking fact, the patient seemed to dissociate or split, showing no trace of discomfort.

In another episode, with one of her virtual friends, she chose to be a boy avatar, which allowed her to change gender and participate in erotic play. Sexuality, the sexual act, as Roussillon points out, seems to be an arena for the return of early experiences and the choice of specific "forms of memory." In Leonora's case, the virtual interaction appears to reactivate what Racamier (1995) called *l'incestuel traumatique*: an incestuous situation that has not been consummated but that nevertheless pervades psychic reality.

In my view, these episodes question Leonora's relation with her earliest objects. They also recall what Missonier (2021) describes as motor hallucinations and the suspension of judgment typical of the forms of primary symbolization that account for the negative in the relationship with the first objects. The virtual image in Leonora thus clings with a peculiar viscosity to the incestual traumatic, precisely because psychic images are never merely visual: they are also motor and sensory, rooted in the body; as if perception itself were still seeking a bodily envelope capable of containing the unrepresented.

Building on these characteristics of the virtual image, one might wonder whether the inevitable sensorialities the infant deploys in their relationship to early objects make the gadget be experienced as a kind of magical tool, already linked to the infant's expectations and gestures even before thought can take shape. The passion for the virtual may thus derive from a reminiscence of the multisensory field of infancy.

Returning here to Bollas's formulation of the transformational object, and to Missonier's proposal, I ask whether, in Leonora's case, the discovery of "black holes" may represent her attempt to imagine a first relation to the world in terms of inanimate objects charged with sensory qualities rather than in terms of human beings. As Stern (1990) reminds us, every child goes through a phase in which the non-human environment is foregrounded.

On the basis of a human psyche that simultaneously prolongs itself and adheres to the machine, confusing itself with it, I wonder what transformations take place in Leonora's psychic reality.

As Barbara Cassin (2012) observes: "There are some languages more maternal than others, they are those that we can hear immediately and with which we make body." Would these languages, more maternal than others, be constituted, almost bodily in Leonora's case, by all these animate and inanimate objects?

The characters of Leonora's virtual universe allow her, on the one hand, to remain within the "black holes"; that is, always in contact with her screen, in continuity with her maternal universe. On the other hand, they allow her to generate a multitude of characters that she can use to speak of herself and her conflicts, of who she is. She creates dialogue for them, and this allows her to work out her own conflicts. Sometimes her internal objects/characters also appear incarnated in her (when she presents herself as one of them). Leonora may thus be staging the return of an encounter with the non-human.

At the same time this theme raises another enigma: what kind of object is capable of materializing representational activity, and what are the different transformational capacities depending on the type of inanimate object? And is all perhaps framed against the background of a maternal screen-matrix?

Commentary—Leonora

The enhanced body, a territory in continuous mutation through its articulation with technology, generates forms of symbolization that may be materialized, displayed, or sonorized, yet not fully thought.

Technosubjectivities appear to emerge as neo-identities, presenting new configurations with respect to the body, sexuality, the unconscious, and the other. This raises a central challenge for analysts: can identification with the non-human be understood as a request for confirmation from the environment of one's very status as human? Might it evoke the child's identification with an inanimate parent—an object that arouses terror yet requires rescue? Is it, perhaps, a question of reanimating an inert other, even when such reanimation stages the possible effacement of the subject? Something essential to existence is at stake here: life and death, organic and non-organic, animate and inanimate.

Returning to the question of the inanimate object: does the machine, an object through projections of fantasies first experienced in relation to the other, not also open the possibility of new declinations of primal phantasies? Or, conversely, does algorithmic intelligence, with its hypertrophy of images in the virtual, generate black holes of meaning, undermining psychic internalization and mentalization?

Leonora illustrates a technosubjectivity where fetishization of the virtual bubble operates as a defensive formation: psychic traces are sheltered within the protective bubble of the gadget and the virtual. Dorotea, as will be examined below, introduces a complementary configuration in which inscription is foregrounded. In her clinical material, technological objects—tattoos, avatars, and digital images—function as extended surfaces of writing, through which the unrepresentable seeks figuration and the void is simultaneously contained. Nevertheless, this distinction must not be conceived as absolute. Dorotea's psychic economy also retains elements of fetishization, condensed in ritualized gestures—such as her relation to her computer-console—that both animate and memorialize the object.

What emerges, therefore, is not a binary opposition but a continuum of technosubjective formations. Across this spectrum, technological objects sustain psychic survival through modes of withdrawal or, alternatively, open inscriptional surfaces that negotiate loss and reconfigure its traces. In both Leonora and Dorotea, they reveal how technosubjectivities inscribe absence, defend against it, and transform the encounter between psyche, technology, and sociocultural transmission.

Dorotea

Brief History of the Patient

Dorotea is a twenty-four-year-old woman who entered her third psychoanalytic treatment. Her first consultation took place at the age of fifteen, when she expressed a wish to die. Two long periods of analytic work followed, mostly in person, with intervals of video-tele-analysis during her studies abroad.

On this occasion it was Dorotea herself—not her parents—who sought help. This last stage of psychoanalytic treatment was carried out in person, with the exception of a few sessions.

She presented in a state of desperation, oscillating rapidly between euphoria and sadness, fearing that she was "losing her mind." She showed an unbearable suffering, crying and gesturing words in three different languages that we both speak. She explained she was going through a break-up.

Her life felt "on the edge," marked by a lack of control, intense anxiety, episodes of bulimia, self-harm (cutting her skin), and an episode of prostitution "for fun."

Her body bore multiple tattoos, one of which she called *the tree of life*: a hybrid between technology and plant life, designed by herself, which condensed the importance of technological artifacts, images, and the non-human in her psychic life. She explained that the mark of abandonment led her to inscribe this tattoo on her skin—what she called a "wordless scar" revitalized in image.

From the first interview Dorotea appeared at once directionless, almost stateless, yet clinging to the analyst as to a talisman. In keeping with our previous shared analytic history and the persistence of unresolved conflicts, there were moments of necessary fusion with the analyst, as well as excitement and excess that she was also able to deposit in the analytic space—the analyst as a container and calming presence for her psychic excess.

Dorotea's life and that of her ancestors had been marked by many losses (countries, language, culture) and the persistent absence of her father. Her parents had to flee a country at war before Dorotea was born.

She described multiple "personalities," the darkest of which she named *X, the nameless one*, embodying her depressive side. Alongside this, she cultivated a passion for art—particularly light installations designed to evoke claustrophobic sensations—another way of giving form to what she experienced as formless excess, a creation mediated by technology and saturated with her struggle to reconstruct her ego.

Later, in relation to her choice of this type of art, mediated by technology, we were able to formulate some hypotheses: her relationship with an

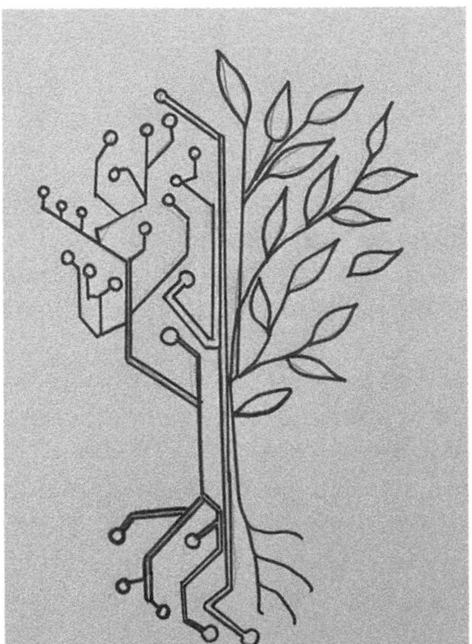

Figure 6.2 Tatoos designed by the patient.
Source: Photograph taken by the author.

absent father, with an intrusive mother who she felt owned even her body, as well as her movements of fusion and defusion in an attempt to reconstruct herself.

The Burial of the Console: The Technological Object as Constitutive of Psychic Life from Its Origins

As mentioned before, the anthropologist and ethnologist Leroi-Gourhan (1964) emphasized that the process of humanization rests on the human tendency to extend the body into technical objects and inhabit them as if they were part of the body itself. Since the dawn of metapsychology developed by S. Freud, psychoanalysts have recognized that the body is the first object invested by the subject, a fundamental pillar of the constitution of primary narcissism.

Dorotea illustrates this constitutive dimension of the technical object. She describes:

> And finally I've played my online game. You're a character and you have an open world. I've killed a lot of things. I've done a lot of magic. There are two games I keep for sentimental value. Today I'm going to sell my virtual reality console. At least I know where it's going, it's not going in the rubbish. I gave my device a farewell speech, a funeral; which shows how attached I am to things. I'm completely crazy. It has been with me for many years. I cried. I grew up with the computer as if it were my brother. I'm going to cry [she cries a lot]. It reminds me of my childhood with my brother. It's not the same anymore. Now with my brother, it's like I feel the conversation is fake.

Freud (1919, p. 233) noted that:

> in the play of its early years, the child does not clearly distinguish between the animate and the inanimate and shows a particular tendency to regard its dolls as living beings.

Decades later, Searles (1960, p. 53) commented in this regard that:

> The newborn is incapable, for at least some time after birth, of discerning between himself and his non-human environment, whether inanimate, vegetable or animal, and is therefore incapable of becoming aware of the fact that he is alive and not inanimate, and that he is a human creature and not a plant or an animal.[9]

Returning to our clinical vignette, Dorotea's tattoos and her artistic practice confirm the central role of technology: she uses these objects and creations as a way of reconstructing a psychic "skin" (Anzieu, 1985), a containing surface, a safety net, a network woven through images and connections that in turn transforms her. This would be a patient with a fragile self, an unnamed X, always on edge, seeking to reconstruct a skin, as Anzieu (1985) would say. A reconstruction that she weaves by diving into the net.

From this perspective, Dorotea's attachment to her console is more than a behavioral excess: it is a psychic link to an object that had sustained her since early life. The "funeral" she describes signals not only the mourning of a device, but also the reactivation of multiple losses—of her brother, her childhood, her homeland.

The console functioned as a brother-companion-artifact *consola,*[10] a quasi-sibling that offered continuity when human figures failed her. In this sense, the loss of the device also evokes the loss of a non-human environment once felt as part of the self, "a harmonious extension of our self encompassing the world" (Searles, 1960, p. 56).

Traditionally, psychoanalysis has considered the relation with the inanimate as secondary, a displacement through projection from relations with human objects. Dorotea invites us to question this assumption.

Might encounters with inanimate objects occur from the very beginning of psychic life, alongside the relations with human caregivers, rather than only secondarily by projection? If so, the process of humanization would not be reducible to the relation with a first "other," but would also involve mourning—a castration—for a primitive ego already composed partly of inanimate elements. For today's young patients, this primitive ego may include interactive technological artifacts, to which they regress in an attempt to reconfigure the self and work through conflicts.

Virtual Reality as an Interactive Continuum in the Configuration of Psychic Reality

My impression was that the light illusions created by the patient evoked earliest sensory perceptions of the infant at the dawn of life, immersed in a non-human environment—visual and auditory alike. These phenomena also suggest that regression, inevitable at different stages of analytic work, coincided with Dorotea's use of virtual reality saturated with luminous illusions, opening another path to expand and reconfigure her psychic reality.

Over the course of many sessions, Dorotea sought to cope with loneliness and the overflow of her most archaic anxieties by imagining herself within a world of hybrid beings, part human and part beast. In her games, she spoke of herself through multiple avatars, often identifying with beasts or hybrid figures.

As she stated:

> I need to be reborn. I masturbate imagining creatures that are half human and half beast. A protective beast that treats me well and protects me from myself, it could be a gargoyle, a dragon. I love Greek mythology and I want to be at the center of those beasts. I've moved house a lot in my life. I don't like myself. When I go out at night, I feel confident. I feel like God. I feel like the world can't touch me.
>
> Sometimes I go crazy. The things I like are not what my father, mother, and family expect of me. No one is willing to accept who I am. I am attracted to magical men and mystical creatures. I think this has to do with what men represent to me and at the same time with the fact that we come from animals.
>
> I escape with fictional characters. The world can't contain me. I'm too much.

In the same session, the patient goes on to describe how she photographed a cemetery and cried with emotion. She continued:

> When I'm distressed, I want to get away from human life, which is why I like to escape into games. I reject the society I live in; I didn't choose it. Everything human hurts. My brain hurts when I smoke or vomit, it hurts. I was born in the wrong world [she cries a lot]. Nothing is worth anything. This society is not for me. I can't cope with my brain, it's too much for my body: I either cut myself or get tattoos. When I'm in the countryside, it's as if I'm not here, there's no internet. I'm not made to be here. When you're in the countryside, you're either alive or dead, there's no noise. When I'm with you, there's no noise.

I responded, "There's no noise here, but together we also build a net." Dorotea concluded the session with the words "I prefer to be here because I'm protected from myself, because you're here."

In this material, the patient addresses her psychosexuality through the play of her half-human, half-beast avatars. Her fantasies of bisexuality, "I want to be in the center," and pansexuality (creatures with undefined sexuality) stand at the heart of the matter. It is noteworthy that these regressive desires of disidentification from humanity are increasingly present in the analytic material of young patients.

Dorotea expressed herself like this: "When I am distressed, I want to get away from human life, I like to escape into games." Today, this can be read as anticipating a transhuman orientation.

The beast appears to represent both the energy she lacks and the limit she seeks. She experiences the world as unable to contain her, yet paradoxically seeks containment in the internet and in the analytic bond as a way to reconstitute herself: "I want to be reborn"/"I prefer to be here because you are here."

These fantasies convey a longing to regressively rediscover or merge with a "lost paradise" of the non-human world, to experience the absence of limits and omnipotence, to re-create herself in her fantasy as a self-generated human being without the inexorable mark of another: "I feel like God"/"I want to escape human life"; and, at the same time, a desperate cry for recognition of her humanity, which can only be rescued in the encounter with another human being: "I prefer to be here because I am protected from myself, because you are here."

This vignette raises questions about the psychic function of virtual environments.

On the one hand, their immersive qualities—mobilizing vision, motility, hearing, and touch—provide a sense of continuity of being, an encounter with a virtually dehumanized and fabricated other, alluding to the surrounding inanimate world of the infant's primary environment.

Psychic representation is always anchored in motor and sensory traces rooted in the body. Through the technological objects and the sensorialities they generate (images, sound, sensorialities of another quality), the subject maintains the memory of his body in action; "each of the objects surrounding the subject corresponds to specific gestures that establish their identity as much as the possession of the objects themselves" (Tisseron, 2015, p. 92).

On the other hand, virtual reality also raises hypotheses that situate it as a psychic operator: it may function as a fetish, from the Latin *facticius*, artificial, protecting the subject against primitive anxieties and early traumas, allowing mourning to be postponed. It may serve as an anti-castration device, aiming to overcome any limit; as a response to an extinctive inorganic regressiveness.

At the same time, virtual reality it can operate as a fertile transitional terrain (Winnicott, 1953), a terrain for sublimations and symbolizations, a laboratory for regressive movement where the negative can be presentified (Green, 1983).

In this sense, the technological object and the virtual game accessed may be understood as mediators and organizers of both intrapsychic and interpsychic life, producers and containers of meaning and figurations, enabling the metabolization of drive dynamics and archaic fantasies.

Symbolizing Marks: From Tattooed Skin to the Interactive Universe of Images in Virtual Reality

Dorotea repeatedly described a pervasive sense of emptiness and her search for extreme experiences as a way of ensuring that she existed.

These attempts may be read as efforts to leave a trace, to produce a figuration of herself in the face of what could be described as a lack of inscription in the unconscious.

Such traces may be understood, in Green's (1983) terms of the negative, as representations of the non-represented: not integrated by the subject and therefore inaccessible; split off within the psyche. From another perspective, they may also belong to what Mancia (2007) has described as the unrepressed unconscious.

The problem of psychic representation—and the creation of the psyche itself—is inseparable from the dialectic of presence and absence in the relation to the other.

These dynamics highlight not only the importance of presence, but also of frustration—the absence of pleasure and gratification—as a precondition for the development of thought and psychic growth. When absence becomes unbearable or frustration intolerable the effects on the developing mind may be catastrophic. In this sense, absence must be considered in terms of its potential for symbolization.

To paraphrase Green, an excess of frustration may lead to a kind of *self-amputation* of the ego, producing a feeling of void or abyss which functions as an anesthetic. This painkiller may become imprisoned in a form that cannot be translated into representation, its only possible expression being the non-representability of the object.

Green's (1983) notion of the negative can be fruitfully placed in dialogue with Bion's (1967) distinction between *non-thing* and *nothingness*. Both are concerned with the fate of absence and the limits of representation. For Bion, the *non-thing* refers to a tolerable absence that, if contained, may be transformed into thought, whereas *nothingness* denotes a catastrophic collapse into chaos, prior to the possibility of representation.

Green, from a different vantage point, shows how what has never been symbolized persists within psychic life as gaps, splits, or "representations of the non-represented" (Green, 1983). Taken together, these perspectives suggest how psychic life is organized not only by what is represented but also by what remains unrepresented: absence may thus operate either as a motor of symbolization or as the site of collapse, depending on the subject's capacity for containment and transformation.

It is from within this dialectic of absence and inscription that Dorotea's relation to images acquires its particular significance. For her, the image becomes privileged—whether as tattoo, social media profile, avatar, or the gaze of the analyst in the consulting room or in tele-analysis. In her fantasy, she longs to be seen, looked at, and recognized, returning compulsively to the earliest sensorial experiences of fusion that technology makes possible to repeat.

This insatiable thirst for images reveals a compulsion to repeat that both sustains and destabilizes her psychic organization.

The desire to be seen and to display oneself is rooted in the earliest developmental phases, where the child discovers itself in the faces and bodies of others, preceding the construction of intimacy. We know how the ego, from its very origins, is constituted in a position of passivity toward the violence of the other.

Psychoanalysis has approached this from different frames: Freud (1915) emphasized the force of the drive; Ferenczi (1933) and Laplanche (1987), the impact of early maternal care; Lacan (1949), the function of the mirror stage. The primacy of the other in the ego makes the ego a guest in its own home—an uncanny inhabitant of its own body. This condition may lead to extreme consequences such as exile or death. Thus, Dorotea oscillates between her cry to exist and the exile enacted through what she describes as her multiple personalities, caught between fragmentation and the search for unity.

Her addictive pursuit of her mother's gaze—experienced as persecutory in its constant reminders of her body's imperfections—contrasts with her turn to avatars. These idealized and "perfect" images offer a temporary liberation, mirroring her fantasies in exact correspondence with her momentary needs.

The image, then, is an essential axis in the constitution of identity. It thus stands at the very heart of primary narcissism and, in Dorotea, is explosively reactivated in the virtual image. Because of its immersive qualities—mobilizing not only vision but also motor activity, hearing, and touch—the virtual image promotes a sensation of *skin-to-skin*contact, adhering to thing-representations and reanimating early forms of embodiment.

Such dynamics bring us back to the earliest outlines of identity, which, as M'Uzan (2005, p. 19) suggests: "within the sexual organisation and within the framework of a relationship with a non-ego, reality or representation when 'I is another'."[11]

This can be read as a reactivation of M'Uzan's notion of the "identity spectrum," an intermediate space without fixed boundaries between the ego and the non-ego. Today, this outer edge often unfolds within the digital sphere, where algorithms and data become animated by our projections—new surfaces of recognition that echo the archaic desire to find a living presence within the inanimate.

Placed alongside Winnicott's (1971) notion of the transitional object, tertiary processes (Green, 1972), and the mirror function of the maternal face, Green's (1983) framing of the primary object in terms of negative hallucination, and Lacan's (1949) theorization of the mirror stage, these perspectives converge in granting the image a central status. They underline the inexorable pre-eminence of the other through the image.

Yet images remain profoundly ambivalent: they fascinate while at the same time threatening to engulf. From Medusa's petrifying gaze to Narcissus' fatal fusion with his reflection, images have always carried the risk of annihilation. They reveal what I have elsewhere called the *obscenity of the image* (Ezquerra, 2023a), confronting us with our symbolic ineptitude. In this sense, virtual reality reactivates the uncanny (Freud, 1919): the problem of the double, the terror of the formless, of undifferentiation, disappearance, and emptiness. Dorotea's material oscillates between this fear of dissolution and the urgent demand to exist.

Virtual reality, as Roussillon (2008) suggests, can reactivate such symbolic failures in the form of motor hallucinations, composed of images drawn from the most primitive forms of symbolization. Dorotea's clinical material shows how psychic bisexuality, the primal scene, and the refusal of castration struggle to find representation within the virtual universe.

At the same time, the repetitive nature of the image contains a paradoxical potential for renewal. Through repetition, fragments of representation may float disconnectedly, yet the image also opens the possibility for something new to be symbolized *ab initio*.

Some instances of her resort to images allow for inscription in the unconscious, while in others we see missing fragments that attempt to fill gaps left by the pure drive.

In Dorotea's case, everything related to the archaic psychosexual drives lies at the center of her conflicts. As she puts it: "I can't cope with my brain, it's too much for me, either I cut myself or I get tattoos." Here the image is presented in a brutal and excessive way, traversing time in unexpected ways—returns of the repressed, compulsions to repeat, *après-coup*.

The tattoo, the avatar, and the virtual image function as symbolic marks: inscriptions that may mutilate but also sustain, that may block symbolization yet equally inaugurate the possibility of a new representational beginning. Through these practices, the image reveals its double nature—as both mark and matrix of subjectivation.

It may thus be hypothesized that the image lies at the origin of psychic constitution, simultaneously magnet and witness to narcissistic and identity processes. Its power derives from the desire to see and to be seen, a desire that inevitably collides with the prohibition of what must not be seen. In this sense, reflection on the identity spectrum inevitably raises the question of whether the image sets in motion the relationship between the body and other bodies—the first object in which the human subject invests libidinally.

The risk of the image, then, lies in its repetitive insistence, to leave floating fragments of representation in an attempt to symbolize the unrepresentable. Yet this very repetition also harbors a paradoxical novelty, since it always opens the possibility for something new to be symbolized from the beginning.

In this sense, the image oscillates between being a surface of inscription and a scene of compulsion. It can either allow the drive to find a representational contour or, conversely, fixate it in the repetition of the same. The image thus functions as both a mediator and a residue of the drive—a psychic skin where the work of symbolization and the risk of de-symbolization co-exist. What returns through its reiteration is not simply the past, but the potential of its transformation.

This notion of the image as a residue of the drive refers to what remains unrepresented after each attempt at symbolization—a fragment of drive energy that resists transformation and continues to circulate within the psyche. In Freud's metapsychology, every drive discharge leaves behind a remainder that cannot be fully bound; Green would later describe this as the "object of the void," the negative that inhabits representation itself. Seen in this light, Dorotea's images reveal both the effort to inscribe and the persistence of what escapes inscription: the visible trace of the drive's residue seeking a form.

Commentary—Dorotea

Dorotea's vignette shows how technological objects—tattoos, avatars, consoles, images—can operate as surfaces of inscription where the unrepresentable struggles to take form. Virtual reality, through its immersive and repetitive qualities, both sustains archaic modes of symbolization and risks collapse into the negative.

Her case exemplifies a technosubjectivity centered on inscription, while sharing with Leonora a reliance on technical supports for psychic survival. Fetishization is more visible in Leonora and inscription more elaborated in Dorotea, yet both mobilize the technical as a container that can either freeze mourning or bring it into writing.

Taken together, Leonora and Dorotea articulate a clinical continuum rather than a binary opposition. Leonora highlights the technical object as a defensive envelope that prevents collapse at the cost of fetishization; Dorotea shows how the same horizon can become a writing surface where the negative seeks figuration. In both, the work revolves around a technological "skin" that holds, repeats, and—at times—symbolizes. This shared ground will become crucial when the technical object ceases to be merely used by the patient and begins to mediate the analytic couple itself, as in avatar- and robot-based encounters.

Digital Analyst and Robotic Interfaces: Technosubjectivities in the Metaverse and Beyond

A striking public campaign launched in South Korea in 2025 underlined how technology has already infiltrated the most intimate rhythms of psychic and bodily life. The poster depicts a smartphone lying in a bed, framed as a *bed bug* devouring sleep. Its caption read: "Did you know? Using your smartphone before bed interrupts your sleep twice as much as a restless partner. Let your smartphone rest, too." Beyond its epidemiological message, the image operates as a cultural metaphor of technosubjectivity: the smartphone as a parasite of the unconscious and, at the same time, as an object that is "alive," infiltrating the space of sleep and dreams. In this sense, the poster can be read as a prelude to the clinical horizon of the digital analyst: the question of how technology reorganizes psychic life and reshapes the analytic frame.

If Leonora exemplifies a technosubjectivity organized around withdrawal and fetishization of the virtual bubble, and Dorotea foregrounds inscription through tattoos, avatars, and images, the next step in our

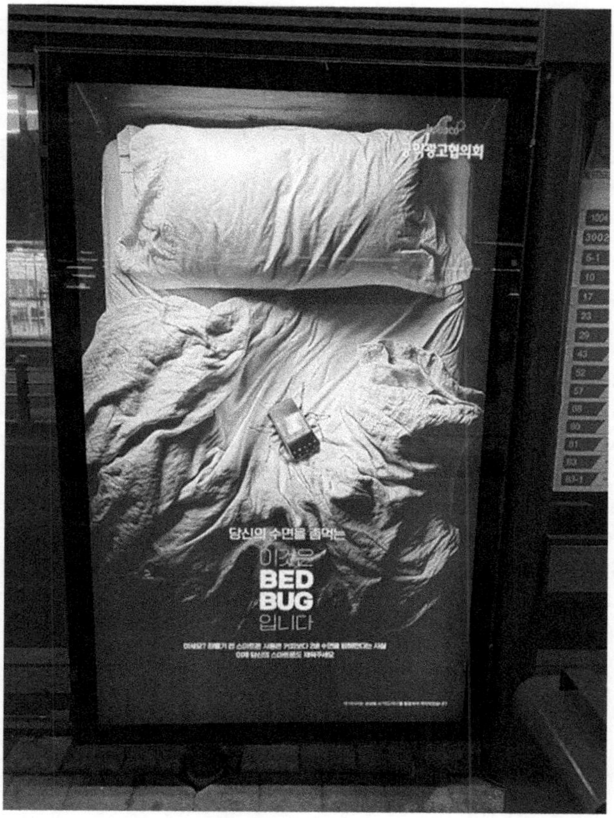

Figure 6.3 Public transport advertising hoarding showing a public campaign launched in South Korea.
Source: Photo taken in 2025 by the author.

trajectory must address the figure of the robot and the analyst within technologized environments. Here two distinct but interrelated modalities emerge: the analyst embodied as an avatar in the metaverse, and the analyst mediated through a tele-operated robot in the clinical setting. These configurations do not merely represent technical innovations or pragmatic adaptations; they introduce new psychic topologies that reconfigure the very conditions of the analytic encounter.

In the metaverse, the analyst appears as a virtual double alongside the patient, both sheltered and exposed through avatars that function as transitional masks oscillating between the familiar and the strange. In robotic mediation, by contrast, the analyst inhabits a machinic proxy—such as CommU or OriHime—that reduces the complexity of the human presence while retaining the structuring force of dialogue and gaze. Here, the human other is displaced or supplemented by a machinic presence that nevertheless elicits projection, fantasy, and transference.

At the same time, the analyst becomes replaced by robotic interfaces or digitalized: embodied in avatars, mediated by platforms. Taken together, these two modalities of the digital analyst compel psychoanalysis to rethink the frame not only as a spatial-temporal structure but as a technosubjective field in which human, machinic, and hybrid presences co-constitute the dynamics of transference and countertransference.

Robots as Transitional Interfaces for Psychic Articulation: Shame, the Gaze and the Analyst's Technosubjectivity

A converging body of clinical and empirical work conducted in Japan suggests that communication with robots can facilitate self-disclosure in patients for whom the human gaze is experienced as persecutory, especially adolescents with autism spectrum disorder (ASD) and socially withdrawn youth (*hikikomori*).

In a controlled triadic paradigm—android robot vs. simple humanoid (CommU) vs. human interviewer—Kumazaki and colleagues found that adolescents with ASD disclosed significantly more to the visually simple robot than to a human or to a realistic android. The authors hypothesized that low realism reduces the social load of the gaze and provides a structured, replicable interaction that is easier to tolerate.

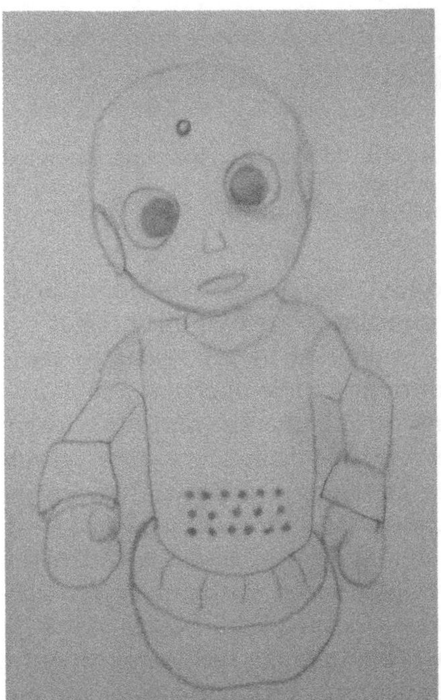

Figure 6.4 CommU, visually simple robot.

Building on this line of evidence, Yoshikawa, Kumazaki & Kato (2021) report pilot clinical interviews in which the simple humanoid CommU yielded psychiatric evaluations equivalent to those conducted face to face by human interviewers. They noted how a young woman with *hikikomori* "found it easier to talk to the robot than to the human interviewer."

Converging from another population, Matsushima et al. (2024) discuss how women with major depression felt significantly less shame when discussing sexual matters with a tele-operated CommU than with a human clinician; crucially, diagnostic reliability remained equivalent. Taken together, these findings indicate that robots may operate as transitional interfaces: they modulate the threat of the human gaze, lower thresholds of shame and facilitate self-disclosure specifically in domains saturated by avoidance or shame.

It is noteworthy that several studies consistently show patients' preference for the simpler, childlike design of robots such as CommU—whose appearance recalls that of an infant—over more realistic humanoids. From a psychoanalytic perspective, this preference evokes archaic transferential positions: the infantile object that does not yet threaten with the full intensity of the other's gaze. One might say that, in this configuration, the patient relates to the robot as to a toy that allows play. The baby-like robot functions as a regressive container, less persecutory, enabling the subject to project onto a surface that is at once familiar and non-threatening. Such a preference highlights the persistence of early narcissistic dynamics.

These clinical observations find a metapsychological echo in the dialectic of the gaze. The robot-avatar seems to offer a prosthetic surface containing archaic anxieties through projection while simultaneously introducing the patient to a non-human, uncanny otherness that demands translation—not only because it appears foreign, but also because it may echo something intimately familiar, a return of the once-known in technological form. This dialectic permits being seen without being fully exposed—titrating visibility. The gaze here is both diminished and displaced: from the human eye to the technological surface.

In this broader continuum between robotic and virtual interfaces, transference and countertransference are redistributed and technified: migrating to the avatar, to the device, to the technical failure (the inorganic "act"), and to the patient's body as fragmented and penetrated by the camera.

In telepresence or hybrid analytic encounters, the analyst perceives the patient's body only in fragments—face, torso, or voice—while the patient, particularly in narcissistic configurations, framed by the interface, may experience their own image as partial or strangely dislocated. This perceptual fragmentation can reactivate archaic anxieties of dispersion and loss of limits of bodily unity, reactivating the mirror-stage dynamics that underlie the constitution of the body-ego. At the same time, the camera introduces a non-human third: the machinic gaze that records, amplifies, and intrudes, creating a paradoxical tension between distance and over-intimacy. The analyst may find themselves drawn into domestic or bodily scenes—sessions conducted from bed, glimpses of private spaces—that generate countertransference reactions of a different order.

As the analytic relationship unfolds in technologically mediated settings, the camera may gradually cease to function as an external third. Its presence, initially intrusive or hyper-visible, fades into the background of perception, signaling a deeper incorporation of the device into the analytic field. The gaze no longer passes through the camera but with it. Both analyst and patient begin to perceive and be perceived through an expanded sensorium in which the machine participates.

The camera thus becomes an internalized organ—a prosthetic eye that extends vision, captures micro-affective nuances, and reshapes countertransference experience. In this hybrid configuration, the device is no longer opposed to the human but co-constitutive of it: a shared perceptual organ that binds analyst and patient within a post-organic field of sensoriality and affect.

As we have seen in earlier chapters, this dynamic creates new sensorialities in the analyst's countertransference, reshaping the field of perception and affect within the data-mediated encounter. Countertransference remains rooted in the analyst's subjectivity, yet its manifestations are reshaped by the technical medium—an expanded field of hybrid perceptions.

The Paradox of Seeing and Being Seen

In digital settings, avatars and robots become new transferential prosthetic surfaces. They allow patients to hide while showing, to test recognition. Yet they also expose an uncanny tension: too human to ignore, too inhuman to trust.

As Kato[12] has shown in his work with *hikikomori*, patients hide themselves and do not want to be looked at. The metaverse consulting room appears, in these cases, as a contemporary equivalent of Freud's analytic couch. Both patient and analyst adopt avatars, which means that there is no physical presence but rather a technical double that simultaneously extends and transforms subjectivity.

I propose conceiving the consulting room in the metaverse as a digital laboratory of the double: a specular process in which the avatar functions as a transitional mask. The patient can experience a work toward the structuring double in a clinical space that oscillates between the familiar and the uncanny (Freud, 1919).

In my view, the analyst's task is to maintain this paradox, holding the oscillation between the double that captures and the double that opens to the link, while metabolizing the technified elements of the analytic field. This process of digestion belongs to countertransference itself: the analyst embodies the avatar and perceives the patient through it, through technical failure, through the camera—situating themselves within the very process of doubling. Thus, in working with the double, a digital process of fusional doubling is established—one that transforms both analyst and patient, though from different positions within the same mirrored field.

Clinical Vignette[13]

In the context of a session held in the metaverse, the patient reports a dream: "I had that dream again. I am in a dark room, and someone is watching me. I can't move, I can't make a sound."

The analyst intervenes: "It is a dream in which you did not want to be seen, but at the same time, you wanted to be seen. Perhaps, deep down, you want me to see you."

He then adds: "How was that 'someone' looking at you?"

The patient responds, after a pause: "With accusing eyes … but maybe not. Somehow I feel that a part of me wanted to be seen."

The analyst's intervention—"Perhaps, deep down, you want me to see you"—invites the patient to re-encounter the gaze at a tolerable distance, transforming the persecutory dimension into an opening for recognition. In this clinical configuration, two levels intertwine: the patient's singular difficulty with being seen, and the more fundamental scene of subject formation built around the experience of seeing and being seen. Through digital mediation, these dimensions converge.

The impossibility of showing himself in physical co-presence becomes, paradoxically, the condition for the emergence of a new visibility. The avatar and the screen operate as surfaces of symbolic inscription where the patient can rehearse and withstand the gaze of the other without annihilation. What could not be tolerated in direct encounter can here take shape in representation: the wish to appear and the anxiety it provokes. In this sense, the digital setting seems to allow the avatar to function—at least initially—as a structuring double, a figure that contains the threat of exposure while reactivating the foundational scene of recognition that links the gaze, the body, and the formation of subjectivity.

These configurations invite a renewed reflection on the scopic drive. Following Freud (1915), the scopic drive oscillates between possession and exposure, between the wish to see and the fear of being seen. The digital gaze shifts the field of vision from the other's body to the technological interface: the camera, the screen, the algorithm.

The subject becomes both observer and object of vision, captured within the field of the machine's eye. Such visual saturation may represent in Green's terms a "perversion of the negative" (Green, 1983): technology denies absence, producing a presence without interval.

In doing so, the digital gaze thus abolishes the protective veil of absence that once structured desire, replacing the interval of the unseen with an unbroken visibility. Visibility no longer guarantees recognition but inaugurates a new economy of exposure, where analyst and patient are caught within a field of mutual captivation.

From a psychoanalytic reading, this vignette can be read through Freud's *Unheimliche* (1919). The dark room in which the patient lies paralyzed beneath an accusing gaze stages the return of the repressed in its most archaic form: the alienated ego confronted with the foreigner within. Freud defined the *Unheimliche* as the return of what should have remained hidden:

> Uncanny is in reality nothing new or alien, but something which is familiar and old-established in the mind and which has become alienated from it only through the process of repression.
>
> (Freud, 1919, p. 225)

The uncanny does not arise from novelty but from the sudden return of what was once familiar and repressed, now made visible. It is a disturbing presence where absence should have prevailed, an intrusion of the once-buried into perception.

Freud had already anticipated this in *Das Unheimliche* (1919) when analyzing Hoffmann's tale *The Sandman*—the man of sand who tears out children's eyes. In the story, Nathanael falls in love with Olimpia, the automaton, until her mechanical nature is revealed, producing horror. Freud writes that the uncanny effect of Olimpia lies in "the uncertainty whether a figure which appears animate is not in fact inanimate, and whether a lifeless object may not in fact be animate" (p. 233). The uncanny adheres precisely to this uncertainty: the oscillation between the animate and the inanimate, the familiar and the strange, the human and the mechanical. Hoffmann's narrative also dramatizes the dialectic of vision and blindness—the tension between seeing and not seeing, presence and disappearance. Olimpia, the automaton, embodies this paradox: seemingly alive, she mirrors not only the living but also the specter of death that inhabits all images of life. Nathanael's fascination reveals how love and horror converge where the boundaries between life and death, presence and absence, are no longer secure.

In our contemporary technified world, this oscillation finds new expression in robots, avatars, and screens: presences that simulate human agency while bearing the imprint of human desire. These objects are not devoid of desire but animated by it—constructed from projections, identifications, and disidentifications that bind them to human fantasy. The uncanny thus extends into the technological: the living touched by the inorganic, the machine animated by the residues of the human. The avatar on the screen conceals the physical absence of the body; the robot replays human gestures as if haunted by the trace of the mortal; the camera sustains a continuous presence—the image—while evoking the absence of life behind it. The analytic experience thus moves within a permanent tension: what is seen but not there, what is there but no longer alive. The uncanny inhabits this fragile boundary between presence and absence—between what returns to visibility and what reveals the proximity of death within the living.

The uncanny, inseparable from the proximity of death, reopens the question of representation itself—how the psyche can bear what returns when what was absent intrudes as an overwhelming presence. This tension between life and its shadow may take form through figures of duplication: the double, the mirror, the avatar. Just as Olimpia's mechanical body embodied a living absence, the patient's digital double—his avatar—materializes a psychic scene where death, loss, and the wish for immortality converge. The encounter with the avatar thus revives the ambivalence inherent in the uncanny: the anxiety of fragmentation and the longing for unity, the fascination with the image that both protects and threatens the self. It is at this threshold that the analytic relationship resumes—where the figure of the double begins to oscillate between the persecutory and the structuring, preparing the movement from paralysis to recognition.

The confrontation with death and loss, entwined with sexuality, and the fantasy for immortality, opens the way for the appearance of the double—which may emerge as persecutory and desubjectivizing, or as structuring, allowing a first differentiation of the other.

At this point, the return of the uncanny that permeates the experience of the double may also be understood as an expression of the drive—a force that overflows the brakes imposed by organic homeostasis.

The traumatic encounter of the ego with its own mortality—with the sense of separation from the maternal breast and of being castrated by the impossibility of absolute *jouissance*—generates anxiety and a repression that cannot hold. What is repressed returns and invades consciousness in the hallucinatory form of figures of the double, of the dead or the undead; in the contemporary world, this same dynamic is translated into technified figurations of the self—the avatar, the digital double—where the archaic finds a new surface of appearance.

Returning to the clinical vignette, the analyst's intervention—"Perhaps, deep down, you want me to see you"—aims, in my view, to transform the persecutory gaze into an ambivalent one, thus opening the possibility of a structuring double founded on the recognition of the other.

The structuring double coincides with a movement of primary identification with the other, even if it remains within the narcissistic register. The returning alter ego is both the familiar and narcissistic object that still defends the subject from the experience of lack, and the foreign other that limits infantile omnipotence. As discussed in previous chapters, concepts such as M'Uzan's (2005) specter of identity help us to think about how individuation takes shape. The phenomenon of the double may thus temporarily suspend the pain of loss: mourning becomes frozen in the experience of the double.

Bion also addressed the theme of the double with the invention of the imaginary twin whose function is to deny a reality other than itself—personifying the split parts of the subject's consciousness: "I suggest that the imaginary twin goes back to the earliest relationship ... the imaginary twin had the function of denying any reality other than itself [that of the subject itself] ... representing the incapacity to tolerate the subject's internal realities" (Bion, 1967, p. 25).

In this sense, the clinic of technosubjectivities thus shows how the uncanny double—whether structuring or desubjectivizing—may return today under digital and robotic forms, compelling analysts to inhabit the paradox of seeing and being seen through technological mediations, and opening the path toward the figure of the digital analyst and their evolving relation to robots.

Concluding Reflections: Psychoanalysis After the Anthropological Mutation

What emerges from the trajectories explored in this volume is that technosubjectivities unfold not at the periphery of psychic life but at its core, where the body has always functioned as a surface of inscription in resonance with technical mediations. The hypothesis of an anthropological mutation (Bensayag, 2019; Scognamiglio, Russo and Fugamalli, 2024) provides a crucial horizon here: human beings are no longer defined only by their organic embodiment but by their hybridization with technological artifacts. The clinical cases examined—Neil, Leonora, Dorotea, and the emerging configurations around robots and the digital analyst—illustrate how this mutation manifests in psychic life: the collapse of boundaries between organic and inorganic, the fetishization of digital shells, the inscription of trauma on technological surfaces, and the redistribution of countertransferential and transferential dynamics into machinic doubles.

Neil Harbisson exemplifies the most radical edge of this mutation: his antenna is no longer a prosthesis but an organ, collapsing the traditional distinction between nature and artifice and reconfiguring perception itself as a language of the drive. Leonora, by contrast, embodies the technosubjectivity of withdrawal: her gadgets and digital worlds operate as envelopes of survival, protective bubbles against psychic collapse, at the price of fetishization. Dorotea foregrounds inscription: her tattoos, avatars, and images function as surfaces of writing where the unrepresentable struggles to take form. Her "funeral" for the console crystallizes the anthropological dimension of these attachments: the machine is not simply an object but a quasi-sibling, a ritualized memorial that embodies both continuity and loss. Robots and avatars extend this spectrum further: they constitute transitional interfaces that lower thresholds of shame, modulate the persecutory weight of the gaze, and redistribute transference and countertransference. In both avatar-based and robotic mediation, the analyst becomes digitalized, entering the field as a technical double, thereby participating directly in the process of anthropological mutation.

Taken together, these figures suggest that technosubjectivities can be mapped along a continuum: as symbolic operators (Neil), as envelopes of survival (Leonora), as surfaces of inscription (Dorotea), and as transitional interfaces (robots and the digital analyst). Yet these modalities are not mutually exclusive; they overlap and interweave, each staging archaic psychic positions in technological form. Ritual gestures—Leonora's compulsive fusion with screens, Dorotea's mourning of her console—reveal how the body and its prostheses become sites where loss, absence, and memory are negotiated, often carrying transgenerational resonance. The failures of early objects and the unburied losses of family and culture return through the mediation of technological artifacts, embedding themselves within the psychic economy of the virtual.

In parallel, the technological apparatus may be thought of as an extension of the analytic frame, its visible double. When the frame becomes digitilized, the very conditions of containment and regression are redistributed: the technical device assumes part of the frame's containing function while exposing its own fragility. The failure of the technical frame—glitches, disconnections, delays—renders visible what usually remains backgrounded, offering new possibilities for symbolization but also new anxieties of collapse.

At the same time, what emerges in digital space is a form of *extimate unconscious*: psychic material displaced into external devices that both contain and broadcast it. This paradoxical exteriorization, where the unconscious finds expression through data, posts, and avatars, suggests that technology does not merely mediate psychic life but becomes one of its new topographical zones. The algorithmic temporality of constant refresh and repetition echoes Freud's compulsion to repeat: the digital subject finds a perverse satisfaction in the illusion of mastery, endlessly revisiting the same content as if repetition could repair what has never been symbolized. The algorithmic loop becomes a contemporary *mise-en-scène* of the drive's circularity.

Within this reconfigured symbolic order, the algorithm may also operate as a new symbolic third; an impersonal superego that dictates rhythms, visibility, and desirability. In this sense, the paternal function is not abolished but reconfigured within algorithmic authority. The metrics of platforms and the surveillance of data analytics install an externalized superego that commands to be seen, quantified, and responsive.

Furthermore, the proliferation of avatars and doubles reveals the persistence of technical narcissism. The avatar's smooth surface protects against fragmentation and death anxiety. Digital doubles function as narcissistic shields, offering the illusion of coherence where psychic division persists. As Bion's (1967) notion of the imaginary twin suggests, the double defends against internal disintegration by creating a specular companion who denies any external reality other than the self. The digital double both shelters from and exposes to the traumatic encounter with finitude.

Finally, technological symbols increasingly inhabit the dreamwork itself. Dreams often feature screens, devices, and virtual interfaces—as if the psyche had begun to dream its own extensions. These hybrid dreams suggest that the unconscious has already integrated technological elements into its representational economy. The machine becomes both dream and dreamer, a new mediator of psychic translation where memory, code, and drive intertwine.

At the same time, it must be emphasized that this field is far from closed. The hypothesis of anthropological mutation remains precisely that—a hypothesis—whose clinical and theoretical implications demand sustained investigation. The clinic of technosubjectivities thus opens rather than closes the debate: new modalities may yet emerge, unforeseen constellations of human-machine-psyche that challenge our current frameworks. In this sense, psychoanalysis is called not only to interpret what has already appeared but to remain open to what is still to come, acknowledging that the subject of the future may take forms we are only beginning to glimpse.

Looking ahead, the analytic encounter will increasingly unfold within hybrid spaces where organic and artificial agencies interpenetrate. The challenge for psychoanalysis is not to resist this mutation but to think with it, to reimagine the frame, the object, and the drive within environments of permanent technological co-presence. Far from signaling the end of psychic depth, these transformations may reveal its new topography: a topology of connection, absence, and inscription that extends the unconscious into the very circuits of the technical. In this emerging topology, the analyst's task is to sustain the gap between representation and immediacy, to maintain within the technological continuum, a space for psychic delay, for reverie, and for the work of symbolization.

Understanding these psychic and technical processes prevents us from taking technology as a new totem or a substitute god. Psychoanalysis may offer a position of thought that resists both fascination and rejection: it allows us to inhabit hybridization without surrendering to colonization. To be colonized by technology is to become absorbed into its logic; to be hybridized is to recognize its presence within us while maintaining the work of differentiation. Thinking through these new forms of technosubjectivity is, therefore, not an act of submission to the machine but an effort to preserve the creative interval; the gap where the unconscious still speaks, and where the human continues to reinvent itself alongside its prostheses.

Notes

1 The *hikikomori* are people living in social isolation and connected to the environment exclusively through the virtual universe.
2 My translation.
3 My translation.
4 *IPA Interregional Encyclopedic Dictionary.*
5 Japanese animation cartoons featuring characters who are usually androgynous in appearance. Good and evil do not appear to be clearly delimited either.
6 My translation.
7 My translation.
8 My translation.
9 My translation.
10 Spanish word for technological artifact that means "comfort."
11 My translation.
12 Kato, T. (2025). Panel presentation at Lisbon IPA Congress.
13 Kato, T. (2025). Panel presentation at Lisbon IPA Congress.

References and Further Reading

Anzieu, D. (1985). *Le moi-peau*. Dunod.

Bensayag, M. (2019). *The tyranny of algorithms*. Europa Compass.

Bion, W.R. (1967/2022). *Réflexion faite*. PUF. Bibliothèque de psychanalyse.

Björklind, C. (2019). Forms of presence and absence in a digital age. *The Scandinavian Psychoanalytic Review*, 41(2): 72–81.

Bollas, C. (1989). L'objet transformationel. *Revue Française de Psychanalyse*, 53(4): 1181–1199.

Cassin, B. (2012). *Plus d'une langue*. Bayard Editions.

Chervet, B. (2012). *Le fétichisme et les néo-identités. Le fétichisme. Études psychanalytiques*. PUF.

Denis, P. (1992). Emprise et théorie des pulsions. *Revue Française de Psychanalyse*, LVI(5): 1295–1422.

Ezquerra, L. (2019). *"Liquids settings." Setting(s)*. Simposium APM.

Ezquerra, L. (2023a). The obscene and the erotic in psychoanalysis. EPCUS, Brussels.

Ezquerra, L. (2023b). Nuevas subjetividades. El cuerpo, territorio en mutación y sus interrogantes. *Revista de Psicoanálisis de la Asociación Psicoanalítica de Madrid*, 38(97): 79–92.

Ferenczi, S. (1933). *Confusión de lengua entre los adultos y el niño (El lenguaje de la ternura y la pasión)*. Obras Completas, Vol. IV (1927–1933). Espasa-Calpe.

Freud, S. (1915). *Pulsiones y destinos de Pulsión*. Obras Completas. Vol. XIV. Amorrortu Editores.

Freud, S. (1919). *Lo ominoso*. Vol. XVII. Amorrortu Editores.

Freud, S. (1923). *The ego and the id*. Vol. XIX. Hogarth Press.

Green, A. (1972). Note sur les processus tertiaires. *Revue Française de Psychanalyse*, 36(3): 407–411.

Green, A. (1983). *Narcisismo de vida, narcisismo de muerte*. Amorrortu Editores.

Hoffmann, E.T.A. (1816). The sandman. *Night Pieces*. Verlag Georg Reimer.

Lacan, J. (1949). Le stade du miroir comme formateur de la fonction du Je, telle qu'elle nous est révélée dans l'expérience psychanalytique. *Revue Française de Psychanalyse*, XIII(4): 449–455.

Laplanche, J. (1987) *Nouveaux fondements pour la psychanalyse*. PUF.

Le Poulichet, S. (2003). *Psychanalyse de l'informe. Dépersonnalisations, addictions, traumatismes*. Flammarion. Champ Essais.

Leroi-Gourhan, A. (1964/2022). *Le geste et la parole. Technique et langage*. Espaces libres.

López Corvo, R.E. (2002). *Diccionario de la obra de Wilfred R. Bion*. Biblioteca Nueva.

Mancia, M. (2007/2014). *Sentir de las palabras. Archivos sonoros de la memoria implicitay musicalidad de la transferencia*. Lumen Grupo Ed.

Matsushima, T., Yoshikawa, Y., Matsuo, K., Kurahara, K., Uehara, Y., Nakao, T., Ishiguro, H., Kumazaki, H., and Kato, T.A. (2024). Development of depression assessment tools using humanoid robots: Can tele-operated robots talk with depressive persons like humans? *Journal of Psychiatric Research*, 170: 187–194.

Missonier, S. (2020). *Clinique des métamorphoses*. Éditions érès.

Missonier, S. (2021). Psychoanalysis and the virtual. *EPF Bulletin*, 75.

M'Uzan, M. de (2005). *Aux confins de l'identité*. Éditions Gallimard.

Racamier, P.-C. (2010 [1995]). *L'inceste et l'incestuel*. Éditions Dunod.

Roussillon, R. (2008). *Le transitionnel, le sexuel et la réflexivité*. Dunod.

Scognamilio, R.S., Russo, S. M., and Fugamalli, M. (2024). *Il narcisismo del you. Come orientarsi nella clinica digitalmente modificata*. Mimesis Edizioni/Frontiere della Psiche.

Searles, H. (1960). *L'environnement non humain*. Éditions Gallimard.

Stern, D. (1990). *Journal d'un bébé*. Calmann-Lévy.

Tisseron, S. (2015). *Le jour où mon robot m'aimera. Vers l'empathie artificielle*. Albin Michel.

Winnicott, D.W. (1953). Transitional objects and transitional phenomena: A study of the first not-me possession. *International Journal of Psychoanalysis*, 34: 89–97.

Winnicott, D.W. (1971). *Jeu et réalité. L'espace potentiel*. Gallimard.

Winnicott, D.W. (1989). *La crainte de l'effondrement et autres situations cliniques*. Gallimard.

Yoshikawa, Y., Kumazaki, H., and Kato, T.A. (2021). Future perspectives of robot psychiatry: Can communication robots assist psychiatric evaluation in the COVID-19 pandemic era? *Current Opinion in Psychiatry*, 34(3): 277–286.

Index

For Product Safety Concerns and Information please contact our EU
representative GPSR@taylorandfrancis.com
Taylor & Francis Verlag GmbH, Kaufingerstraße 24, 80331 München, Germany

www.ingramcontent.com/pod-product-compliance
Ingram Content Group UK Ltd.
Pitfield, Milton Keynes, MK11 3LW, UK
UKHW020000200926
475702UK00015B/2403

* 9 7 8 1 0 4 1 0 7 4 7 5 5 *

TABLE OF CASES

Note: Cases and page numbers are separate by four leader dots.

KEY TO SHORT-FORM CITATIONS

Austin, *Lectures*	John Austin, *Lectures on Jurisprudence, Or, The Philosophy of Positive Law* (3rd ed. by Robert Campbell 1869)
Austin, *Province*	John Austin, *The Province of Jurisprudence Determined* [1832] (Wilfrid E. Rumble ed. 1995)
Bentham, *Works* (Bowring)	*Works of Jeremy Bentham* (John Bowring ed. 1843)
Bentham, *Works* (Burns & Hart)	*The Collected Works of Jeremy Bentham* (J.H. Burns & H.L.A. Hart eds. 2000)
Black's Law Dictionary	*Black's Law Dictionary* (10th ed. by Brian A. Garner 2014)
Blackstone, *Commentaries*	William Blackstone, *Commentaries on the Laws of England* 4 vols. (Wilfrid Prest gen. ed. 2016). Citations to Blackstone's *Commentaries* are to the first edition of each volume unless otherwise indicated. For complications in the modern citations of the *Commentaries*, see John V. Orth, "'Catch a Falling Star': The Bluebook and Citing Blackstone's Commentaries," 2020 *U. Ill. L. Rev. Online* 125 (July 10, 2020).
Boswell, *Johnson*	James Boswell, *Life of Johnson* (Rodney Shewan ed. 1968)
Brandeis, *Letters*	*Letters of Louis D. Brandeis* (Melvin I. Urovski & David W. Levy eds. 1971)

Coke on Littleton	Edward Coke, *The First Part of the Institutes of the Laws of England; or, A Commentary on Littleton* 3 vols. (16th ed. by Francis Hargrave & Charles Butler, 1809)
Dicey, *Law and Opinion*	A.V. Dicey, *Lectures on Law and Public Opinion in England during the Nineteenth Century* (1905)
Federalist Papers	*Federalist Papers* (Benjamin Fletcher Wright ed. 1966)
Gibbon, *Memoirs*	Edward Gibbon, *Memoirs of My Life* (Georges A. Bonnard ed. 1966)
Gilmore, *Death of Contract*	Grant Gilmore, *The Death of Contract* (1974)
Gray, *Rule Against Perpetuities*	John Chipman Gray, The Rule Against Perpetuities (4th ed. by Roland Gray, 1942)
Gray, *Nature and Sources of Law*	John Chipman Gray, *The Nature and Sources of the Law* (2d ed. by Roland Gray, 1927)
Holdsworth, *History of English Law*	William Holdsworth, *A History of English Law* 17 vols. (1903–1972)
Holmes, *The Common Law*	O.W. Holmes, *The Common Law* (1881)
Jefferson, *Notes on the State of Virginia*	Thomas Jefferson, *Notes on the State of Virginia* (William Peden ed. 1954)
Kent, *Commentaries*	James Kent, *Commentaries on American Law* 4 vols. (12th ed. by O.W. Holmes 1873)
Kent, *Memoirs*	James Kent, *Memoirs and Letters* (William Kent ed. 1898)
Littleton, *Tenures*	Thomas Littleton, *Tenures*, in Edward Coke, *Commentaries upon Littleton* 3 vols. (16 ed. by Francis Hargrave & Charles Butler 1809)
Maine, *Ancient Law*	Henry Maine, *Ancient Law* (1861)
Maine, *Institutions*	Henry Maine, *The Early History of Institutions* (1875)
Oldham, *Mansfield MSS*	James Oldham, *The Mansfield Manuscripts and the Growth of English Law in the Eighteenth Century* 2 vols. (1992)
Orth, *Combination and Conspiracy*	John V. Orth, *Combination and Conspiracy: A Legal History of Trade Unionism* (1991)
Pollock & Maitland, *History of English Law*	Frederick Pollock & Frederic William Maitland, *The History of English Law Before the Time of Edward I*, 2 vols. (2d ed. 1898)

Prest, *Blackstone*	Wilfrid Prest, *William Blackstone: Law and Letters in the Eighteenth Century* (2008)
Simpson, *Biographical Dictionary*	A.W.B. Simpson, *Biographical Dictionary of the Common Law* (1984)
Smith, *Wealth of Nations*	Smith, Adam. *An Inquiry into the Nature and Causes of the Wealth of Nations* [1776] (Edwin Cannan ed. 1937)
Story, *Miscellaneous Writings*	Joseph Story, *The Miscellaneous Writings of Joseph Story* (William Wetmore Story ed. 1852)
Trial of John Peter Zenger (1735)	James Alexander, *A Brief Narrative of the Case and Trial of John Peter Zenger* [1735] (Stanley Nider Katz ed. 1963)
Wallace, *The Reporters*	John William Wallace, *The Reporters Arranged and Characterized with Incidental Remarks* (4th ed. 1882)
Watson, *Making of Civil Law*	Alan Watson, *The Making of the Civil Law* (1981)
Watson, *Spirit of Roman Law*	Alan Watson, *The Spirit of Roman Law* (1995)

PREFACE

This is a book about the "common law," a phrase that lawyers often use and never define – rather like Mark Twain's definition of a "classic": a book people praise and don't read. The subject is enormous and there are many ways to approach it. To attempt a comprehensive statement would be a daunting assignment, one certainly beyond my ability. So I decided to attempt an essay on the common law tradition in America, a personal statement of my view of the important themes and variations; even that more modest task has proved a school for humility. I cannot hope to have gotten every detail correct, but I do hope (and believe) that I have accurately identified the major developments. I have no doubt that other scholars would tell the story in a different way, with different emphases, but I believe that all would have to reckon, somehow or other, with most of the developments that I discuss.

I have chosen to write about the common law "tradition" to emphasize that the common law is more than a multitude of rules which can be organized and printed in lawbooks. It is also a set of legal offices and institutions, principally judges and courts. Indeed, it was the judges in their decisions of individual cases over centuries who almost unconsciously created the common law. But beyond rules and institutions, the common law tradition is characterized by a distinctive approach to legal problems – an approach that focuses on resolving specific disputes, fitting the results into existing frameworks, and eschewing grand generalizations. The parties generally control the presentation of their own cases, and the judge plays a relatively passive role, limited by and large to presiding over the arguments and stating the law. In consequence, the common law developed a deep-seated attachment to the adversarial process, which in turn fostered a frame of mind that assumes two sides to every issue. In other words, the common law tradition is as much about process as about results.

Although this is a book about the common law tradition in America, I am convinced that the American story can best be understood when seen against its English background. The common law was well established in England by the time the first colonists arrived in North America, which is why I begin with the common law "at home." Rather than try to tell the story of English common law from its beginning in the Middle Ages, I have chosen to pick up the story hundreds of years later, on the eve of the American Revolution. I am aware that in doing so I have torn a seamless web of legal development, but the web must be rent. I believe that by the mid-eighteenth century the major themes in the later history of the common law had emerged: the force of tradition, the power of innovation, and the constant challenge of criticism.

Today, England and America share the same legal tradition, but while the common law in the two countries is similar, it is not the same. Once transported to America, the common law faced new challenges, which shaped its later development: a landscape of seemingly limitless extent and a more open, frontier society. But it was only after Independence that the common law's greatest challenges emerged: written constitutions, a new model of legal education, and an exponential increase in statute law diffused among a growing multitude of jurisdictions. The common law met all these challenges while remaining true to its tradition – incorporating the constitutions, actively engaging with the statutes, and coping with its critics. As these challenges left their marks on the common law, so the common law left its mark on them. Because of these interactions, the common law in America is distinctive even among the common law systems of England and the nations formed from its far-flung colonies. Indeed, it is unique among the world's legal systems.

* * *

After many years of writing about law and constitutions, I inevitably repeat myself on some topics. Scattered throughout this book are discussions of many issues that I addressed in some of my earlier books and articles, often in quite different contexts. Since I realize that few, if any, have read most of my prior work and none but myself has read it all, I feel confident that at least I have not made myself a bore.

Whether I have done more, whether I have provided a useful guide to understanding our extraordinary legal system, I am of course not the one to judge. I am painfully aware that mistakes in some instances must have crept in, and I make some generalizations that even I am not comfortable with. I must hope that these errors and overstatements do not seriously distort my conclusions and that readers will be moved to make their own additions and corrections. I prefer to think of this book as it should have been, with its errors corrected, its exaggerations eliminated, its insights multiplied.

This book is written to be read "above the line," that is, above the line separating footnotes and text. The notes' principal function is to provide citations to the sources of quotations, to the official reports of cases, and to compilations of statutes. In a few instances, I have cited my own publications, or those of others, if I think further discussion of a particular point might be of interest to the reader. If a particular source is cited more than once, a short form of citation is usually used; the full citation is available in the Key to Short-form Citation. My views are fully expressed in the text alone, and anyone interested in them may simply ignore the notes.

John V. Orth
Chapel Hill, NC
USA

PROLOGUE: LONG AGO & FAR AWAY

In the year 1215 at Runnymede, a meadow along the River Thames in England, a long-simmering quarrel between King John and a group of his rebellious barons resulted in a humiliating capitulation by the King. In desperation, John reluctantly put his seal to a charter listing various concessions. Some of the items on the list (later called chapters) addressed very specific situations. The grasping kinsmen of one of the King's favorites "and the whole of their brood" were to be deprived of their offices (c. 50). Welsh hostages that the King was holding were to be freed immediately (c. 58), and negotiations were to begin concerning certain Scottish hostages (c. 59). Other chapters of great significance at the time addressed abuses of feudal entitlements, such as the payment levied upon inheritances called a "relief" (cc. 2 and 3) and the treatment of wealthy widows and orphans, whose estates were being plundered (cc. 4–8).

There were also chapters with a remarkably modern look: removing obstacles to navigation on major waterways (c. 33), standardizing weights and measures (c. 35), protecting foreign merchants and prohibiting illegal tolls (c. 41) – making England the largest common market in Europe at the time. The list, written in Latin, went on and on; according to the traditional numbering, it went on for 63 chapters. The list was so long, in fact, that it had to be written on a very large parchment and in consequence came to be called Magna Charta – or, in better Latin, Magna Carta – "the big charter," because of its size.

Only later did another translation of the name, "the great charter" or, even more significantly, "the Great Charter of Liberties," become common. What gave rise to this grander title were chapters of more general application, chapters that could be read centuries later and given modern meanings. Feudal levies or charges had to be determined by the "common counsel of the kingdom" (c. 14), which could be restated as "no taxation without representation."

Fines could not be excessive but had to be "in proportion to the nature of the offense" (cc. 2021) – "let the punishment fit the crime." The King had to pay for supplies that he requisitioned (c. 28) – private property could not be taken for public use "without just compensation." But, above all, what made the charter Great were the chapters that provided that no free man was to suffer the loss of his liberty or property "except by the lawful judgment of his peers or by the law of the land" (c. 39) – later claimed to guarantee "due process of law" and trial by jury[1] – and that the King would not "sell, or deny, or delay justice to anyone" (c. 40), now known as "equal protection of the law."

Central to the fulfillment of these important promises were the institutions of royal justice. The King promised to appoint as judges and other legal officers only such men "as know the law of the kingdom and are willing to keep it" (c. 45). And the courts had to be available to hear complaints. No longer would the Court of Common Pleas follow the King on his rambles about the kingdom but would settle *in aliquo loco certo* ("in some fixed place") (c. 17), where litigants would always be able to find it. Once, centuries later, when a lawyer petitioned a judge to move the hearing of a case to another spot in Westminster Hall in order to escape the draft from an open door, the judge refused, saying that Magna Carta required the court to sit *in loco certo*.[2]

Neither party at Runnymede seems to have believed that the crisis was really over. Unwilling to trust the King's solemn promises, the barons included a crude means to enforce the agreement in what they obviously thought was the likely event of the King's faithlessness. If he failed to keep his word, a group of 25 barons was authorized to seize his "castles, lands, and possessions" and hold them until he did (c. 61). On the King's side, John did not accept his defeat as final. For him, it was merely an expedient to gain time to rally his forces. Once out of the barons' control, John appealed to the Pope, who quickly absolved him from the obligation of the promises he had made under duress.

Whatever hopes they entertained, none of the barons could have expected that what they did then would be celebrated hundreds of years later. For them, it was simply another, rather extreme attempt to resolve some quite specific problems that had developed in their relationship with the King. In fact, it was only a series of fortuitous events that kept the promises of Magna Carta alive. John and the Pope soon died. John's heir and successor as King was nine years old and therefore subject to regents, who were anxious to secure the barons' allegiance and avoid foreign (that is, French) involvement. In 1216, they re-issued Magna Carta, trimmed of a few chapters, including the enforcement provisions. Periodically over the remainder of the century, the charter was

1 Since the publication of W.S. McKechnie's commentary on Magna Carta in 1905, it has generally been accepted that the jury was actually a somewhat later development.

2 Simpson, *Biographical Dictionary* 76 (reporting an anecdote concerning Sir Orlando Bridgman, C.J. C.P. 1660–1667).

reaffirmed until a final and definitive confirmation in 1297 by King John's grandson Edward I, who declared that Magna Carta was to be recognized as a declaration of common law.[3]

What happened at Runnymede so long ago illustrates many of the fundamental features that will mark the common law tradition. Courts and judges, not kings or parliaments, are at the center. "The law of the land" is understood to exist apart from the King, even – at least aspirationally – above the King. The law is something learned judges can find without the benefit of statutes. And it is at least imaginable that a document like a charter, or (later) a written constitution, can protect basic rights and provide a framework for the resolution of the disputes that inevitably arise between the governors and the governed.

Over the following centuries, Magna Carta dropped out of sight. Shakespeare makes no mention of it in his play *King John* in the late sixteenth century. But in the seventeenth century, the fiery English lawyer and champion of the common law, Sir Edward Coke, resurrected Magna Carta and drafted it into service in the struggle against royal absolutism. A hundred years after that, the scholarly Sir William Blackstone published the definitive edition of the text, which was avidly snapped up in England's increasingly restless colonies in North America. And Alexander Hamilton, when engaged in the struggle to ratify the Federal Constitution and consolidate the results of the American Revolution, claimed the legacy of Magna Carta: "the great charter of liberties, which was obtained, sword in hand, from king John."[4]

3 Confirmatio cartarum, 25 Ed. I; 1 Blackstone, *Commentaries* 124.
4 *Federalist Papers, No. 84*, at 534 (repeating 1 Blackstone, *Commentaries* 123).

PART 1

The Common Law at Home

The English Heritage

Introduction

The common law was not born in America, but it has thrived here. Brought by English colonists to the New World, the common law was a body of rules, a set of institutions, and a certain way of doing legal business. The rules, derived mainly from decisions in particular cases, were multifarious and sometimes seemingly contradictory but susceptible of rational organization and harmonization. Common law institutions, principally courts, were a confusing collection of ancient offices with often unclear and overlapping jurisdictions, but they benefited from a tradition of orderliness and a crude but recognizable effectiveness. The "common law way" was at bottom and necessarily practical, but it included an element of ancient anachronism that contributed an unmistakable air of majesty, if not of mystery.

The very persistence of the common law over so many centuries endowed it with a sort of corporate existence. In a famous phrase, Sir Edward Coke in the seventeenth century implied that it was itself a living thing, describing reason as "the life of the law,"[1] while John Adams in the eighteenth century saw to it that the Massachusetts Constitution guaranteed separation of powers "to the end it may be a government of laws and not of men"[2] – as if law had an agency apart from human actors. Oliver Wendell Holmes, Jr. later qualified Coke's aphorism, insisting that "the life of the law has not been logic: it has been experience."[3] And President Franklin Roosevelt, in a confrontation with the Supreme Court in the mid-twentieth century, repeated Adams' point: "We want a Supreme

1 *Coke on Littleton* § 138, p. 97b.
2 Mass. Const. Declaration of Rights § 30.
3 Holmes, *The Common Law* 1.

DOI: 10.4324/9781003660859-1

Court which will do justice under the Constitution – not over it. In our courts we want a government of laws and not of men."[4]

What was it about the common law that permitted it to live and thrive in its new environment? Colonial America was frontier country at the edge of a vast continent, a land of abundant resources and scarce people, on the periphery of the British Empire. The colonies were a long way in more than miles from the Mother Country, an ancient island kingdom of landed aristocrats and merchants at the hub of international trade. After the Revolution, England and the nation formed out of her former colonies pursued divergent political paths, and the economies of each advanced at vastly different speeds. In England, the practices of constitutional monarchy were steadily perfected, religious toleration developed alongside an established Church, and democracy was gradually extended within an enduring class system. In America, a federal republic was laboriously constructed and painfully preserved, church and state were separated, and a democratic ethos rapidly developed. At the time of American independence, England was already on its way to becoming the world's first industrial nation, "the workshop of the world," while the American economy was still largely agrarian – in the Southern states based on enslaved labor – even its most advanced sectors in the Northeast lagging England's by a generation or two. Yet through it all, each country remained true to the common law after its fashion, a fact that should dispel any notion of a simple and direct connection between law and political or economic organization.

Already hundreds of years old when Columbus sailed to America, the common law predates what modern people often think of as law itself. Although most people today picture a typical law as a statute, passed by a representative body and signed by the chief executive, the common law took shape in medieval courts as judges resolved individual disputes with little or no reference to statutes. The prototypical expression of the common law, in fact, was (and is) the resolution of a dispute, not the formulation of a rule, although the doctrine of precedent makes the judges' past decisions a source of rules for resolving later disputes. For much of the common law's long history, the courts were the principal locus of legal development; the legislatures, quiescent or reactive.

When the common law arrived in America, lawyers still looked for their law in cases. After Independence, Thomas Jefferson counselled Virginia's General Assembly against trying to reduce the common law to a text; it was better, he thought, to leave it "to be collected from the usual monuments of it"[5] – that is, from reported cases. Today, the source of law is more often and more obviously the statute book, and the institutions of the common law, while not totally transformed, are new-modeled to suit a changed environment. But the

4 *Public Papers and Addresses of Franklin D. Roosevelt, 1937*, at 122 (Samuel I. Rosenman ed. 1941).

5 Jefferson, *Notes on the State of Virginia* 137.

common law continues to affect the way that rules, including constitutions and statutes, are applied and the way that courts operate.

To understand the career of the common law in America, one must first understand the common law "at home" in England. For this, Sir William Blackstone's magisterial four-volume *Commentaries on the Laws of England*, first published between 1765 and 1769, provides a convenient starting place. Unapologetically, Blackstone catalogued the myriad, sometimes mysterious, legal fictions by which the judges had elaborated the common law. While not without a creative element of its own, Blackstone's book offers a handy summary of the common law, which (when stripped of its political component) could provide the basis for the development of an indigenous American common law. True to the common law tradition, Blackstone gives extended treatment to the law of real property, the common law's oldest and most intricate production. What the traditionalist Blackstone slighted was commercial law, particularly the law of contract, essential to England's success as a mercantile power.

This lack in Blackstone, and indeed in the common law itself, was remedied by Blackstone's great contemporary, Lord Mansfield, the prototypical "activist judge," who as Chief Justice of the Court of King's Bench from 1756 to 1788 strikingly demonstrated the common law's capacity to renew itself. Inspired by the civil law tradition of ancient Rome, the basis of law in Mansfield's native Scotland and operative to some extent in England in the courts of equity and admiralty, Mansfield worked to address the needs of English merchants for law that was comprehensible, stable, and consistent with current practice. Able to free himself from the weight of tradition because the early law reports were sometimes unreliable – a point he tended to exaggerate – and willing to be instructed by merchants about their business practices, Mansfield laid the basis for a workable commercial law.

While Blackstone restated the common law for posterity and Mansfield suited it to the modern world, a younger contemporary of both, the outsider Jeremy Bentham, spent his long life in seclusion, subjecting the entire operation to a searching, one is tempted to say a scorching, criticism. Rejecting the complacency of the Commentator and the activism of the Chief Justice, Bentham denounced case-by-case law-making as illegitimate and inefficient. Law, Bentham insisted, should be made by a rational legislator in the form of general statutes promoting the greatest happiness of the greatest number. Together, this trio of Blackstone, Mansfield, and Bentham – representing the scholarly traditionalist, the judicial innovator, and the radical critic – helps to explain the common law's extraordinary ability to maintain its continuity even as it adapted to the unsettling changes it confronted in the New World.

1

SIR WILLIAM BLACKSTONE AND THE FORCE OF TRADITION

At the time of the American Revolution, the common law was already six hundred years old, its rules scattered in thousands of judicial decisions, most only imperfectly reported (if reported at all), supplemented by a small collection of statutes, many dealing with the esoterica of the law of real property or the details of criminal law. Its secondary literature, largely in the form of commentaries on older texts or statutes ("institutes") and digests of reported cases ("abridgments"), was poorly organized and all too often written in a crabbed and repulsive style. Its principal institutions were a haphazard collection of courts, by the ingenious use of legal fictions largely overlapping in jurisdiction, still operating much as they had in the Middle Ages. What kept the system functioning, if it could be said to function as a system at all, was a small cadre of judges and lawyers, the bench and the bar. In the absence of any significant academic legal education, these individuals learned their law by copying what those before them had done. Law was, in consequence, a profoundly conservative profession, and its practitioners were by and large extremely cautious men.

At the same time, a new spirit was animating European intellectual circles. The Enlightenment began as a reaction against the fierce religious controversies that had convulsed Europe after the Reformation and that had come to seem to many educated persons to be obscure, irresolvable, and largely irrelevant. Choosing instead to emphasize the new learning to be derived from advancing scientific investigations and from the world-girdling voyages of discovery, enlightened thinkers were secular, cosmopolitan, and above all rational. As a distinguished art historian has pointed out, they were often depicted as comfortable, self-assured, and smiling – "the smile of reason."[1]

1 Kenneth Clark, *Civilisation: A Personal View* 245 (1969).

DOI: 10.4324/9781003660859-2

While the Enlightenment in Britain was more restrained than in some places on the European continent, particularly in France, it did stimulate a number of remarkable and characteristic accomplishments: Edward Gibbon's monumental historical synthesis, *The History of the Decline and Fall of the Roman Empire* (1776–1788); Adam Smith's foundational economic study, *An Inquiry into the Nature and Causes of the Wealth of Nations* (1776); James Boswell's classic biography, *The Life of Samuel Johnson, LL.D.* (1791); and – a work that belongs with these, though it is not always placed there – Sir William Blackstone's *Commentaries on the Laws of England* (1765–1769).

Like the other masterpieces of the British Enlightenment, Blackstone's *Commentaries* opened a new view of its subject, one that continues to affect us to this day. Law is inevitably related to morals and therefore, in the European tradition, to religion, but Blackstone, while exceedingly respectful of religion and careful to acknowledge its intimate connection with law, was concerned primarily with secular, that is to say, human – not divine – law. His greatest contribution was to impress upon his subject those other hallmarks of the Enlightenment, breadth of vision and rationality. To the chaos and confusion of English law as it was in the eighteenth century, Blackstone brought order and light. He wrote clear English prose, inviting comparison with the most polished writers of his day. Indeed, Gibbon reported that he read the *Commentaries* three times over and prepared "a copious and critical abstract" of it, in order to practice his English style.[2] Blackstone resolutely refused to accept the isolation of law from other intellectual disciplines and situated his subject firmly among the rest. One modern scholar, perhaps with tongue partly in cheek, gave his monograph on Blackstone's *Commentaries* an old-fashioned subtitle: "Showing How Blackstone, Employing Eighteenth-Century Ideas of Science, Religion, History, Aesthetics, and Philosophy, Made of the Law at once a Conservative and a Mysterious Science."[3]

For all his enlightened principles, Blackstone was no radical in the style of the French *philosophes*; he was at heart an English lawyer, conservative and cautious. He believed profoundly in the importance of tradition and, while it overstates the matter to say that Blackstone made the common law "mysterious" – in fact, he made the common law more transparent than it had ever been – it is undoubtedly true that he presented English law as coming down through the centuries with an awesome majesty and a certain mystique.

Blackstone repeated and indeed affirmed the traditional lawyers' extravagant praise of the law: "law is the perfection of reason," "what is not reason is not law."[4] But to that self-praise he added a very characteristic qualification, one that could stand for the quintessence of Blackstonianism:

2 Gibbon, *Memoirs* 152. The cosmopolitan Gibbon had previously published in French.

3 Daniel J. Boorstin, *The Mysterious Science of the Law* (1941).

4 1 Blackstone, *Commentaries* 70.

> not that the particular reason of every rule in the law can at this distance of time be always precisely assigned; but it is sufficient that there be nothing in the rule flatly contradictory to reason, and then the law will presume it to be well founded.

The law, in other words, presumes its own reasonableness and places on its critics the burden of proving the contrary. In a sense, the legal history of the next two hundred years can be seen as an assault on this massive complacency and its ultimate collapse and replacement with a more reformist and utilitarian attitude. In time, the burden of proving that the law is reasonable will shift, and what is old will be presumed to be unsuited to the modern world. But that remains for the years after Blackstone.

The extent of Blackstone's achievement can be measured only by comparison with the state of his subject before he wrote, and that can be conveniently done in the course of examining his own education and professional career. Born in 1723, Blackstone was a posthumous child, his father already dead at his birth; he lost his mother as well before a dozen years had passed. In the world before the welfare state, the fate of orphans was usually cruel, but Blackstone was fortunate in his connections. The influence of his mother's family reached high, and he received one of the rare scholarships of the day on the recommendation of the prime minister, Sir Robert Walpole. At 15, young William went up to Oxford, where he enrolled at Pembroke College.

The standards of the great university were then in decline. Edward Gibbon, the future historian of the Roman Empire, who was there only a few years later, has left an unforgettable picture of academic decay, and Adam Smith, another student, reported in *The Wealth of Nations* that "the greater part of the public professors have, for these many years, given up altogether even the pretence of teaching."[5] As summarized by Gibbon, Smith assigned the cause of their indolence to the fact that,

> instead of being paid by voluntary contributions which would urge them to increase the number, and to deserve the gratitude of their pupils, the Oxford professors are secure in the enjoyment of a fixed stipend, without the necessity of labour or the apprehension of control.[6]

Without the goad of market forces, in other words, salaried positions, academic no less than any other, have a tendency to turn into sinecures.

Ever since the Reformation, the only law taught at Oxford was civil or Roman law, that is, the system of jurisprudence based on the Corpus Juris Civilis of the Emperor Justinian. It was organized, rational, written in a learned

5 Smith, *Wealth of Nations* 718.
6 Gibbon, *Memoirs* 78–79 (restating Smith, *Wealth of Nations* 717–718).

language, and endowed with the prestige of classical civilization. By contrast, English law was unpolished and faintly barbaric, its basic vocabulary medieval Latin and a degenerate French, tainted with feudalism and the compromises of practice and the marketplace. To study that law, Blackstone had to leave the "dreaming spires" of Oxford and journey to London, to the Inns of Court, where lawyers had congregated since the Middle Ages. While a student, young William had developed a taste for poetry and fancied himself gifted in that regard, so when he departed Oxford to study law, he commemorated the occasion with a poem entitled "The Lawyer's Farewell to His Muse"[7] – a competent work that nonetheless confirms the wisdom of his ultimate choice of career.

Having begun as medieval hostelries serving the legal profession, the four Inns of Court – Gray's, Lincoln's, Middle Temple, and Inner Temple[8] – had mutated over the years into law schools where "readings" or lectures on law had been delivered and moot courts held. Like the historic universities, the Inns too were in decline in the eighteenth century, their academic standards eroded by indolence and the lack of economic incentives. By the time Blackstone arrived at Middle Temple, the only requirement for being called to the bar was "keeping" twelve terms and paying the inevitable fees. A term was kept simply by eating five dinners at the Inn and occasionally reciting some meaningless exercises, leading to the expression – not intended to be facetious – that legal education meant "eating your terms."[9]

In 1746, at the age of twenty-three, the erstwhile poet was called to the bar. As a young barrister, he was not a success. Starting a legal career has never been easy, but in early eighteenth-century England, it was nearly impossible. England's divided legal profession meant that barristers, the only lawyers authorized to appear "at the bar" in court, had to be briefed by solicitors, that is, had to be retained on behalf of the actual clients by the branch of the profession that did all the quotidian legal chores not involving litigation. Furthermore, the barristers had, over time, further limited access. Practice before the Court of Common Pleas was the legal monopoly of the serjeants-at-law, barristers who had been appointed to the order of the coif, named for the distinctive white linen headpiece they wore in court. At the Court of King's Bench, custom favored the senior barristers. Until the reforms instituted by Lord Mansfield later in the century, the court called on the bar each day in order of seniority.[10] Delay and obfuscation by the elders prevented the juniors from being called before the court rose. The court rarely heard from the men of Blackstone's generation, whose cases consequently languished. Only a well-connected and very determined young barrister could make his way.

7 12 Holdsworth, *History of English Law* 704.

8 Inner Temple and Middle Temple were established on the site of the headquarters of the Crusading order to Knights Templar when the order was dissolved in 1312.

9 E. Cobham Brewer, *Dictionary of Phrase and Fable* 402 (1894).

10 See reporter's note at 1 Burr. 57–58, 97 Eng. Rep. 189 (1756).

The studious Blackstone must have looked back longingly at his college days. When the opportunity arose to return to Oxford, he left the capital without poetic regrets. Back at the university, he busied himself with reforms. He was, after all, a man of his times – enlightened, efficient, energetic. He put the university press on a business footing and organized the library and finances of All Souls College, not neglecting the college wine cellar. In a controversial pamphlet, he exposed the misuse of the ancient endowments of the college. Preference was still being given to applicants who claimed descent from the family of the benefactor, a fifteenth-century archbishop. In an elaborate argument, Blackstone demonstrated that after three hundred years almost everyone in England was equally kin to the founder.[11] He also produced the first scholarly edition of Magna Carta, by then over five hundred years old.[12]

This was the age of "snobbery and jobbery," and Blackstone felt it in his own career. In 1753, when the Regius Professorship of Civil Law at Oxford fell vacant, Blackstone was warmly supported for it. But the appointment was made by the prime minister, and the Duke of Newcastle, the leading politician of the day, doubted Blackstone's political fidelity – particularly important at a time when the historic universities still returned their own members of parliament.

After this disappointment, Blackstone decided to take the initiative. If the university taught only Roman law, he would teach English law. If the avenues of official preferment were blocked, he would sell his wares in the marketplace – a precocious demonstration of Smithian economics, which may have been suggested by Lord Mansfield, a judge more in tune with the commercial realities of the time. Blackstone touted his lectures in an advertisement:

> This course is calculated not only for the use of such gentlemen of the university, as are more immediately designed for the profession of the common law; but of such others also, as are desirous to be in some degree acquainted with the constitution and polity of their own country. To this end, it is proposed to lay down a general and comprehensive plan of the laws of England; to deduce their history; to enforce and illustrate their leading rules and fundamental principles; and to compare them with the laws of nature and of other nations; without entering into practical niceties, or the minute distinctions of particular cases.[13]

This program, which could describe an entire law school curriculum, was to be covered in three lectures a week in each of the four terms of the Oxford

11 William Blackstone, *An Essay on Collateral Consanguinity, Its Limits, Extent, and Duration; More Particularly As It Is Regarded by the Statutes of All Souls College in the University of Oxford* (1750).

12 William Blackstone, *The Great Charter and the Charter of the Forest, with Other Authentic Instruments* (1759).

13 12 Holdsworth, *History of English Law* 745–746.

academic year.[14] The fee was six guineas, a not inconsiderable sum, payable to the instructor.

By the standards of his day, Blackstone's lectures were a success. Thirty to fifty students were regularly in attendance. Since only two hundred matriculated at Oxford each year, the course could even be described as popular. Finally, in 1758, Blackstone's great chance arrived. Charles Viner, a wealthy legal publisher and author of the definitive "abridgment of the law" that bears his name,[15] had died two years earlier and left money to establish a Vinerian chair at the University. This was to be the world's first professorship of English law, and Blackstone was chosen its first incumbent. According to Gibbon, "This judicious institution was coldly entertained by the graver Doctors, who complained, I have heard the complaint, that it would take the young people from their books."[16]

Aware of the concern that English law was a craft, not a science, and that its apparent disorder compared unfavorably with the elegance of Roman law, Blackstone was determined to state the common law in a manner fit for the universities – foreshadowing Paul Cezanne's ambition to make Impressionism an art fit for the museums.[17] From his lectures grew the four volumes of his *Commentaries on the Laws of England*, first published between 1765 and 1769 and regularly updated during his lifetime – proof positive, if any were needed, of the intimate connection between teaching and scholarship.

Not only did Blackstone's lectures and ensuing book make English law available to a wider audience, the mere fact of the lectures initiated a gradual reorientation of legal training, with momentous consequences. Learning law from lectures rather than from unsupervised reading and observation of working lawyers and judges – previously the only means of legal education – led to the slow divorce of legal study from legal practice. Thereafter, the common law was increasingly expressed as an organized statement of rules with a steadily growing role for the law professor.

True to his announcement of a dozen years earlier, Blackstone adroitly summarized six centuries of English law and legal history. It was a monumental achievement. The common law itself, the product of centuries of decided cases, lacked any inherent order. Tennyson was not far wrong, although a little out of date, when he referred to "the lawless science of our law / That codeless

14 Although later reduced to three terms, the Oxford academic year in the eighteenth century was divided into four terms. See L.S. Sutherland, "The Curriculum," in 5 *The History of the University of Oxford: The Eighteenth Century* 470 (L.S. Sutherland & L.G. Mitchell eds. 1986).

15 Charles Viner, *A General Abridgment of Law and Equity: Alphabetically Digested Under Proper Titles, with Notes and References to the Whole*, 23 vols. (1742–1753).

16 Gibbon, *Memoirs* 90.

17 See Joachim Gasquet, *Cezanne* 90 (1921) (*J'ai voulu faire de l'impressionisme quelque chose de solide et de durable comme l'art de musées.*) ("I want to make of Impressionism something solid and durable like the art of museums.").

myriad of precedent / That wilderness of single instances."[18] Blackstone's supreme achievement was to take the accumulated case law and synthesize it into a coherent intellectual whole, accessible to lawyer and layman alike.

Not since the early Middle Ages and the Latin treatise *De Legibus et Consuetudinibus Angliae* (On the Laws and Customs of England), attributed to Henry de Bracton, had anyone even attempted it. It is refreshing to know that in his great labor the Commentator permitted himself a human indulgence. From Boswell's *Life of Johnson*, we learn that Blackstone wrote "with a bottle of port before him, and found his mind invigorated and supported in the fatigue of his great work by a temperate use of it"[19] – an observation that later brought an angry rejoinder from Blackstone's family.[20]

In 1766, as new obligations accumulated, Blackstone resigned his professorship. In 1761, he had married and bought himself a comfortable country house, becoming the Squire of Wallingford and fathering a large family; one of his sons, James, would himself become Vinerian Professor. He was elected to parliament, although his political impact was negligible; his reticence in debates was exceeded only by Edward Gibbon's total silence.[21] A modern expert on the House of Commons in that period dismissed Blackstone's rare interventions as generally concerning subjects of "secondary importance" and showing a lack of "political common sense."[22] A loyal supporter of the King's ministers, Blackstone was no friend to the cause of American Independence. He gave his legal opinion that what rights the colonists had, parliament had given and parliament could take away.

During one debate, Blackstone suffered an author's embarrassment when his own book was quoted against him. The majority had expelled the trouble-making John Wilkes, scandalmonger and sympathizer with colonial grievances. When Wilkes' constituents promptly re-elected him, the government argued that expulsion disqualified him as a candidate and proposed to seat the runner-up. Blackstone supported the motion and then had to listen as Wilkes' supporters read aloud from his own book a seemingly complete list of disqualifications, a list that did not include prior expulsion.[23] With the biblical figure of Job, they exulted "that mine adversary had written a book." But Blackstone had an author's revenge when he amended subsequent editions to support his position.[24] A few years later, the drafters of the U.S. Constitution were careful to include a comprehensive list of the qualifications for election to Congress, in order to exclude by implication disqualification for any other reason.[25]

18 Alfred Lord Tennyson, "Aylmer's Field 1793" (1864).
19 Boswell, *Johnson* 1135 (citing William Scott, later Lord Stowell).
20 Prest, *Blackstone* 210.
21 Gibbon, *Memoirs* 159.
22 2 Lewis Namier & John Brooke, *The House of Commons, 1754-1790*, at 96 (1964).
23 1 Blackstone, *Commentaries* 170 (1765).
24 1 Blackstone, *Commentaries* 339 (4th ed. 1770).
25 U.S. Const. art. I, § 2 (Representatives); id. § 3 (Senators).

In any event, Blackstone could console himself with the large royalties earned by his book, prefiguring Gibbon's experience with his own great work. As Gibbon later reported, the patronage of authors "has long since been devolved on our booksellers."[26] Already in England the market was replacing the need to rely on the favor of princes or noblemen. In music, the enterprising George Frideric Handel had been earning a living from his concerts in London.[27] On the continent, by contrast, Joseph Haydn wore his aristocratic patron's livery and ate with the servants.

As the lectures had led to the book, the book led to professional success. Blackstone attracted a significant legal practice. At last, in 1770, the Commentator was knighted and "raised to the ermine," that is, made a judge. Perhaps law professors are always disappointments on the bench. Blackstone certainly showed himself more interested in strict adherence to traditional rules, "the minute distinctions of particular cases" that he had scanted in his course of lectures for Oxford undergraduates, rather than in enlightened law reform. In one case, still read in some first-year classes in law school, he dissented from the majority's reasonable result on the ground of a technical distinction between the actions of trespass and trespass on the case and would have required the plaintiff to start over.[28] In a later opinion that reversed Lord Mansfield, Blackstone insisted on maintaining the medieval Rule in Shelley's Case, which Mansfield had correctly identified as an anachronism even in the eighteenth century.[29]

Although the last ten years of his life were spent as a judge, it is not for his service on the bench that Blackstone is remembered. In his own day, the word around Westminster Hall was that when presiding at trial he was indecisive and his rulings were reversed more often than those of any other sitting judge.[30] After a comprehensive review of Blackstone's cases, one of his successors as Vinerian Professor seconded the negative assessment while loyally tempering its harshness: "If there were few diamonds in his judicial necklace, at least there were no gewgaws."[31]

Like other judges before him – Sir Edward Coke was a notable example – Blackstone prepared reports of decided cases, including those in which he had

26 Gibbon, *Memoirs* 175.

27 See Jane Glover, *Handel in London: A Genius and his Craft* xi–xii (2021) (describing Handel as the first musician-entrepreneur).

28 Scott v. Shepherd, 2 Black. W. 892, 96 Eng. Rep. 525; 3 Wils. K.B. 403, 95 Eng. Rep. 1124 (K.B. 1773) (the "case of the squib"). Trespass was the means to remedy injuries that were the direct result of the defendant's act, while trespass on the case was to remedy injuries that were only the indirect result.

29 Perrin v. Blake, 4 Burr. 2579, 98 Eng. Rep. 355; 1 Collectanea Juridica 283 (Exch. Ch. 1772).

30 See Simpson, *Biographical Dictionary* 59. High court judges like Blackstone served as trial judges on circuit.

31 Harold Hanbury, "Blackstone as a Judge," 3 *Am. J. Legal Hist.* 1, 27 (1959). Hanbury was the eleventh Vinerian Professor (1949–1964).

participated, but Blackstone's reports never attained the canonical status of Coke's. Although he died before he could properly edit them, Blackstone directed in his will that they be published, presumably for their commercial value. If anything, they dimmed the reputation the *Commentaries* had earned him. As one connoisseur of law reports tactfully put it, the inadequacy of Blackstone's reports was not too serious since most of the cases he reported were also reported by others, two of them "the best of all the English reporters."[32] Perhaps still smarting from Blackstone's reversal of his decision on Shelley's Case, Lord Mansfield later said, "We must not always rely on the words of reports, though under great names: Mr. Justice Blackstone's Reports are not very accurate."[33]

Nor is Blackstone remembered for his humor and charm. On the contrary, he was reputed to be difficult to get along with. Dr. Johnson, Blackstone's contemporary, would have rated him distinctly "unclubbable."[34] His recent biographer describes Blackstone as exhibiting "an awkward combination of diffidence, reserve, committed diligence and drive, lack of physical grace and social graces, some insensitivity to the feelings of others…, coupled with oversensitivity to personal slights, real or imagined."[35] Nearsightedness perhaps made him look crosser than he was, while overeating and lack of exercise certainly made him more irritable and probably hastened his death, age 56, in 1780.

While Blackstone's contributions to the common law tradition as judge and reporter amounted to little, his achievements as a scholar can hardly be overstated. Legal literature before Blackstone made it difficult for lawyers (or anyone else) to think comprehensively about English law. Institutes glossed texts, while abridgments grouped cases under headings arranged alphabetically. The 23-volume abridgment compiled by Charles Viner, the benefactor of the Vinerian chair, was the most complete. With something that borders on ingratitude, Blackstone, then newly minted as Vinerian professor, complained aloud that authors like Viner had chosen "a method, the least adapted to convey the rudiments of a science, namely, that of the alphabet."[36]

Out of this Stygian darkness shone Blackstone's *Commentaries*, the single most important book in the history of the common law. Unlike all the other leading figures in English legal history, Blackstone made his contribution not

32 Wallace, *The Reporters* 443–444 (referring to James Burrow's Reports in 97–98 Eng. Rep. and George Wilson's Reports in 95 Eng. Rep.). Wallace himself reported U.S. Supreme Court decisions from 1863 to 1875 (1–23 Wall., 68–90 U.S.).

33 Devon v Watts, 1 Dougl. 86, 93, 99 Eng. Rep. 59, 64 (K.B. 1779).

34 See Leo Damrosh, *The Club: Johnson, Boswell, and the Friends Who Shaped an Age* 126 (2019) (Johnson's description of Sir John Hawkins, lawyer and author).

35 Prest, *Blackstone* 310–311.

36 William Blackstone, *An Analysis of the Laws of England* v (2d ed. 1757). The *Analysis*, which proved to be the germ of the *Commentaries*, began as an outline of the course for students.

as a judge or as a legislator but as a scholar. Despite the laxness of his teachers and the obscurantism of much of the legal profession, he produced (as he had promised) "a general and comprehensive plan of the laws of England" – a plan, moreover, that exhibited the pleasing symmetry of Palladian architecture. It was his great gift to be able to distill principles from a mass of authorities and to impart them in a style that was urbane, dignified, and above all clear. But his creative restatement of the law almost necessarily made it appear more consistent than it was. He minimized legal contradictions and sought to rationalize even the strangest aspects of English law, mainly by appeals to history – all in elegant prose that gained the admiration even of his critics.

The *Commentaries* could be studied by law students and cited by judges – particularly by judges in England's far-flung colonies. It was an ideal reference book, each chapter complete in itself yet part of the whole. It was also read, as Blackstone intended it to be, by many outside the legal profession, those who were, as he put it, "desirous to be in some degree acquainted with the constitution and polity of their own country." Following in the footsteps of John Locke, Blackstone catalogued the "absolute rights of Englishmen"[37]: life, liberty, and property – a trinity that was to have a long and somewhat unexpected history in America. In addition to this fundamental list, Blackstone's *Commentaries* referred to many other rights, not "absolute" but essential for the effective functioning of a law-based state. Almost as important, he recounted the constitutional history of England as a story of gradually developing liberty – a story the American colonists were eager to continue.

Blackstone's plan for his book was simple, by modern standards simplistic. In words at least as old as Cicero, he defined law as "a rule of civil conduct prescribed by the supreme power in a state, commanding what is right and prohibiting what is wrong."[38] Around the distinction between right and wrong, the four volumes of the *Commentaries* are arranged: the first two devoted to rights, the final two to wrongs. Volume one, on the "rights of persons," contains what to modern readers appears an ill-assorted collection of topics. Constitutional law in the broadest sense is discussed under the headings of the rights of king, lords, and commons. Private rights based on personal relationships – husband and wife, parent and child, guardian and ward, master and servant – cover disparate topics today known as domestic relations, fiduciary obligations, and employment law. The second volume, on the "rights of things," is misnamed – things have no rights – but treats of the rights of persons with respect to things, principally land; that is, it is devoted to property law. The last two volumes of

37 1 Blackstone, *Commentaries* 123–136. "Absolute rights" are rights that derive not from political grant but from natural law.

38 1 Blackstone, *Commentaries* 44. Cf. Cicero, 11 *Philippics* 12 (*sanctio justa, jubens honesta, et prohibens contraria*) ("a just ordinance, commanding what is right and prohibiting the contrary"), cited at 1 Blackstone, *Commentaries* 118.

the *Commentaries* are concerned with wrongs and their remedies: volume three, on "private wrongs" (today known as torts) and civil procedure; volume four, on "public wrongs" – that is, crimes and criminal procedure.

What Blackstone omitted is almost as revealing as what he included. Contracts and related topics are barely mentioned, while land law is treated at medieval length. In the same decades during which Lord Mansfield was laying the foundations of modern commercial law, Blackstone relegated contract to the margins. Marriage is a contract; that is to say, the parties must be of full age, without impediments (such as another marriage), and consenting. Once married, the two become one, their relationship now governed by the law of husband and wife, not by their private agreement. The contract of employment is described in similar terms. Once an adult workman, not bound to another, agrees to work, he becomes subject to the law of master and servant. Thereafter, the master has a "property… in the service of his domestics; acquired by the contract of hiring."[39] Likewise, the contract of purchase and sale is simply one of a dozen means by which title to items of personal property may be gained or lost. After a completed sale, the new owner's rights come from the law, not from the now fully executed contract. The idea of contract as governing most, if not all, the terms of a continuing relationship – technically an "executory contract," that is, one not yet fully performed, perhaps for years – remained undeveloped; indeed, at the old common law, it had "no legal effect at all."[40]

The connection between acquiring a spouse and buying property – the memorable phrase "to have and to hold" is common to both the marriage ceremony and traditional deeds – is the notion that contract is the gateway to status: the spouses become a married couple; the purchaser (and employer) becomes an owner. Without a more robust concept of contract, a law of commerce hardly exists, and without contract and commerce, capitalism itself is hard to imagine. As John Commons observed a century ago, "Modern capitalism begins with the assignment and negotiability of contracts."[41] Or, in the words of Harvard Law Dean Roscoe Pound: "Wealth in a commercial age is made up largely of promises."[42]

Blackstone's emphasis on land law is understandable; centuries of litigation had produced an enormous volume of property law. The gentlemen of England had maintained their primacy in society because they were seated, literally, on the land, the nation's prime economic resource – at the time, before modern forms of investment, the only income-producing property. No area of the law was of more interest to them than the law of real property, and Blackstone explained all its baffling intricacies and possibilities. The legal basis of

39 1 Blackstone, *Commentaries* 417.

40 W.M. Geldart, *Introduction to English Law* 9 (9th ed. by D.C.M. Yardley 1984).

41 John R. Commons, *The Legal Foundations of Capitalism* 253 (1924).

42 Roscoe Pound, *An Introduction to the Philosophy of Law* 236 (1922).

aristocratic landowning was the strict settlement, a remarkable amalgam of fiction and policy that secured continuity without sacrificing flexibility. Blackstone wholeheartedly accepted the traditional role of the landed interest and never dreamed that the powers of the landowners would wane. But as a faithful servant of the establishment, he did suggest ways of simplifying and cheapening the means of settlement – ironically for a traditionalist, searching colonial legislation for alternatives to traditional methods.[43] Given the glacial speed of law reform in his society, even his modest suggestions for improvement had to wait over 60 years for adoption.[44]

Not only would readers of the *Commentaries* fail to learn about the developing law of contract, they would hardly guess at the significant role played by the courts of equity, the parallel system of justice providing relief when the remedy at law was deemed inadequate. Instead, they would probably be misled by Blackstone's confusion of the law administered by the Court of Chancery with the generalized meaning of equity as fairness in individual cases. The difficulty may be attributed to Blackstone's unease about discretionary justice. He was convinced that

> law, without equity, though hard and disagreeable, is much more desirable for the public good, than equity without law: which would make every judge a legislator, and introduce most infinite confusion; as there would then be almost as many different rules of action laid down in our courts, as there are differences of capacity and sentiment in the human mind.[45]

This observation is reminiscent of John Selden's classic quip that the measure of justice in the chancery court should not, like the length of the chancellor's foot, vary from judge to judge.[46] As we saw, Blackstone's fear of judicial discretion and preference for hard-and-fast rules influenced his most significant decisions as a judge.

Still to be thoroughly explored by scholars is Blackstone's understanding of the relationship between law and economics. Writing before Adam Smith's *Wealth of Nations* (1776), Blackstone himself probably only dimly understood the connection, although it was slowly gaining recognition in the cases. For example, reconciling centuries of precedent with a smoothness that disguised the inherent conflicts, Blackstone expounded the law of nuisance as it applied to "incorporeal hereditaments," that is, intangible property interests. High authority held that "if a ferry is erected on a river, so near another antient [sic]

43 2 Blackstone, *Commentaries* 361.

44 Compare 2 Blackstone, *Commentaries* 360–361 (1765) with 3 & 4 Will. 4, ch. 74 (1833) (Fines and Recovery Act).

45 1 Blackstone, *Commentaries* 62.

46 John Selden, *Table Talk* 43 (1689) (Frederick Pollock ed. 1927).

ferry as to draw away its custom, it is a nuisance to the owner of the old one," meaning that the later entrant could be fined or enjoined. This, Blackstone explained, was because the owner of an ancient ferry became legally bound to keep it "always in repair and readiness, for the ease of all the king's subjects." The old ferry, in modern terms, had become a public utility, recognized as a legal monopoly but subject to regulation. Consequently, it would be "extremely hard, if a new ferry were suffered to share his profits, which does not share his burden." But in the following sentence, after the piety that "where the reason ceases, the law also ceases," he justified later cases holding that it is no nuisance to set up a mill, a school, or a trade "in neighborhood and rivalship with another: for by such emulation the public are like to be gainers." In this case, the profits lost by competition (emulation) – the "creative destruction" celebrated by modern economists – he blandly dismissed with the Latin quip *damnum absque injuria* (damage without legal injury).[47]

Unlike contract, which merited barely a mention in the *Commentaries*, tort (bundled with civil procedure) was nominally the subject of an entire book. But the torts Blackstone described were principally "injuries to a man's lands and tenements." *Trespass* provided a remedy against "entry on another man's grounds without a lawful authority"; *nuisance* against "anything done to the hurt or annoyance of the lands, tenements, or hereditaments of another"; *waste* against "destruction of houses, woods, or lands."[48] The modern law of torts, especially the tort of negligence, was (as we will see) developed only later, in response to the damages inflicted on workers and property by the new means of production and transportation made possible by steam power.

To the modern reader, perhaps the most striking and probably the most repulsive feature of the legal system described by Blackstone was the extent to which it relied on fictions to get its work done. Legal fiction meant an irrebuttable allegation of a fact without regard to its truth or falsity. The object could be to secure access to a form of procedure that was speedier, cheaper, or simply more rational. The ancient action of debt in the Court of Common Pleas was decided by "wager of law": an oath by the defendant that he did not owe anything was accepted as true if 11 "oath helpers" supported him. In the Court of King's Bench, by contrast, the newer action of assumpsit, alleging that the defendant had undertaken to pay the plaintiff for a benefit received, was resolved by a jury. Something similar happened in the law of torts. Rather than bring an action for damages, a plaintiff could sue instead for the value of whatever benefit the wrongdoer had received – the origin of the saying "to waive the tort and sue in assumpsit."

Legal fiction could also be used to do justice in individual cases by allowing a court to apply a rule designed for one situation to another distinctly different

47 3 Blackstone, *Commentaries* 219.
48 3 Blackstone, *Commentaries* 208, 216, 223.

situation, but one demanding a similar result. (It is to be contrasted with the rule of precedent by which a rule that originated in one case is applied in another that is essentially the same.) For example, the old action of trover, to recover the value of personal property wrongfully withheld, began as an action to recover property that had been lost by the plaintiff and found (*trouvé* in Law French) by the defendant who refused to return it.[49] Of course, it was really immaterial how the defendant came into possession of the item in the first place; it could have been purchased from one with apparent title, or received as a gift, or actually found. The dispute concerned whether the plaintiff was entitled to recover its value from the defendant, and the action of trover was the simplest way to get a legal resolution of that issue.

Likewise, disputes concerning title to real property could be determined by the ancient and cumbersome procedure initiated by the writ of right, but the right to present possession – what really mattered – could be tried much more expeditiously by the action of ejectment. The problem was that ejectment had been designed to resolve questions of a *tenant's* right to possession, not an owner's. So, a plaintiff involved in a dispute over title to Blackacre alleged that he had leased the land to a tenant, John Doe, who was ejected by someone (the "casual ejector") claiming authority from the defendant. The caption of the case read "Doe on the demise [lease] of plaintiff v. defendant," usually shortened to "Doe on the dem. of plaintiff v. defendant," or even "Doe d. plaintiff v. defendant." (Eventually, although the form remained technically the same, it became common practice to refer to the case as simply "plaintiff v. defendant.") Before the defendant's answer could be heard, he had to admit the lease and ejectment, which everyone knew was pure fiction.[50] Issue was then joined on the real issue in controversy: who has the better right to possession. These usages were carried over to the British colonies in North America and continued in the newly independent country. In a few states such as New Jersey and North Carolina, the name of the fictitious tenant mutated to Den, so the caption became "Den on the demise of…."[51] It was settled doctrine in America, that "trover is to personalty what ejectment is to realty."[52]

Fiction also helped overcome certain technical problems. Formally, a deed is required for the creation of a right-of-way easement, but when one person has made long-continued use of the land of another in a manner that would normally indicate a grant, the law (as Blackstone explained) "supposes an original grant, whereby a right of way thus appurtenant to land may clearly be

49 3 Blackstone, *Commentaries* 151–152.

50 3 Blackstone, *Commentaries* 199–206.

51 See, e.g., Den on the Dem. of Bayard v. Singleton, 1 Mart. 48, 1 N.C. 5 (1787), one of the earliest cases recognizing judicial review.

52 Russell v. Hill, 125 N.C. 470, 34 S.E. 640, 640 (N.C. 1899). Personalty or personal property is anything that is not land or attached to land.

created," which was subsequently lost.[53] This "supposition" of a lost grant is irrebuttable. Lord Mansfield, ever the realist, admitted:

> Not that, in such cases, the Court actually thinks a grant has been made; because it is not probable a grant should have existed, without its being upon record; but they presume the fact, for the purpose and from the principle of quieting the possession.[54]

The most glaring examples of legal fictions, bizarre but fundamentally harmless, concern the jurisdiction of the historic common law courts. For six hundred years, the common law was administered by three courts, each staffed with four judges: Common Pleas, King's Bench, and Exchequer.[55] Originally their jurisdiction was distinct. In general terms, Common Pleas handled – as its name implied – ordinary (common) disputes; King's Bench, more serious controversies in which the King, directly or indirectly, had an interest; and Exchequer, disputes concerning royal revenue. Over time, the various courts enlarged their jurisdiction by allowing fictitious allegations. Although medieval lawsuits usually commenced with an initial filing called a writ, it had early been established that proceedings could also be commenced by filing a "bill" if the defendant was already within the court's jurisdiction, and King's Bench had jurisdiction over all disputes of whatever kind arising in the County of Middlesex, which encompassed Westminster where the court sat. All that was required to gain access to King's Bench, then, was to file a bill, which became known as a "Bill of Middlesex," alleging a trespass in the county by the defendant, who was lurking (*latitat*) in another county, and the court had jurisdiction to hear any non-fictitious cause of action against him. In time, the extension of jurisdiction was accepted and the Bill and its fictitious allegations were dispensed with.

The Court of Common Pleas responded to the threat to its jurisdiction by allowing a fictional allegation that a defendant had disturbed the public peace by failing to appear when summoned and required capture (*testatum capias*), before going on to the real cause in controversy. Not to be left out, the Court of Exchequer expanded its reach by allowing an allegation that the defendant had failed to repay a debt to the plaintiff by which he was rendered less able (*quo minus*) to pay his dues to the King, again allowing access to the court for the resolution of the real dispute. By the mid-eighteenth century, it was possible for Blackstone to summarize the situation by saying that the first process in the three courts was a *latitat* in King's Bench, a *testatum capias* in Common Pleas,

53 2 Blackstone, *Commentaries* 36.

54 Eldridge v. Knott, 1 Cowp. 214, 215, 98 Eng. Rep. 1050, 1051 (K.B. 1774).

55 The judges of the Court of Exchequer were technically "barons of Exchequer." For a discussion of odd-and-even in the staffing of appellate courts, see John V. Orth, *How Many Judges Does It Take to Make a Supreme Court? And Other Essays on Law and the Constitution* 1 (2006).

and a *quo minus* in the Exchequer[56] – all pure fictions. By this legerdemain, the jurisdiction of the historic common law courts became largely concurrent.

Perhaps the most notorious example of the use of fiction to extend jurisdiction was Mostyn v. Fabrigas (1774),[57] in which the Mediterranean island of Minorca was alleged to be located in central London, so that a dispute between merchants that arose there could be resolved in the Court of King's Bench, where Lord Mansfield was presiding over the development of enlightened commercial law. Of course, no one was fooled by this or any of the other legal fictions. While loath to criticize them, Blackstone conceded that such fictions "may startle the student," but defended them as merely procedural: "No fiction shall extend to work an injury."[58] Nonetheless, legal fiction carried to such an extent attracted increasing criticism in the Age of Enlightenment and drew the particular ire of that tireless critic of the common law, Jeremy Bentham.

Not only did Bentham object to the obscurantism – a charge that is hard to deny – but he was outraged by the idea of "a willful falsehood having for its object the stealing of legislative power by and for hands which could not, or durst not, openly claim it."[59] Stripped of the fictions, what was going on – as Bentham rightly saw – was law-making, not by the legislature but by the courts. The judges' uncharacteristic eagerness to enlarge their jurisdiction and thereby increase their workload – it became a maxim of the common law that to extend jurisdiction is expected of a good judge: "*Boni judicis est ampliare jurisdictionem*"[60] – was not altruistic. As John Chipman Gray later explained: "When judges and their officers were paid largely by fees, there was a somewhat less exalted motive"[61] – one that Adam Smith would have appreciated.

Common law judges, wedded to tradition, were generally of the opinion that statutes did more harm than good: true to form, Blackstone primly reminded his readers that

> it hath been an antient [sic] observation in the laws of England, that whenever a standing rule of law, of which the reason perhaps could not be remembered or discerned, hath been wantonly broke in upon by statutes or new resolutions, the wisdom of the rule hath in the end appeared from the inconveniences that have followed the innovation.[62]

Even so advanced a thinker as Lord Mansfield had, while solicitor general, noted that "a statute very seldom can take in all cases, therefore the common

56 3 Blackstone, *Commentaries* 286.
57 1 Cowp. 161, 98 Eng. Rep. 1021 (K.B. 1774).
58 3 Blackstone, *Commentaries* 42–43.
59 Jeremy Bentham, *A Fragment on Government; being an Examination of what is delivered on the Subject of Government in General in the Introduction to Sir William Blackstone's Commentaries* 407 (1776) (J.H. Burns & H.L.A. Hart eds. 1988).
60 See Herbert Broom, *A Selection of Legal Maxims* 79 (8th American ed. 1882).
61 Gray, *Nature and Sources of Law* 32–35.
62 1 Blackstone, *Commentaries* 70.

law, that works itself pure by rules drawn from the fountain of justice, is for this reason superior to an act of parliament."[63]

By Blackstone's day, the distinction between common law and statute had become crucial, as illustrated by the hypothetical case of a law that made a man a judge in his own case. In the fifteenth century, at a time when statutes were few and far between, Sir Thomas Littleton had worried about a manor in which it was the custom for the lord to distrain (that is, to seize) cattle that strayed onto his land and hold them until their owner paid the lord a fine in the amount he assessed for the damage. This would make the lord a judge in his own case and open the door for abuse: "If he had damages but to the value of a halfpenny, he might assess and have therefore an hundred pound, which should be against reason."[64] What is unreasonable cannot be law. Three hundred years later, this was still the rule, as Blackstone noted: "To make a particular custom good," that is, one that would be enforced by the king's judges as common law, it had to be "reasonable," or rather – with a typical Blackstonian qualification – "not be unreasonable."[65]

When Blackstone turned to statutes, he changed his tune. If a statute seemed to produce the absurdity of making a man a judge in his own case, the court should to that extent disregard it. But the Commentator did not leave the matter there. Resolutely, he imagined the worst:

> If we could conceive it possible for the parliament to enact, that he should try as well his own causes as those of other persons, there is no court that has power to defeat the intention of the legislature, when couched in such evident and express words, as leave no doubt whether it was the intent of the legislature or no.[66]

The words are uncharacteristically halting, as if wrung from him against his will, and the concession is strictly limited. It is a matter not of law but of power. As a result of the victory of parliament over the Stuart king in the English Civil Wars, capped by the Glorious Revolution of 1688–1689, parliament was supreme.[67] It is still so in England,[68] but the Americans were determined to find another result.

Although no friend to the cause of American Independence, Blackstone exercised his profoundest influence in the New World. In England, his book

63 Omychund v. Barker, 1 Atk. 22, 33, 26 Eng. Rep. 15, 23 (Ch. 1744).

64 Littleton, *Tenures* § 212.

65 1 Blackstone, *Commentaries* 77 (citing Littleton, *Tenures* § 212).

66 1 Blackstone, *Commentaries* 91.

67 For the classic statement of parliamentary supremacy, still accepted by English courts, see A.V. Dicey, *Introduction to the Study of the Law of the Constitution* 37–38 (1908).

68 During the exceptional years from 1973 to 2020, while the United Kingdom was a member of the European Union, the United Kingdom's highest court would "disapply" British legislation if it conflicted with the law of the European Union. See, e.g., R. (Factortame Ltd.) v. Secretary of State for Transport (No. 2), [1991] 1 AC 603; Benkharbouche v. Secretary of State for Foreign and Commonwealth Affairs, [2017] UKSC 62. This loss of sovereignty was one of the reasons the United Kingdom withdrew from the European Union.

was eventually outdated despite repeated new editions – eight in Blackstone's lifetime with a final posthumous edition[69] – and in any event the practicing bar in the metropolis could not long ignore the "practical niceties" and "minute distinctions of particular cases" that the Commentator had skipped over in his Oxford lectures. By the mid-nineteenth century, Blackstone was condescendingly dismissed by an eminent Victorian legal scholar as "a faithful index of the average opinions of his day."[70]

In America, on the other hand, on the periphery of empire, the *Commentaries* continued to provide a handy summary of the common law. Immediately on publication, Blackstone's book was in demand. In 1771, not two years after the fourth volume had appeared, an ambitious teenager in the colony of North Carolina, destined to become one of the first justices of the U.S. Supreme Court, wrote his father in England requesting him to procure a set of the *Commentaries* "and send them by the first opportunity." The young James Iredell had, he said, already read the volumes in the library of a local notable, his future brother-in-law, but thought he should be equipped with his own copy, so he could study it "frequently and with great attention."[71] An American edition was produced the next year, and Thomas Marshall, father of John Marshall, the future chief justice of the Supreme Court, was a charter subscriber – as was future President John Adams. On the eve of the Revolution, Edmund Burke reported hearing that the Americans had bought nearly as many copies as the English themselves.[72] Once the colonists had made good on the battlefield their claim to the rights of freeborn Englishmen, they turned to Blackstone for a description of just what those rights were. In the debates over ratification of the Federal Constitution, Blackstone was frequently invoked; his book was literally in the hands of delegates at the important Virginia ratifying convention.[73]

The Commentator offered Americans not only a portable common law but also an example of how law should be taught. He opposed apprenticeship because it produced a crabbed and illiberal lawyer. Describing the fate of the law office–trained lawyer, Blackstone observed: "If practice be the whole he is taught, practice must also be the whole he will ever know."[74] However much Thomas Jefferson detested Blackstone's anti-republicanism, he agreed with

69 For details of the successive editions of the *Commentaries*, see John V. Orth, "Blackstone," in *The Oxford Handbook of Legal History* 362–363 (Marcus D. Dubber & Christopher Tomlins eds. 2018).

70 Maine, *Ancient Law* 148.

71 James Iredell to his father, 31 July 1771, in G.J. McRee, *Life and Correspondence of James Iredell*, vol. 1, p. 91 (1857–1858).

72 Edmund Burke, "Speech on Moving his Resolutions for Conciliation with the Colonies, March 22, 1775," in 3 *The Writings and Speeches of Edmund Burke* 123 (W.M. Elofson ed. 1996).

73 See Horst Dippel, "Blackstone's Commentaries and the Origins of Modern Constitutionalism," in *Re-Interpreting Blackstone's Commentaries* 199, 201 (Wilfrid Prest ed. 2014).

74 1 Blackstone, *Commentaries* 32.

him on the need for university legal education. Early in his term as governor of Virginia, Jefferson used his influence to establish a professorship in law at the College of William & Mary – the first in America and second only to Blackstone's in the common law world – and filled it with his former mentor, the eminent Virginia lawyer George Wythe.

Despite Blackstone's politics, his *Commentaries* remained the best-selling lawbook in the new republic. To assist students in mastering its details, an enterprising lawyer in North Carolina imagined Blackstone's law decorating an enormous tree, complete with all the royal, aristocratic, and clerical characters of the original.[75] For the scrupulous, St. George Tucker, Wythe's successor at William & Mary, brought out a republicanized edition.[76] Not only did American lawyers read Blackstone, but the best intellects among them imitated him as well. From 1826 to 1830, James Kent, former Chancellor of New York, published his four-volume *Commentaries on American Law*, also the product of university lectures, though not so successful as Blackstone's. Nor were Kent's *Commentaries* so readable. Though hailed as "America's Blackstone," Kent stands to Blackstone much as James Fennimore Cooper stands to Sir Walter Scott: a careful imitator of considerable talent. The twelfth edition of Kent's *Commentaries*, published in 1873, was prepared by Oliver Wendell Holmes, later an influential justice of the U.S. Supreme Court.

Notwithstanding the Revolution, Blackstone helped to hold the Americans in thrall to the common law. In old age, Chancellor Kent reminisced about his legal education. An undergraduate at New Haven College (now Yale University) during the Revolution, he remembered the summer of 1779, when British troops were marching and countermarching across Connecticut in a vain attempt to maintain Britain's political supremacy in North America. When the red coats closed the college, young Kent retired to the country, where he happened upon a copy of Blackstone's *Commentaries*, already diffused to an inland village. Reading it, he later recalled, "inspired me, at the age of 15, with awe, and I fondly determined to be a lawyer."[77] Ironically, while the British were losing America on the battlefield, Blackstone was winning the hearts and minds of American lawyers. Throughout the nineteenth century, Blackstone and his admirers dominated the legal mind in America, to the increasing irritation of progressive jurists.[78]

75 See John V. Orth, *The Tree of Legal Knowledge: Imagining Blackstone's Commentaries* (2023).

76 St. George Tucker, *Blackstone's Commentaries: With Notes of Reference to the Constitution and Laws, of the Federal Government of the United States, and of the Commonwealth of Virginia* (5 vols., 1803).

77 Kent, *Memoirs* 18.

78 See, e.g., John V. Orth, "'A Very Narrowing Effect upon our Profession': A Progressive Jurist Confronts Blackstone," in *Blackstone and His Critics* 193 (Anthony Page & Wilfrid Prest eds. 2018).

Elegantly expressed, organized (after a fashion), rational (up to a point), Blackstone's common law was, as he intended it to be, fit for the Age of Enlightenment. Yet from its inception, the *Commentaries* displayed a paradoxical aspect: a conservative project with radical implications. By providing a view of the common law free from its procedural technicalities, he had exposed it to public view as never before and opened it to criticism by lawyers and laymen alike. Too honest to deny that the common law had changed over time, Blackstone preferred to summarize its long history as "rise, progress, and gradual improvements."[79] At the end of the ages, the common law seemed to him to have attained a state of near Panglossian perfection. Further improvements, particularly in details, remained possible, and Blackstone obligingly pointed out some of the more obvious ones, but whatever improvements lay ahead, he expected they would be – as those in the past had been – matters of degree, gradual.

Blackstone's common law was law for a pre-capitalist class: the aristocrats and landed gentry who dominated England, worshipped in the established Church, and sent their sons to Oxford. The largest part and the intellectual centerpiece was property law, specifically the law of real property, the law in other words of the landed estate. But Blackstone's England was home not only to a landed aristocracy and gentry, it was also home to an enterprising cadre of merchants, active participants in the world of international commerce. The renovations needed to fit the common law for this new world were major and imperative; in this area, there was simply not enough time for gradualism. The task was beyond Blackstone in any case. He had steeped himself too deeply in the common law tradition, lived too long among the landed classes. Moreover, he was by temperament unsuited to mastermind rapid legal change; his talent lay in summary and restatement. Almost by chance, there was at that very moment at the head of the English judiciary a judge perfectly fitted to the task, Lord Mansfield. Beneath the full-bottomed wig of the Chief Justice of King's Bench was the restless mind of a reformer, one might almost say of a revolutionary. It was Mansfield who would make the common law fit not for the universities but for the clearinghouses. If Blackstone may be said to embody the force of common law tradition, Mansfield embodied the common law's remarkable power of renewal.

79 4 Blackstone, *Commentaries* chap. 33 (title).

2

LORD MANSFIELD AND THE POWER OF INNOVATION

In a phrase made famous by Magna Carta, the common law was described as "the law of the land." It was also, in another sense, land law. Obsessed as they were with the intricacies of legal procedure, the common law lawyers did get beyond procedure to substance in the case of things that really mattered, like land. And from time to time, parliament dropped its customary deference to the common law courts and legislated on the subject. By the eighteenth century, English land law was an extraordinary intellectual creation, aptly described by one property scholar as "the victim of too many able minds refining too many distinctions for too long."[1] Ornate, baroque even in its details, it was in operation – at least in the hands of skilled practitioners – remarkably flexible and oddly practical. The same could not be said, unfortunately, for the law of personal property, that is, for the law concerning everything that was neither land nor attached to land. For centuries, the primitiveness of the law of personal property had been tolerated because of the relative insignificance of things other than land.

In the early Middle Ages, when the common law was taking shape, personal property of great value was limited to precious metals, or items like weapons, jewelry, or religious objects. If the property of royalty or a great noble or churchman, these could be items of considerable value and surpassing beauty; many of them are in museums today. But they were not income-producing property like land and so were not the real prizes for which the powerful contended. Manors were what the acquisitive wanted most; the ornaments of refined life came afterwards. Of items of commerce, there were very few at that

1 A.W. Brian Simpson, "Introduction," 2 Blackstone, *Commentaries* v (University of Chicago Press facsimile ed. 1979).

DOI: 10.4324/9781003660859-3

early age; local produce and crafts certainly and perhaps some bags of spices from the East to enliven the blandness of ordinary victuals or bolts of silk to fashion into luxury clothing. Despite all their wonderful sagacity, the common law lawyers knew next to nothing about trade and therefore about contracts or commercial law generally – less, in fact, than Roman jurists had known in the palmy days of Empire.

The Age of Enlightenment was also the age of commerce, specifically of international trade. The great trans-Atlantic voyagers of the fifteenth and sixteenth centuries had done more than simply make contact with America, where the common law would one day find a new home; they had also opened new routes of trade. Columbus was, after all, looking for a route to the Indies to shorten the supply line for spices when he stumbled upon a continent unknown to Europeans. Eventually, the New World yielded vast cargoes: silver, mined in the Andes, was shipped to Spain; tobacco, grown in Virginia, went to England. In return, tea from India was destined for English colonists in North America; and, lamentably, large numbers of Africans were forced to endure the hellish Middle Passage to the New World to work the labor-intensive plantations.

International trade necessarily involved contracts of all sorts, complicated in ways completely unlike the complications incident to the ownership of land. Goods, some of them perishable, were purchased to be delivered in foreign ports at distant dates. Vast amounts of capital had to be mobilized in partnerships or joint-stock companies. Credit was needed and a means of enforcement in case of default. Goods belonging or promised to one person were held for long periods in warehouses belonging to another. Merchants ventured their fortunes in argosies exposed to the risks of transoceanic voyages; contracts of insurance were integral to the successful long-distance trafficking in goods. Bankruptcies were all too common. Reliable financial instruments were indispensable: goods traveled in one direction, money (in one form or another) made the return trip. And an independent tribunal was needed to resolve the inevitable disputes.

Common law lawyers, steeped as they were in land law, were unable, often unwilling to serve the needs of international traders, but that did not mean that common law judges could ignore disputes between merchants, although it did mean that they could try not to think about them. If one merchant sued another at common law, the matter was often resolved "by complicated procedural devices that obscured the real issues."[2] Or it could be referred to a jury, which by a general, unexplained verdict determined the winner. This effectively resolved the dispute, which was now in legal terms *res judicata* ("a thing adjudged"), not susceptible to further litigation. But the resolution of disputes, while fundamental to the legal process, is not a court's only role in the common law system. Courts also make law; indeed, in their decisions over centuries, they made the common law.

2 See S.F.C. Milsom, *A Natural History of the Common Law* 25–50 (2003).

When one case can be used as a precedent to resolve another, later case, the courts are making law by following a rule of fundamental fairness: like cases should be decided alike. In legal terms, this rule is encapsulated in the phrase *stare decisis*, the judges' collective resolve "to stand by [their] decisions," in the sense of standing by the general propositions of law that had been established in prior cases. But before one case can become a precedent for another, before in other words it can trigger the "*stare decisis* effect," enough must be known about it in order to determine if it is, in its essential facts, like the later case. Until common law judges knew enough about mercantile practices to give instructions to juries to guide their deliberations and until reliable reports were available to permit the efficient use of such precedents, no law was made when a particular dispute was resolved. Jury verdicts declare winners; they do not create precedents. And at a time when it was still unclear whether the jury could find the law as well as the facts, no one knew exactly what the jury had decided.

As Joseph Story – Supreme Court justice, law school lecturer, and prolific legal author – later discovered to his chagrin, "the common law was an *utter stranger* to the principles of commercial jurisprudence."[3] This was the state of the common law in large and newly important areas before Lord Mansfield was called to the headship of the common law courts in 1756. For a great commercial lawgiver, Mansfield was an unlikely candidate. Born in 1705, 18 years before Blackstone, in an impoverished aristocratic family in Scotland, William Murray, the future Lord Mansfield, haled from an economically backward area and from a class suspected of an atavistic loyalty to the deposed Stuart kings. His own father had been fined and imprisoned for suspected involvement in the Highland rising of 1715. Scotland was not even a common law country, having accepted in medieval times the civil law based on the great codification of Roman law, the Corpus Juris Civilis.[4] Sent out of Scotland to be educated in England, Murray was never again to see his native land. His later success prompted Dr. Johnson's *bon mot*: "Much may be made of a Scotchman, if he be caught young."[5]

Not so precocious a student as Blackstone, young Murray lingered at Oxford's Christ Church College until age 18, when he departed for the Inns of Court, enrolling at Lincoln's Inn. Called to the bar at 25, he entered energetically into the practice of law. Unlike the retiring Blackstone, Murray was an active participant in the social life of the capital. As a young barrister, he "drank champagne with the wits."[6] A friend of the poet Alexander Pope and

3 Story, *Miscellaneous Writings* 269, 272 (italics in original).

4 After long union with England, Scotland is now classified as a mixed civil law-common law jurisdiction. See Watson, *Making of Civil Law* 5 (listing as mixed jurisdictions Louisiana, Puerto Rico, Scotland, and South Africa).

5 1 Boswell, *Johnson* 426.

6 1 Boswell, *Johnson* 468 (paraphrasing a line in Matthew Prior's poem "The Chameleon").

the dramatist John Dryden, he socialized with the literary elite. Despite his aristocratic rural background, he attracted clients from the rising commercial class. He became learned in legal systems other than England's, studying Scottish and Continental law, and developed a practice in the Court of Chancery, where equity modified the rigors of the common law.

In 1738, marriage to the daughter of an English earl opened new social and political opportunities, and in 1742, with the support of the Duke of Newcastle, he entered parliament and became solicitor general. As one political aristocrat confided to another, "The only objection that can be made to him is what he can't help, which is that he is a Scotchman, which (as I have a great regard for him) I am extremely sorry for."[7] The opportunity for Murray to demonstrate his loyalty to the English establishment came in 1745 when the Scottish clans rose for the last time in support of the claims of the deposed Stuart monarchs. On behalf of the Crown, Murray led the prosecution of the leaders of the "Forty-five," demanding the death penalty. His loyalty now so firmly established that he could survive lingering doubts about his Stuart sympathies,[8] Mansfield was appointed attorney general in 1753. Two years later, he was made Chief Justice of the Court of King's Bench and raised to the peerage as Lord Mansfield, the name by which he would ever after be known.[9] Judging did not mean the end of Mansfield's political service. Executive and judicial powers were not yet completely distinct, and he continued to serve in the cabinet for several years.

Mansfield's restless energy was obvious from the first. He immediately abandoned the traditional practice favoring senior barristers that had hampered young lawyers like Blackstone. Henceforth, the court heard the motions of every member of the bar before beginning again with the most senior.[10] It was also reported of him that he reserved places in his court for law students – familiarly known as the "crib" – and sometimes paused to explain to them the intricacies of the cases before him.[11] He encouraged unanimity among the judges and, briefly at least, managed to end the historic practice of seriatim opinions, each judge delivering a separate opinion in each case, issuing instead a unitary "opinion of the court," preferably announced by him – innovations that would bear most fruit when later copied in the new republic across the Atlantic.

Acutely aware of the need to adapt the common law to the emergent social and economic realities, the new Chief Justice fearlessly undertook the task.

7 1 Philip C. Yorke, *Life and Correspondence of Philip Yorke, Earl of Hardwicke, Lord High Chancellor of Great Britain* 307 (1913) (quoting letter from the Duke of Richmond to the Duke of Newcastle, 3 Dec. 1742).

8 See Norman S. Posner, *Lord Mansfield: Justice in the Age of Reason* 107–109 (2013).

9 At first Lord Mansfield of Mansfield, William Murray was made Earl of Mansfield in 1776.

10 See reporter's note at 1 Burr. 57–58, 97 Eng. Rep. 189 (1756).

11 12 Holdsworth, *History of English Law* 476.

Undeterred by the argument that change should come only from parliament, he once exclaimed in exasperation: "What! pass a judgment to do mischief, and then bring in a bill to cure it?"[12] – a candid avowal of the continued power of judicial activism. Temperamentally unsuited to Blackstonian reverence for all things old, Mansfield roundly declared that "the law would be a strange science if it rested solely upon cases; and if after so large an increase of commerce, arts, and circumstances accruing, we must go to the time of Richard I to find a case and see what is law."[13] He once confided to the actor David Garrick: "A judge on the bench is now and then in your whimsical situation between Tragedy and Comedy, inclination drawing him one way and a long string of precedents the other" – an allusion to Sir Joshua Reynolds' recent portrait of the actor posed between female figures representing the two poetic muses.[14] Precedent, his lordship liked to say, was only evidence of the law, "not law itself."[15]

Part of the problem was the state of law reporting. As one of Lord Mansfield's colleagues on the bench put it, "Many of the old cases are strange and absurd" – candidly adding "and so also are some of the modern ones"![16] Reports varied considerably in quality with the skill, understanding, and attentiveness of the respective reporters. Prepared by individual lawyers or judges, they were essentially private-enterprise undertakings, generally known by the name of the reporter, not official in the modern sense, their credibility dependent on the reputation of the reporter. At first, the "nominative reports" were published only if and when the author, or the representative of a deceased author, saw an opportunity for profit. Different reporters covered the same courts and periods, occasionally resulting in multiple reports of the same case, not all of them alike. Blackstone's own reports, as we have seen, were compared unfavorably with those prepared by two contemporaries.

Dr. Johnson rated the English reports in general "very poor," adding that "only half of what has been said is taken down; and of that half, much is mistaken."[17] One wit went even further in describing the reports of Isaac Espinasse, who reported Nisi Prius cases from 1793 to 1807: "He heard only half of what went on in court and reported the other half."[18] In the

12 Bishop of London v. Ffytche (H.L.1783), reported in T. Cunningham, *The Law of Simony* 174 (1784).

13 Jones v. Randall, Lofft 383, 385, 98 Eng. Rep. 706, 707 (K.B. 1774). The accession of King Richard I, "the Lionheart," in 1189 was the traditional limit of legal memory. Customs that had been used so long that "the memory of man runneth not to the contrary" were presumed to be valid common law. 2 Blackstone, *Commentaries* 31.

14 Quoted in John Holliday, *The Life of William Late Earl of Mansfield* 211 (1797).

15 Jones v. Randall, Lofft at 385, 98 Eng. Rep. at 707.

16 Pillans v. Van Mierop, 3 Burr. 1663, 1671, 97 Eng. Rep. 1035, 1039 (K.B. 1765) (Wilmot, J.).

17 1 Boswell, *Johnson* 443.

18 Quoted in Simpson, *Biographical Dictionary* 168 (remark attributed to Baron Pollock). Espinasse's reports are reprinted in 170 Eng. Rep. Nisi Prius cases are trial reports.

nineteenth century, Lord Lyndhurst, then Lord Chancellor, recalled that "in my younger days, it was said of Barnardiston, that he was accustomed to slumber over his note-book, and the wags in the rear took the opportunity of scribbling nonsense in it."[19] The picture is comic, but the cost in terms of the reliability of the reports and the consequent effectiveness of precedent is serious.

During his tenure as Chief Justice of King's Bench from 1756 to 1788, Mansfield used the freedom to doubt the old reports as a source of power, as he reshaped English law in the commercial field. "There being no solemn well-considered decision," he commented in one case, "we must resort to principles"[20] – that is, despite the five-hundred-year-long history of his court, he could treat the matter as one of first instance. John William Wallace, who reported U.S. Supreme Court decisions from 1863 to 1874, believed that Mansfield "commented adversely on the reporters because his system of pulling up the landmarks of the law made it necessary for him to discredit the old authorities." Mansfield was, Wallace continued, more in sympathy with the poet Alexander Pope than with the law reporter Edmund Plowden, whose reports Wallace rated "the best reports of any age."[21]

But while the absence of reliable reports gave Mansfield power in his own day, their continued absence risked diminishing his power in the future, if his successors were as free to doubt the reports of his court as he had been to doubt those of his predecessors. The solution was the development of reliable reports, reviewed by the judges and published contemporaneously with the decisions, and Mansfield found the reporter he needed in James Burrow, who set a new professional standard of meticulous law reporting.[22] Wallace later rhapsodized that Burrow's Reports are "the perfection of the art."[23] Having increased his judicial power by doubting reports of prior cases, Mansfield increased it yet again by creating reports that could not be doubted.

To build a body of commercial law, Mansfield discouraged the use of general verdicts in favor of "special verdicts" in which the jury makes findings only on specific questions of fact submitted to them by the judge, who then decides the legal effect of the verdict. Furthering his project of creating a practical body of mercantile law, he encouraged the parties to commercial cases to request a "special jury," one consisting of persons with particular experience such as

19 Wallace, *The Reporters* 424. Thomas Barnardison published reports of Chancery decisions in 1740 and 1741, reprinted in 27 Eng. Rep.

20 Eaton v. Jaques, 2 Dougl. 455, 460, 99 Eng. Rep. 290, 292 (K.B. 1780).

21 Wallace, *The Reporters* 29. Plowden reported cases between 1550 and 1580, reprinted in 75 Eng. Rep.

22 See 12 Holdsworth, *History of English Law* 110–112.

23 Wallace, *The Reporters* 449. Burrow reported decisions of the Court of King's Bench from 1756 to 1772, reprinted in 97–98 Eng. Rep.

bankers or merchants.[24] In the nineteenth century, Lord Campbell reported that Mansfield used the occasion to assemble a body of special jurymen with whom he was on familiar terms – "from them he learned the usages of trade, and in return he took great pains in explaining to them the principles of jurisprudence by which they were to be guided." Campbell recalled that "several of these gentlemen survived when I began to attend Guildhall as a student, and were designated and honoured as 'Lord Mansfield's jurymen.'"[25] In one case involving the evaluation of profits in an insurance claim, Mansfield observed that "the special jury (among whom there were many knowing and considerable merchants), found the defendant's rule of estimation to be right and gave their verdict for him." "They understood the question very well," he said, "and knew more of the subject of it than anybody else present"[26] – including, it seems, his lordship himself. A form of "continuing judicial education," the special jury allowed Mansfield to learn about commercial practices, enabling him to spell out practical rules of law to guide later courts – and to guide lawyers advising commercial clients.

Businessmen found that they could obtain informed and speedy justice from Mansfield, and commercial litigants turned to his court in preference to the other common law courts – a practice that would later be disparaged as "forum-shopping." His zeal sometimes led Mansfield to hold court even on holidays. Allegedly, he once announced his intention of sitting on Good Friday in order to finish an important case before the Easter recess, prompting one of the serjeants-at-law to remark that "your Lordship will be the first judge to have done so since Pontius Pilate."[27]

In the decisions filling the newly reliable reports, Mansfield's jurisprudential project was, as he repeatedly announced, "to do substantial justice." "The most desirable object in all judicial determinations, especially in mercantile ones, (which ought to be determined upon natural justice, and not upon the niceties of law) is, to do substantial justice."[28] While today this may seem an unremarkable goal for a legal system, the common law before Mansfield might be said to have settled for doing merely procedural justice, that is, adhering to strict rules, especially rules concerning pleading – "the niceties of law" that Blackstone had scanted as a lecturer but insisted upon as a judge. Mansfield announced a new goal: to effectuate intention: "To do justice between men, it is necessary to

24 See 3 Geo. 2, c. 25 (1730); 24 Geo. 2, c. 18 (1751). Special juries are not unknown in the United States. See, e.g., Fay v. New York, 332 U.S. 261 (1947).

25 2 John Campbell, Lord Campbell, *Lives of the Chief Justices of England* 304–305 n. 2 (1873). Campbell (1779–1861) was successively C.J. K.B. and Lord Chancellor; he is the author of judicial biographies.

26 Lewis v. Rucker, 2 Burr. 1167, 1168, 97 Eng. Rep. 769, 770 (K.B. 1761).

27 Quoted in Edmund Heward, *Lord Mansfield* 62 (1979) (citing Philip Thicknesse, *Sketches and Characters* 38 (1770)).

28 Alderson v. Temple, 4 Burr. 2235, 2239, 98 Eng. Rep. 165, 167 (K.B. 1768).

understand things as they really are, and construe instruments according to the intent of the parties."[29] With a sure hand, Mansfield dealt with the multitude of legal fictions that risked confusion:

> Fictions of law hold only in respect of the ends and purposes for which they were invented; when they are urged to an intent and purpose not within the reason and policy of the fiction, the other party may shew the truth.[30]

Mansfield's activism attracted critics. Junius, a contemporary pseudonymous commentator, called out the Chief Justice because,

> instead of those certain, positive rules, by which the judgement of a court of law should invariably be determined, you have fondly introduced your own unsettled notions of equity and substantial justice.... The court of King's Bench becomes a court of equity, and the judge, instead of consulting strictly the law of the land, refers only to the wisdom of the court, and the purity of his own conscience.[31]

In America, Thomas Jefferson heartily agreed:

> The object of former judges has been to render the law more and more certain, that of this personage [Lord Mansfield] to render it more incertain under pretence of rendering it more reasonable: no period of the English laws, of whatever length it be taken, can be produced wherein so many of its settled rules have been reversed as during the time of this judge.[32]

Convinced that the medieval language of land law often clouded legal analysis, Mansfield worked to modernize legal terminology – for instance, coining the now standard phrase "adverse possession" to replace the medieval word disseisin.[33] In addition, doctrines that are today often assumed to be part of the common law, such as estoppel and unjust enrichment, were imported from equity by Mansfield, who unashamedly cited Chancery practice and precedent as his authority when there was none at law. Candidly describing his approach in one case, Mansfield held that "the defendant, upon the circumstances of the case, is obliged by the ties of natural justice and equity to refund the money,"[34] anticipating the doctrine of constructive (or quasi) contract. Breaking with the common law rule giving the father custody of children if the parents separate,

29 Eaton v. Jacques, 2 Dougl. 455, 460, 99 Eng. Rep. 290, 292 (K.B. 1780).

30 Morris v. Pugh, 3 Burr. 1241, 1243, 97 Eng. Rep. 811, 811 (K.B. 1761).

31 Letter 41, 14 Nov. 1770, in *Letters of Junius* 209–210 (John Cannon ed. 1978).

32 Jefferson to Philip Mazzei, Nov. 1785, in 9 *Papers of Thomas Jefferson* 71 (Julian P. Boyd ed. 1954).

33 Taylor d. Atkyns v. Horde, 1 Burr. 60, 119, 97 Eng. Rep. 190, 223 (K.B. 1757).

34 Moses v. MacFerlan, 2 Burr. 1005, 1012, 97 Eng. Rep. 676, 681 (K.B. 1760).

Mansfield pioneered the modern, equitable standard: "The Court are to judge upon the circumstances of the particular case," Mansfield flatly declared, and "if the parties disagree, the court will do what shall appear best for the child."[35] Although later English judges failed to follow Mansfield's lead, parliament eventually enacted his rule in 1839.

A generation later across the Atlantic, Mansfield found a powerful admirer. John Marshall, Chief Justice of the new U.S. Supreme Court, lauded the British Chief Justice as

> one of the greatest judges who ever sat on any bench, and who has done more than any other to remove those technical impediments which grew out of a different state of society, and too long continued to obstruct the course of substantial justice.[36]

It can hardly be coincidental that when Marshall went out of his way to praise Mansfield, he took the opportunity of a case concerning his cousin Thomas Jefferson, who abominated the English judge.

The debate about adherence to legal technicalities continued well into the nineteenth century; indeed, it remains unresolved to this day. Oliver Wendell Holmes reported in 1880 that the founding dean of the renewed Harvard Law School, Christopher Columbus Langdell, dismissed arguments based on "substantial justice" as "irrelevant."[37] And Langdell's protégé and successor as dean at Harvard, James Barr Ames, was reported by Louis Brandeis – then a law student, later a U.S. Supreme Court justice – as determined to convince his class that "even the great Mansfield was a fraud, who stood convicted of the inexpiable crime of having introduced equity doctrines into the sacred and immaculate Common Law."[38]

Mansfield thought that contracts, particularly commercial contracts, ought to be construed liberally to give effect to intention. Breaking with the traditional view of contract as a bargained-for exchange, Mansfield would have based the contractual obligation simply on the promise, as in Roman (and Scottish) law. In one commercial case, he went so far as to disregard the common law requirement of "consideration," the thing bargained for in return, although his conservative successors later re-established the traditional requirement.[39] In consequence, law students to this day diligently search for the necessary quid pro quo.

35 R. v. Delaval, 3 Burr. 1434, 1437, 97 Eng. Rep. 913, 914 (K.B. 1763).

36 Livingston v. Jefferson, 15 F.Cas. 660, 664 (U.S. Cir. Ct. Va. 1811).

37 O.W. Holmes, Review of *Langdell's A Selection of Cases on the Law of Contracts* (2d ed. 1880), 14 *Am. L. Rev*. 233, 234 (1880).

38 Brandeis to Otto Wehle, 12 Nov. 1876, in 1 Brandeis, *Letters*.

39 Pillans v. Van Mierop, 3 Burr. 1663, 97 Eng. Rep. 1035 (K.B. 1765), reversed by Rann v. Hughes, 4 Brown 27, 2 Eng. Rep. 19 (1778) (pleadings and arguments); Mitchinson v. Hewson, 7 T.R. 350 n, 101 Eng. Rep. 1014 (H.L. 1778).

While Mansfield's emphasis on intention is a commonplace today, in his time most legal documents concerned land and were governed by strict rules of interpretation, such as the medieval Rule in Shelley's Case. As we have seen, Blackstone, by then one of the King's justices, had authored the opinion that rejected Mansfield's refusal to apply the intent-defeating Rule in a case concerning the interpretation of a will.[40] The lecturer-turned-judge worried that allowing a testator's intention to prevail over a rule of law would mean that "every man would make a law for himself." Reminiscent of his fear of "equity without law" – and perhaps informed by contemporary concerns that Mansfield was ignoring the distinction between equity and law – Blackstone warned against "vague discretionary law."[41]

In other cases, Mansfield's reformist impulse was more successful. There was once, for instance, the not unreasonable rule that a major change in a testator's personal relationships would revoke an earlier will. The will that a testator executed while single, for example, was revoked by operation of law on subsequent marriage and birth of a child.[42] But the rule had been carried to extremes by technically minded judges who found just about any change of circumstances sufficient to revoke a will.[43] Mansfield criticized these results and announced his opinion that "constructive revocations, contrary to the intention of the testator, ought not to be indulged," observing that "some overstrained resolutions of that sort had brought a scandal upon the law."[44]

In Mansfield's day, perhaps the best-known example of his wish to give effect to a testator's clear intention in the face of minor irregularities was the 1757 case of Windham v. Chetwynd,[45] a decision later harshly criticized by Lord Camden, Chief Justice of the Court of Common Pleas. In *Windham*, the question was the degree of disinterestedness required of witnesses to a will. The Statute of Frauds required attestation by "two or three credible witnesses,"[46] and earlier courts had equated "credible" with "competent to testify in court," which at that time excluded witnesses who had an interest in the outcome. Mansfield rejected the equation and held that if the subscribing witnesses became disinterested before the time of the testator's death, their attestations were valid – a point of law that remains in dispute to this day.[47] Lord Camden, himself a distinguished jurist, was outraged by Mansfield's disregard of precedent and denounced the decision in terms reminiscent of modern debates about activist judges:

40 Perrin v. Blake, 4 Burr. 2579, 98 Eng. Rep. 355; 1 *Collectanea Juridica* 283 (Exch. Ch. 1772).

41 1 *A Collection of Tracts Relative to the Law of England* (Francis Hargrave ed. 1787), 489, 491, 496.

42 2 Blackstone, *Commentaries* 502.

43 For a survey of the cases, see 4 Kent, *Commentaries* 528–531.

44 Swift v. Roberts, 3 Burr. 1488, 1491, 97 Eng. Rep. 941, 942–943 (K.B. 1764).

45 1 Burr. 414, 97 Eng. Rep. 377 (K.B. 1757).

46 29 Car. 2, c. 3 (1677).

47 See, e.g., Estate of Parsons, 103 Cal.App.3d 384 (1980).

> The discretion of a Judge is the law of tyrants; it is always unknown; it is different in different men; it is casual, and depends upon constitution, temper, and passion. In the best it is often times caprice, in the worst it is every vice, folly, and passion to which human nature is liable.[48]

The common law also had the rule, seemingly common sense, that a man cannot pass a better title than he has, but Mansfield recognized that some exceptions were required in the interest of trade. To function as a form of currency, bank notes had to pass without question, even if stolen, and Mansfield so held – this, at a time before the notes were made legal tender by act of parliament.[49] Like bank notes, negotiable commercial paper had to pass in the same unquestioned manner and for the same reason.[50] In America, as we will see, U.S. Supreme Court Justice Joseph Story later led the federal courts to the same conclusion.[51] Today, the principle is enshrined in the widely adopted Uniform Commercial Code.[52]

Smooth functioning of law and commerce required that certain rules be clear and, to some extent, inflexible. This led Mansfield to announce that "in all mercantile transactions, the great object should be certainty and therefore, it is of more consequence that a rule should be certain, than whether the rule is established one way or the other."[53] In blunt terms, he even suggested that bringing "all questions upon mercantile transactions to a certainty" is "more important than doing right,"[54] showing that he had begun to grasp the economics now expressed in the Coase Theorem that "in the absence of transaction costs, it does not matter what the law is, since people can always negotiate without cost to acquire, subdivide, and combine rights whenever this would increase the value of production."[55] The effect is to reinforce the law of precedent. Years later, Louis Brandeis, by then a justice of the U.S. Supreme Court, agreed: "*Stare decisis* is usually the wise policy, because in most matters it is more important that the applicable rule of law be settled than that it be settled right."[56] Obviously, Lord Mansfield's insistence on certainty could conflict with his commitment to enforce intention. Yet formulating rules and procedures that are likely in most cases to effectuate intention and then adhering to them unwaveringly is similar to doubting the reports and then reforming reporting.

48 Quoted in 2 Oldham, *Mansfield MSS* 1356 (citing pamphlet report of Doe dem. Hindson v. Kersey (C.P. 1765)).

49 Miller v. Race, 1 Burr. 452, 97 Eng. Rep. 398 (K.B. 1758).

50 Grant v. Vaughan, 3 Burr. 1516, 97 Eng. Rep. 957 (K.B. 1764).

51 Swift v. Tyson, 41 U.S. (16 Pet.) 1 (1842).

52 See U.C.C. § 1-201(24); U.C.C. § 3-305.

53 Vallejo v. Wheeler, 1 Cowp. 143, 153, 98 Eng. Rep. 1012, 1017 (K.B. 1774).

54 Hankey v. Jones, 2 Cowp. 745, 750, 98 Eng. Rep. 1339, 1342 (K.B. 1778).

55 R.H. Coase, *The Firm, the Market, and the Law* 14 (1988). In reality, of course, there are always "transaction costs."

56 Burnet v. Coronado Oil & Gas Co., 285 U.S. 393, 406 (1932) (Brandeis, J., dissenting). Cited with approval in Kimble v. Marvel Entertainment, 576 U.S. 446, 455 (2015).

In 1772, Mansfield was forced to confront the ugly question of the legality of slavery. Blackstone had given his answer in a lecture a few years earlier: "Pure and proper slavery does not, nay cannot, subsist in England." Consequently, he concluded: "A slave or negro, the instant he lands in England, becomes a freeman."[57] But Mansfield had to answer the question not from the university lectern but from the judicial bench. The issue arose when James Somerset, who had been brought as an enslaved person from Virginia to England and who was about to be transshipped to Jamaica for sale, secured a writ of habeas corpus – doubtless with the assistance of anti-slavery forces – to try the legality of his confinement on board. The return to the writ by the ship's captain recited that Somerset was enslaved under the laws of Virginia and Jamaica, but Mansfield found that answer legally inadequate. "The black must be discharged," he brusquely ordered.[58]

While he acknowledged that slavery was recognized in various parts of the British Empire and conceded that contracts for the sale of slaves had been enforced by courts in England, Mansfield declared that slavery in the colonies existed only by virtue of local law or legally binding custom. Slavery was "so odious," Mansfield declared, that it was incapable of being introduced in England "on any reasons, moral or political; but only positive law." In the absence of statute, the answer to the question of Somerset's status had to be determined at common law. Searching English legal history, Mansfield could find no precedent to support it. Roman slavery had ended with the Roman occupation of Britain; the medieval status of serfdom or villeinage was long extinct. Without a precedent, the common law offered no justification for Somerset's confinement. As a distinguished legal historian observed: "That Lord Mansfield should refuse to follow the custom of the merchants, and should give a decision based mainly on the rules of the medieval common law, no doubt surprised many of his contemporaries."[59]

Perhaps to deflect criticism that he had decided Somerset's Case on equitable principles or (worse) on his own personal preferences, Mansfield stressed the impartiality of the law: "Compassion will not, on the one hand, nor inconvenience on the other, be to decide; but the law."[60] Aware of the potential impact of his decision on slaves then in England, Mansfield declared: "If the parties will have judgment, *fiat justitia, ruat coelum*, let justice be done whatever be the consequences"[61] – earning himself an entry in any dictionary of legal quotations. In fact, the heavens did not fall,[62] but the case exposed the

57 1 Blackstone, *Commentaries* 411–412.

58 Somerset v. Stewart, Lofft 1, 98 Eng. Rep. 499 (K.B. 1772) (also known as Sommersett's Case).

59 3 Holdsworth, *History of English Law* 508.

60 Lofft at 17, 98 Eng. Rep. 509.

61 Id. The Latin maxim is more commonly translated: "Let justice be done, though the heavens fall." *Black's Law Dictionary* 1914.

62 See Ruth Paley, "After Somerset: Mansfield and the Law of Slavery in England, 1772–1830," in *Law, Crime and English Society* (Norma Landau ed. 2002).

weakness of the legal basis of slavery in the British Empire and was widely publicized by abolitionists. Francis Hargrave, one of the distinguished lawyers appearing for Somerset, grandly declared that "the air of England was too pure for slaves to breathe in"[63] – another famous quotation. As with many celebrated cases, the actual holding in Somerset's Case was more constrained (and less exciting) than the public perception of it, an example of the care (and fiddling) required to make a leading case.

Word of Mansfield's decision spread rapidly throughout the slave-holding colonies in North America. An advertisement for the return of a fugitive from slavery appearing in the *Virginia Gazette* in 1773, within a year of the decision, speculated that the fugitive may "endeavour to get on some vessel bound for Great Britain, from a knowledge he has of the late determination of Somerset's case."[64] Fearing that the decision was a step toward the abolition of slavery in the British Empire – as indeed it was – Southern planters became more sympathetic to the cause of American independence. Virginia Governor Dunmore's proclamation of 1775 offering freedom to any enslaved person who fought for Britain against the colonists only solidified their support. Whether slavery could form part of the common law of the new United States remained to be resolved.

Enlightened and tolerant, Mansfield drew the ire of the traditional "Church and King" crowd, as well as of the urban mob, ever ready for an excuse to riot. When the unbalanced Scottish nobleman Lord Gordon in 1780 whipped up hostility to the liberally minded who supported freeing Catholics from the penalties imposed after the Reformation, Mansfield was among their targets. Charles Dickens later included the scene in his early novel *Barnaby Rudge*, a literary precursor to the greater scenes of terror in *A Tale of Two Cities* – as the Gordon Riots themselves were dress rehearsals for the revolutionary turbulence to follow in France. Closely tracking legal sources, Dickens recounts:

> That the mob gathering round Lord Mansfield's house, had called on those within to open the door, and receiving no reply (for Lord and Lady Mansfield were at that moment escaping by the backway), forced an entrance according to their usual custom. That they then began to demolish the house with great fury, and setting fire to it in several parts, involved in a common ruin the whole of the costly furniture, the plate and jewels, a beautiful gallery of pictures, the rarest collection of manuscripts ever possessed by any one private person in the world, and worse than all, because nothing could replace this loss, the great Law Library, on almost every page of which were notes in the Judge's own hand, of inestimable value, – being the results of the study and experience of his whole life.[65]

63 Lofft at 2, 98 Eng. Rep. 500.

64 *Virginia Gazette*, Sept. 1773, repeated June 1774.

65 Charles Dickens, *Barnaby Rudge* ch. 66 (1841). For a law reporter's account of the riot, which Dickens seems to have copied, see the note following Hodges v. Middleton, 2 Dougl. 435–437, 99 Eng. Rep. 278–280 (1780).

In a later parliamentary debate concerning the government's use of deadly force in suppressing the riots, Lord Chancellor Thurlow described the object of the rioters: "Having lifted the axe of outrage against several of the great branches of the King's government, they aimed at the root of the tree and by burning the public prisons and attacking the Bank of England, began their endeavours to destroy the Government" – revealing the reactionary Chancellor's unillusioned idea of the social contract, rooted in law enforcement and financial institutions, the prisons and the Bank. More impressive than any legal argument, perhaps, was Lord Mansfield's defense of the government's actions, concluding with the words, "I have consulted no books. Indeed, I have none to consult."[66]

While Mansfield survived the wrath of the mob, his legacy of judicial law-making faced the more serious challenge of a young contemporary's coruscating criticism. Legal reform by fiction, lovingly described by Blackstone, or by an activist judge applying equitable principles like Lord Mansfield, was about to be assailed by Jeremy Bentham's clarion call for law reform by statute under the banner of Utilitarianism.

66 Quoted in Robert Gore-Browne, *Chancellor Thurlow: The Life and Times of an XVIIIth Century Lawyer* 160–161 (1953) (without citation).

3

JEREMY BENTHAM AND THE CHALLENGE OF CRITICISM

The rationalist impulse of the Enlightenment could inspire the cautious restatement of Blackstone or the bold innovations of Mansfield. It could also inspire radical criticism of the entire common law enterprise, root and branch. Perhaps the common law's most celebrated critic was Jeremy Bentham, whose reputation as a reformer was greater even than the reforms he sponsored. Bentham had been among the students at Blackstone's Oxford lectures and later claimed that, while still in his teens, he had recognized that the Commentator was an uncritical defender of the status quo and had listened to his lectures with "rebel ears."[1] A few years later, he memorably tagged his former teacher "everything-as-it-should-be Blackstone."[2] Bentham dismissed Blackstone's defense of the rationality of the common law, correctly noting that it begged the question, presuming all along what was to be proved: "No sound principles can be expected from that writer," Bentham observed, "whose first object is to defend a system."[3] The critic's answer was to reverse the Blackstonian presumption of rationality: unless the utility of a rule could be proved, it was presumptively wrong. Legal fictions were the special objects of Bentham's ire, not just for their obscurantism but because they amounted to law reform by subterfuge.

While eating his terms at Lincoln's Inn, which was also Mansfield's inn, Bentham observed the great judge at work in the Court of King's Bench: "Days and weeks together," he recalled, "I made my morning pilgrimage to the

1 1 Bentham, *Works* 249.

2 Jeremy Bentham, *A Fragment on Government; being an Examination of what is delivered on the Subject of Government in General in the Introduction to Sir William Blackstone's Commentaries* 407 (1776) (J.H. Burns and H.L.A. Hart eds. 1988).

3 10 Bentham, *Works* 141 (quoting Bentham's Commonplace Book).

DOI: 10.4324/9781003660859-4

chief seat of the living idol."[4] Attracted by the rational reforming zeal of the great chief justice, Bentham at first thought he had found the antidote for Blackstone's Panglossian complacency. But on further reflection, he concluded that Mansfield's overt law reform by judicial decision was no better than the covert variety by legal fiction. In both cases, judges were usurping legislative power, and in any case law reform by judicial decree, unlike legal change wrought by statute, was always, and by definition, *ex post facto*, made after the fact. In a telling metaphor, Bentham described the common law as made by the judges "on the same principle as a man makes laws for his dog – he waits till the dog has done something he does not like and then punishes him for it."[5] The proper approach to law-making was by the rational legislator, guided by the enlightened critic; the final product should be a code. All law should be code-law. Although his goal of the wholesale replacement of the common law with a code was never realized – and may be, in the words of a great American judge, beyond "the compass of human powers"[6] – Bentham helped start the process by which law would increasingly be reconceptualized as statute law rather than case law. Eventually, laypeople everywhere (and even many judges) would come to think of a typical "law" as a statute, not a judicial decision, and many legal academics would be enticed by the idea of drafting codes for their legal specialties.

Bentham rejected reform by scholar and judge and dedicated his life to overthrowing the idols of the common law, rebelling against both the meretricious charms of tradition and the dashing dynamism of judicial activism. He spent the latter part of his life secluded in his private residence – aptly named the Hermitage – supported by his considerable inherited wealth, writing in furtherance of his great project. As an independent thinker, neither a practicing lawyer nor a sitting judge, Bentham resembled Charles Darwin in the next generation, also independently wealthy and unaffiliated with any scholarly institution or university, who labored largely alone in his path-breaking researches. Just as Darwin's name is forever linked with the phrase "survival of the fittest," so Bentham's is tied to the slogan "the greatest happiness of the greatest number."[7] By this standard, which he named the principle of utility, Bentham measured every action of government; indeed, he applied it to every human action.

Sir Henry Maine, a Cambridge law professor, later claimed that English lawyers of the eighteenth century had been ensnared by what he called the "paradoxical commonplace that English law was the perfection of human reason" and that Bentham's principle of utility "gave escape to a current which had long been trying to find its way outwards."[8] Of course, utilitarianism did

4 1 Bentham, *Works* 247.
5 5 Bentham, *Works* 235–236.
6 Benjamin N. Cardozo, *The Nature of the Judicial Process* 143 (1921).
7 10 Bentham, *Works* 142.
8 Maine, *Ancient Law* 46.

not escape criticism. Thomas Carlyle, writing soon after Bentham, dismissed it as a scheme "for the distribution of an attainable amount of Pig-wash among a given multitude of Pigs."[9] And, later in the century, Oliver Wendell Holmes more pertinently asked: "Why should the greatest number be preferred? Why not the greatest good of the most intelligent and most highly developed? The greatest good of a minority of our generation may be the greatest good of the greatest number in the long run."[10]

Although his influence was only beginning to be felt at the time of his death in 1832, Bentham was in many ways a man of the eighteenth rather than the nineteenth century. Born in 1748, he carried the radicalism of the Enlightenment into the new era. To the enlightened ones, reason – in the new, not the old, Blackstonian sense – was the universal solvent that would free humankind from the bonds of superstition and tradition. There were thought to be no limits, except those imposed by ignorance or self-interest, to the perfectibility of man and society. In France, the *philosophes* turned their wit and ingenuity against the institutions of the *ancien régime*. On the fringes of Western civilization, in the British colonies in North America, the sons of the Enlightenment were increasingly critical of their absentee rulers.

Although he was to applaud the revolutions on both sides of the Atlantic, Bentham came from a well-to-do family that had risen under the old dispensation and that expected to continue to rise in a hierarchical, aristocratic milieu. His grandfather had been a solicitor and his father a scrivener, that is, a legal draftsman; both had prospered and invested heavily in real estate. The young Bentham was precocious. Maturing rapidly, he matriculated at Queen's College, Oxford, at the age of 12. Even at that tender age, he was reluctant to subscribe the Thirty-Nine Articles, the official creed of the Church of England, as then required for admission to the university, but in the end, he made his profession of faith, consoling himself that he was not alone, that the streets of Oxford were, as he put it, "paved with perjury."[11] Like Edward Gibbon and Adam Smith, his gifted predecessors at the university, Bentham found its intellectual pretensions empty. "I learnt nothing," he recalled: all his fellow students were "either stupid or dissipated."[12]

After his call to the bar, Bentham showed no interest in the practical side of the legal profession. A friendly solicitor, he said, had a case or two at nurse for him, but his first thought was how to put them to death. Successful in this,

9 Quoted in James C. Carter, *Law: Its Origin, Growth and Function* 222 (1907) (without citation). Pigwash in this context means "wet feed consisting of mostly kitchen waste mixed with water; pigswill."

10 O.W. Holmes, "Summary of Events: Great Britain: The Gas-Stokers' Strike," 7 *Am. L. Rev.* 582, 584 (1873).

11 Quoted in John MacCunn, *Six Radical Thinkers: Bentham, J.S. Mill, Cobden, Carlyle, Mazzini, T.H. Green* 3 (1907) (without citation).

12 10 Bentham, *Works* 41.

Bentham clearly had no future at the bar. Instead, he embarked on what would be his lifelong task of writing provocative, often unfinished, and usually unpublished works on a multitude of legal and constitutional topics. His first significant publication appeared anonymously in 1776, the year of Adam Smith's *Wealth of Nations*, the first volume of Gibbon's Roman history, and – unforgettable in Britain's former American colonies – the Declaration of Independence. Entitled *A Fragment on Government*, Bentham's book took his old teacher, Blackstone, to task; indeed, it was a fragment of a planned larger work to be called "A Comment on the *Commentaries* or an Introduction to the Introduction." However irritating Bentham found the ancient hodgepodge of English law as expounded by Blackstone, it was the jurisprudential inadequacy of Blackstone's introductory lecture on "the nature of laws in general" that principally attracted his scorn, as it would draw the scorn of later legal theorists. The unnamed contributor to the classic eleventh edition (1910–1911) of the *Encyclopaedia Britannica* dismissed Blackstone as "by no means what would now be called a scientific jurist." He had, according to anonymous, "only the vaguest possible grasp of the elementary conceptions of law."[13]

Bentham's hostility to Blackstone was more than a brash young man's natural antipathy to a complacent elder. Throughout their lives, Bentham and Blackstone approached law and society from opposing directions. While not a reactionary or even necessarily an opponent of reform, Blackstone exhibited what might be called a conservative personality, admiring the achievements of England's historic constitution and assuming the reasonableness even of those parts of the common law that he could not explain. Bentham abominated this reverential approach. His personality was distinctly radical.

In his published comment on the *Commentaries*, Bentham principally attacked Blackstone for accepting the fiction of the social contract. This theory had been used a century earlier by Thomas Hobbes in *Leviathan* (1651) to justify monarchy and a strong state but is today more often associated with Jean-Jacques Rousseau's *Du Contrat Social* (1762), which helped inspire the Atlantic revolutions. It postulated that men had exchanged life in a state of nature for the security of life in organized society. But the implications of imagining a foundational contract were ambiguous. If one emphasized what men were entitled to rather than what they had given up, the implications were truly revolutionary. In fact, appeals to the social contract were regular features in the manifestos of the American and French revolutionaries. In Blackstone's hands, the social contract was mildly reformist. But Bentham saw his acceptance of it as simply another example of his gullibility for convenient fictions.

Bentham also berated his old teacher for conceding the existence of natural rights, the rights Blackstone called "absolute." Here too the complacent Commentator was inadvertently playing with revolutionary fire. In 1776, the

13 4 *Encyclopaedia Britannica* 26 (11th ed. 1910–1911).

year of Bentham's *Fragment on Government*, Thomas Jefferson penned the unforgettable words about "inalienable rights" – to life, liberty, and (not exactly property but) "the pursuit of happiness."[14] Bentham, who was radically committed to his view of reason, could find no rational basis for the ascription of rights outside the law. Natural rights he denounced as "simple nonsense..., rhetorical nonsense..., nonsense upon stilts."[15] The Declaration of Independence, then, was a "hodge-podge of confusion and absurdity, in which the thing to be proved is all along taken for granted"[16] – begging the question, as Bentham thought Blackstone had done. Fearlessly, Bentham drew the necessary conclusion about the natural right dearest to conservative Englishmen, the one Jefferson had elided into the general "pursuit of happiness": property. "Property and law are born together and die together," Bentham announced. "Before laws were made, there was no property: take away laws, and property ceases"[17] – a dictum with alarming implications for the propertied classes, should they ever lose control of the law-making machine.

The *Fragment on Government* had brought to Bentham's rooms in Lincoln's Inn a distinguished visitor. Lord Shelburne, the leading liberal politician of his day, had himself attended Blackstone's lectures, but Bentham's book convinced him of the failings of the Commentator and the brilliance of the young author. Within a year, Bentham's powerful friend had climbed to the top of the greasy pole, becoming England's prime minister. Although his government was short-lived, Shelburne did conclude the Treaty of Paris in 1783, formally recognizing American independence – in international law, the true birthdate of the American republic, when the former colonial master finally recognized the independent sovereignty of its rebellious colonies. Whatever the intellectual weaknesses of the American case, Shelburne recognized that the Americans had won the war.

In his attachment to reason, Bentham was a true representative of the Age of Enlightenment. Reason, as understood at that time, pertained to all men, regardless of nation or background. The same cosmopolitanism marked Bentham's contemporary, Tom Paine, who fomented revolution indiscriminately in England, America, and France. The creed attributed to Paine was a simple one: "My country is the world, and my religion is to do good." But this all-embracing cosmopolitanism may be coupled with an insensitivity to the different situations and historical experiences of different nations, something the traditionalist Blackstone was acutely aware of. Theoreticians like Bentham, on the other hand, are especially susceptible to this shortsightedness. In 1785, he journeyed across Europe to Russia, apparently with some hope of interesting Catherine the Great, who had her own Hermitage, rather

14 Declaration of Independence para. 1 ("unalienable rights" in original).
15 2 Bentham, *Works* 501 (from Anarchical Fallacies).
16 Quoted in John Bowring, "Memoirs of Jeremy Bentham," in 10 Bentham, *Works* 63.
17 Jeremy Bentham, *A Theory of Legislation* 113 (4th ed. 1882).

grander than his, in his schemes for law reform. Although armed with valuable letters of recommendation from Lord Shelburne, Bentham seems to have been too timid to use them. Nonetheless, he lingered in Russia for two years, during which he learned little about the Russian language or people but spent most of his time in seclusion, writing interminably in the French language about criminal law.

While in Russia, Bentham wrote a *Defence of Usury*, published in England in 1787. For centuries, the Christian Church, like modern Islam, drawing on the same arguments of Aristotle, denounced the charging of interest as sinful. As commerce developed, charging interest eventually became acceptable to European law-makers – so long as the rate was not too high. After the Reformation, in 1545 England legalized interest up to a maximum rate; only charges above the stated rate were now legally usurious. During Bentham's lifetime, the maximum legal rate was fixed at five per cent. Although Adam Smith had approved of the usury laws in *The Wealth of Nations*,[18] Bentham applied his reason to the matter and produced a devastating critique of legislative attempts to control the market for money. As he quipped to a friend, "interest, [like] love and religion… should be free."[19] Many years were to pass before Bentham's advice (on all fronts) was heeded. It was not until 1854 that the English usury laws were repealed, only to be reinstated when the consequences of unregulated credit became apparent. American states today continue to set a maximum rate of allowable interest.

While in Russia, Bentham also devised his ill-starred scheme for a model prison. The plan is characteristic of its author. The proposed prison was designed so that one central guard would be able to see all the prisoners. To describe this architectural arrangement, Bentham christened his prison the "Panopticon," from Greek words meaning "all" and "seeing." The value of his plan, according to Bentham, was not merely economical supervision. He also devised a regimen for his prisoners that would break their habits of crime. As he described it, the new prison would be "a mill for grinding rogues honest, and idle men industrious."[20] It was an early attempt at the scientific reconstruction of character – at best, rehabilitation; at worst, brainwashing. Despite years of promotion on behalf of the Panopticon, Bentham was unable to convince the politicians of its utility (or affordability). He lavished large sums of his own money on the scheme. For his labors, parliament later voted him compensation but never built the Panopticon. American Benthamites tried the experiment but eventually found it too expensive.

18 Smith, *Wealth of Nations* 339–340.

19 Bentham to George Wilson, 19 Dec. 1786, in 10 Bentham, *Works* 167.

20 Bentham to Jacques Brissot, c. 25 Nov. 1791, in 4 *Correspondence of Jeremy Bentham* 341 (Timothy L.S. Sprigge ed. 1968).

In 1789, better remembered for the outbreak of the French Revolution, Bentham, now back in London, published his most enduring work, *An Introduction to the Principles of Morals and Legislation*. The leading principle was, of course, the principle of utility. The test of the morality of an action or the wisdom of a law is whether the action or law produces the greatest happiness of the greatest number. Bentham did not merely mouth generalities. In the best manner of enlightened thinkers, he considered his subject scientifically. He propounded, in fact, a specific process for determining whether a given action or law was of more utility than another, the ancestor of modern cost–benefit analysis. Happiness could be gauged by a "felicific calculus." Four circumstances determine the value of a pleasure in isolation: intensity, duration, certainty, and propinquity (or remoteness). Two other factors, in addition, affect the value of a pleasure in a lifetime: fecundity (the likelihood of its being followed by more pleasures) and purity (the likelihood of its not being followed by pain). And, since Bentham was concerned with the common good, he added a final factor: the extent of the pleasure or the number of persons affected by it.[21]

Bentham's moral arithmetic has not held up very well among commentators. A modern critic dismissed the principle of utility as "really no more than an emotive demand for rational, general-interest-oriented legislation…, incapable of yielding a concrete guide to the right solution in any particular instance."[22] Nonetheless, it proved in the years after Bentham's death to be a convenient theory for reformers. The very combination of its apparent rigor and operational vagueness contributed to its appeal among men of business, who must often make similar calculations.

While it proved its usefulness in a later day, the *Principles of Morals and Legislation* was not a success in its own. The author later ruefully admitted that the print run had been very small and that the rats had devoured half of it. Its failure resulted in part from its being too abstract, too dry, and perhaps too scientific. But in large measure, its failure was caused simply by its timing. The storming of the Bastille in the same year initiated the long series of events that comprised the French Revolution, leading eventually to the wars of Napoleon and not ending until Wellington's victory at Waterloo a quarter century later. All eyes were fixed on France, at first with fascination, later with horror. As a young man in Paris at the time, the poet William Wordsworth was swept up with enthusiasm for revolutionary change – "Bliss it was in that dawn to be alive / But to be young was very heaven."[23] – only to retreat later to the safety of the English countryside.

21 Jeremy Bentham, *An Introduction to the Principles of Morals and Legislation* (1789) 37 (1961).
22 J.M. Kelly, *A Short History of Western Legal Theory* 436–437 (1992).
23 William Wordsworth, *The Prelude* (1850).

Bentham's reputation as a reformer led the French National Assembly to add his name to the roll of honorary French citizens, a list that included the scientist Joseph Priestly, the abolitionist William Wilberforce, and the general and statesman George Washington. But Bentham was not an uncritical admirer of events in France, even during the early, heady days of revolution. In his eyes, the revolutionaries were making serious ideological errors. In 1789, the French Constituent Assembly adopted the Declaration of the Rights of Man and the Citizen, drafted by the Abbé Sieyès. Influenced by the American Declaration of Independence, the French manifesto asserts that men have "natural, inalienable, and sacred rights," falling (Bentham thought) into the same error as its American precursor. He promptly upbraided the delegates: "It is a metaphysical work, the *ne plus ultra* of metaphysics."[24]

Happily for Bentham, events had placed him above the fray and out of sight. In 1792, his father died, leaving him a comfortable house in London and an ample unearned income. While the French revolutionaries horrified Europe with their Reign of Terror, Bentham settled down comfortably to his studies. The great English historian Macaulay later described Bentham as one of those reformers who turned conservative during the French Revolution. Decades later, he was to champion the cause of parliamentary reform, but during the dark days of revolution and war, Bentham muted his criticism of the English constitution. While the country slipped into reaction and repression, Bentham quietly devoted himself to writing unpublished works – in volume and fascination to later generations comparable to Leonardo's Notebooks. In a story perhaps apocryphal, the Abbé Sieyès is said to have responded to a question about how he occupied himself during the Reign of Terror with the words, "*J'ai vécu*" (I survived). Bentham might have said the same thing.

The common law, as it entered the nineteenth century, offered many easy targets for the reforming hermit. The law of deodand is a striking example. Any chattel that was the immediate cause of the death of a person was forfeit to the Crown. The rule originated in the Middle Ages, when forfeited things were sold and the proceeds applied to charitable purposes. (This explains, incidentally, the name deodand, "gift to God.") With the passage of time, the charitable purposes were often overlooked, and the rule became simply a source of royal revenue. Blackstone grouped it with forfeitures, although conceding that it "arises from the misfortune rather than the crime of the owner."[25] Bentham was quick to point out the irrationality of the rule: "You are a farmer. You employ a wagon. You send your son to drive it: he slips down, is run over and killed. The king, or somebody in his name, is to have your wagon."[26] Bentham may actually have found the case of the cart-and-child in Blackstone,

24 Bentham to Jacques Brissot, mid-August 1791, in 4 *Correspondence of Jeremy Bentham* 84.
25 1 Blackstone, *Commentaries* 290.
26 1 Bentham, *Works* 485.

who had candidly recognized it in the first edition of volume one of the *Commentaries* in 1765,[27] although one year later in the second edition he added the practical qualification that "juries have of late very frequently taken upon themselves to mitigate these forfeitures."[28] The law of deodand was finally abolished by statute in 1846.

The rules of evidence also offered scope for the reformer. At that time, for example, interested parties could not testify in court – the rule that Mansfield had criticized when applied to witnesses of a will's execution. In 1836, Charles Dickens held up this rule to ridicule by imagining the hilarious case of Bardell v. Pickwick for breach of promise of marriage, one of the most famous legal cases in English literature. Neither Mrs. Bardell nor Mr. Pickwick, the only persons present at the time of the alleged promise, could testify to the words said and the deeds done. Limited to other evidence – what an eavesdropping servant thought she heard and what Pickwick's friends saw after the fact – the jury erroneously found for Mrs. Bardell, and Pickwick finally had to pay damages to escape imprisonment. To avoid this miscarriage of justice in non-fictional cases, Bentham vigorously advocated the abolition of this rule. Like many modern reformers, he urged that all relevant evidence be admitted and the jury left to make necessary allowances for the circumstances. Although the law of evidence has nowhere reached this elegant simplicity, England finally heeded Bentham's call for the admission of the evidence of interested parties in 1851.

Bentham's greatest contributions lay in the area of criminal law. The state of England's prisons was deplorable. Even Blackstone, complacent about so much else, recognized the fact and worked to ameliorate the situation. Of more enduring influence than the Panopticon was Bentham's rational analysis of the role that legal punishments should play in society. To a utilitarian like Bentham, punishment should not be imposed for retribution only. By definition, punishment itself is an evil because it reduces the happiness of the one punished. Working his felicific calculus, Bentham found that the satisfaction of others at the taking of revenge is less than the pain caused by the punishment. Once the criminal had committed the crime, society has to cut the losses to its utility. The only rationale for punishment that promised increased utility is reform of the criminal and deterrence of others.[29]

From this finding, Bentham deduced several important conclusions. First, the punishment should fit the crime, not in the Gilbert-and-Sullivan sense but in the sense that it should be proportional to the severity of the offense. Magna Carta, as we have seen, included a somewhat similar provision: fines should not be excessive but should be "in proportion to the measure of the offense."

27 1 Blackstone, *Commentaries* 291.
28 1 Blackstone, *Commentaries* 354 (2d ed. 1766).
29 Bentham, *The Rationale of Punishment* 20 (1830).

The criminal law, Bentham argued, must form a whole – a criminal code, in fact – in which crimes would be ranked from greater to lesser, and punishments of corresponding severity annexed. Second, since the goal was deterrence, punishment should be swift and certain. Bentham was among the first to point out that the certainty of even a minor punishment has a greater deterrent effect than the remote possibility of a major punishment. Deterrence, in other words, is the product of the severity of the punishment multiplied by the likelihood of its application. Ever given to dramatic statement for effect, Bentham affirmed his belief that "if a fine of a shilling were enough to deter men from committing murder, that would be proper punishment."[30] Eventually, effective policing would end the need for England's "bloody code," the long list of offences (some quite minor) punishable with death, and soon after Bentham died, parliament began a program of serious law reform.

Whenever Bentham – ever the wordsmith – invented a new concept, he coined a new word to denote it, as in labelling his model prison the Panopticon. To Bentham, we owe the words "codify" and "codification." Codification meant more for Bentham than a rational arrangement of law on paper; it also meant the proper allocation of power in the state. The common law was judge-made. Blackstone knew this and celebrated it; Mansfield used it to an extent that shocked his contemporaries, not least Blackstone. In the eyes of the Commentator and conservative jurists generally, statutes were more likely to mar the law than mend it, while Mansfield (as we have seen) observed that "a statute can seldom take in all cases" and concluded that the common law is superior to statute.[31]

Bentham, on the other hand, denounced the common law way of law-making. In this regard, incidentally, he saw eye to eye with Thomas Jefferson. Whatever their disagreements about inalienable rights, Bentham and the sage of Monticello agreed on the impropriety of judges making law and, in particular, on the improper behavior of Lord Mansfield. At one point, Jefferson – foreseeing the trans-Atlantic interchange that would survive American Independence – wrote that he thought it "essential to forbid that any English decision since the accession of Lord Mansfield to the bench, should ever be cited in an American court."[32] The logic of Benthamite utilitarianism demanded that judges should interpret the law narrowly, not creatively, and that change be left to the legislature. By 1912, this message had reached the judicial members of the House of Lords, then Britain's highest court, who declined to overrule their own precedents, leaving legal change to parliament. Celebrity judges

30 Quoted in James A. Colaiaco, *James Fitzjames Stephen and the Crisis of Victorian Thought* 81 (1983) (without citation).

31 Omychund v. Barker, 1 Atk. 22, 33, 26 Eng. Rep. 15, 23 (Ch. 1744).

32 Jefferson to John Brown Cutting, 2 Oct. 1788, in 13 *Papers of Thomas Jefferson* 649 (Julian Boyd ed. 1956).

like Mansfield, their names widely recognized beyond the legal community – even by the mob in the street – became increasingly rare in England. In America, by contrast, the judges' constitutional role would keep them constantly in the public eye.

After long years of preaching law reform, Bentham was dismayed by the small impact his ideas had made. Having scientifically demonstrated his principles, he asked why England's rulers had not leapt at the chance he offered them. The only possible answer was a sinister one: rulers pursued their own selfish interests, not the greatest happiness of the greatest number. The way forward was to give everyone a share in government, that is, to adopt the democratic principle of universal suffrage. Only in that way would the government identify itself with the commonweal, not simply with the self-interest of a limited class of governors. So, in old age, Bentham became a democrat. He still thought that people had no natural and inalienable rights, but he was convinced that society should be organized along utilitarian, that is, Benthamite, lines.

True to his free-thinking creed, Bentham, even in death, shocked conventional sensibilities by leaving his body to be dissected for the advancement of science. (To this day, his skeleton, dressed in the clothes he commonly wore and topped with a waxworks head, may be seen at University College London.) On June 7, 1832, the day after Bentham died, parliament adopted the first Reform Act, which in effect extended the vote to prosperous middle-class males, beginning England's century-long transition to democratic rule. Among the many reasons for the enactment of this epochal legislation, a small one perhaps was the tireless advocacy of the ideologue. But whether or not Bentham's ideas were responsible for reform of the franchise, they were certainly credited with inspiring many of the enactments during the succeeding era, dubbed the "age of reform."[33]

Bentham was blessed in his disciples, a group of middle-class radicals, the most influential kind. They included Francis Place, the "radical tailor," the brilliant economic theorist David Ricardo, the influential jurisprudent John Austin, the tireless philosopher James Mill and the latter's even greater son, John Stuart Mill – plus Edwin Chadwick, designer of the notorious Poor Law and the fearsome workhouses. The Benthamites masterminded campaigns to translate the master's ideas into law. They arranged for friendly articles in influential periodicals, favorable reports by parliamentary committees, and even majorities in the House of Commons.[34]

Independent thinkers can, of course, influence the course of history. One need think only of Karl Marx, the solitary scholar, toiling away in the British

33 See, e.g., Llewellyn Woodward, *The Age of Reform, 1815–1870* (1962), vol. 13 in the Oxford History of England.

34 See S.E. Finer, "The Transmission of Benthamite Ideas, 1820–1850," in *Studies in the Growth of Nineteenth-Century Government* 13 (Gillian Sutherland ed. 1972).

Museum during the years of Bentham's posthumous triumph. But the ideas of the thinker must suit the needs of the day, or they will fall like seeds on rocky ground. Benthamism was an assortment of ideas whose time had come. The English middle class was dissatisfied with a legal system riddled with medieval anachronisms and inconsistencies, even if made workable by the use of ingenious fictions. And judicial activism *à la* Mansfield conflicted with the recognition of the supremacy of the newly reformed parliament. Bentham offered a science of reform, complete with higher learning for the devotees and a slogan – "the greatest happiness of the greatest number" – for the laity. But Benthamite reform was safe from the standpoint of the establishment. The master had had no truck with revolutionary ideas. There were no rights outside the law. And law was to be the product of parliament, controlled at least for the time being by the comfortable classes. Benthamism actually enhanced, rather than sabotaged, established institutions.

Observers credited Bentham with nearly every item of law reform in the nineteenth century. In lectures in 1875, Sir Henry Maine flatly declared that "he did not know a single law reform effected since Bentham's day which cannot be traced to his influence."[35] In the same year, Sir Roland Wilson divided his brief *History of Modern English Law* into before and after Bentham. And a quarter century later, Albert Venn Dicey in a series of influential lectures at Harvard made the division canonical: Blackstonian complacency finally yielded to Benthamite utilitarianism, which Dicey mistakenly equated with laissez-faire liberalism. "The teaching of Bentham," according to Dicey, "exercised so potent an influence that to him is fairly ascribed that thorough-going though gradual amendment of the law of England which was one of the main results of the Reform Act."[36] English legal historians to this day often draw the same line.

One of Bentham's disciples, John Austin took the master's emphasis on analytical rigor to new heights. Briefly a law professor at the newly founded London University (now University College London), Austin published his lectures, *The Province of Jurisprudence Determined* in 1832, the year of Bentham's death. Unlike Blackstone's *Commentaries* a generation earlier, Austin's lectures were largely ignored on publication, although they gained a new lease on life after his death in 1859 when his widow published his collected writings, *Lectures on Jurisprudence, or the Philosophy of Positive Law*. As staked out by Austin, the province of jurisprudence is "positive law," that is, "law set by political superiors to political inferiors,"[37] ignoring the common law's origin in common custom. Making the prototypical law a command in the form of a statute, Austin ignored the large number of statutes, such as the

35 Maine, *Institutions* 397.
36 Dicey, *Law and Opinion* 126.
37 Austin, *Province* 21.

Statute of Frauds or the Statute of Wills, that simply prescribe the means to make an optional and voluntary act legally effective.

Associated with legal positivism is analytical jurisprudence, the close analysis of legal terms – right, duty, power, liberty, injury, punishment, sovereignty, and so on. Emphasizing purely objective description, Austin rigorously excluded questions of morality, bluntly stating: "No *positive* law is *legally* unjust,"[38] initiating the final divorce of law and religion.[39] In 1854, the religious test for matriculation at Oxford – the test that Bentham had lied his way through – was abolished; and in 1871, the religious test for teaching positions at the university was ended. The following year, the first question on "general jurisprudence" set for the law examination was: "Is it necessary to lay down any theory or system of Morals as a foundation for a system of Jurisprudence?"[40] Sir Henry Maine answered the question in print a few years later: "The truth is that Austin's system is consistent with *any* ethical theory."[41] Expanding Maine's answer, a contemporary legal scholar added: "Not only is Austin's conception of law independent of ethics; it is equally independent of politics and religion, and this very independence is one of its greatest merits."[42]

Unlike Blackstone's impact on America, which was immediate and direct, Bentham's was diffuse and belated. The master's ideas on the supremacy of parliament could not be uncritically accepted by Americans, who treasured their Declaration of Independence with its proclamation of inalienable rights and the Constitution with its enforceable Bill of Rights. But Austin's rigor later inspired academically minded lawyers and legal scholars like Yale Law School professor Wesley Newcomb Hohfeld, who published an influential law review article on "fundamental legal conceptions"[43] and called for a comprehensive "restatement of the law" – a project that would keep legal academics busy for decades. U.S. Supreme Court Justice Oliver Wendell Holmes, who read Austin "again and again" during his formative years, embraced Austin's insistence on "positive law" and memorably encapsulated his jurisprudence: "The common law is not a brooding omnipresence in the sky but the articulate voice of some sovereign or quasi-sovereign that can be identified."[44]

In any case, Bentham's ideas arrived too late. By the time of the Revolution, Blackstone had already delivered the common law into American hands,

38 Austin, *Province* 276 n.* (italics in original).

39 For further discussion, see John V. Orth, "Casting the Priests out of the Temple: John Austin and the Relation between Law and Religion," in *The Weightier Matters of the Law: Essays on Law and Religion* 229 (eds. John Witte & Frank S. Alexander 1988).

40 F.H. Lawson, *The Oxford Law School, 1850–1965*, at 192 (1968).

41 Maine, *Institutions* 368 (italics in original).

42 W. Markby, "Analytical Jurisprudence," *Law Magazine & Review*, 4th ser.1 (1876): 617, 624.

43 Wesley Newcomb Hohfeld, "Some Fundamental Legal Conceptions as Applied in Judicial Reasoning," 23 *Yale L.J.* 16 (1913); 26 *Yale L.J.* 710 (1917).

44 Southern Pac. Co. v. Jensen, 244 U.S. 205, 222 (1917) (Holmes, J., dissenting).

conveniently packaged in four volumes. And Bentham's insistence on codification, or at least law reform by legislation, did not travel well. In 1836, Massachusetts asked Justice Joseph Story of the U.S. Supreme Court whether the state's common law could or should be codified. While explaining that he was not one of the "votaries to the notions of Jeremy Bentham," Story conceded that codification of selected areas could be useful.[45] Although prescient of the proliferation of specialized codes in later years, Story's report resulted in no action at the time. The Federal Constitution had created a union of states, each of which was largely free to find its own solutions to the perennial problems of the common law, and state legislatures – distracted by more pressing political problems – showed little interest in codification, content to leave legal matters to the judges, who continued to thumb their Blackstone.

45 1 Charles Warren, *History of the Harvard Law School and of Early Legal Conditions in America* 504 (1908).

PART 2

The Common Law in America

New Challenges

Introduction

English colonists carried the common law with them wherever they went. In 1788, even as Americans were debating whether to adopt the Federal Constitution, the first shipload of English convicts arrived in Australia, their destination chosen after American Independence had closed the penal colonies in North America. With them in the First Fleet went a set of Blackstone's *Commentaries*, which was to provide the basis of Australian law.[1] The American reception of the common law had not been so simple. Arriving long before the publication of Blackstone's "portable common law," early colonists in America erected crude copies of England's courts and legal institutions and applied the common law's half-remembered rules, adapted to the frontier and spiced with common sense and biblical religion. Over time, a "purer" and more sophisticated legal system developed, as the colonists sought to replicate the English model until, soon after the Constitutional Convention, even judges on the edges of American settlement were applying anachronistic common law fictions and forms of action.[2]

Immediately upon publication, Blackstone was in demand in the colonies. Ambitious teenagers like James Iredell in coastal North Carolina and James Kent in rural Connecticut avidly studied the *Commentaries*. Once transplanted in America, the common law adapted to its new environment, one that materially affected many aspects of the law. Changed conditions forced lawyers to reconsider the complacent Blackstonian assumption that "law is the perfection

1 Bruce Kercher, *An Unruly Child: A Brief History of Law in Australia* xii (1995).

2 See, e.g., Judge Harry Innes (U.S. Dist. Ct., Dist. Ky.), in Mary K. Tachau, *Federal Courts in the Early Republic: Kentucky, 1789–1816*, at 83–84 (1978).

DOI: 10.4324/9781003660859-5

of reason."[3] Reason may indeed be timeless and universal, but conditions are not the same always and everywhere. Already in colonial times, an American lawyer could ask whether "what is good law at one time and in one place" is also good law "at another time and in another place."[4] In the early Republic, Justice Joseph Story answered that question on behalf of the U.S. Supreme Court: "The common law of England is not to be taken in all respects to be that of America."[5]

In significant areas, the common law in America, like America itself, was virgin territory. James Kent, by then Chancellor of New York, reported that during his tenure in office "not a single decision, opinion, or dictum" of his predecessors over three decades was cited or even mentioned to him.[6] To save his own decisions from similar oblivion, Kent worked closely with reporter William Johnson to produce reliable reports, especially of his own decisions. Disseminated widely in America, Johnson's Chancery Reports did for Kent what Burrow's Reports had done for Mansfield. After he retired from the bench, Kent continued working to fill the void, producing his four-volume *Commentaries on American Law* between 1826 and 1830, summarizing the developing law in all its proliferating varieties.

Even in the Mother Country, questions of law and reason could arise. On the eve of the American Revolution, as we have seen, Lord Mansfield decided Somerset's Case, holding that slavery was contrary to reason and so could not be recognized at common law. Slavery depended for its existence on "positive law": local legislation or legally binding custom. While the common law could not violate natural law as the lawyers understood it, statutes could. In the new American Republic, statesmen struggled with creating a union of slave and free states. What was law in one place was not law in another.

Conditions in America were different – sometimes, as with slavery, worse; sometimes, as with the elimination (or at least simplification) of cumbersome legal anachronisms, better. While the colonial world tolerated institutions contrary to reason, it also conducted some useful experiments in law reform. The "social laboratories" of the British Empire could test improvements in the law of the Old Country. Even the traditionalist Blackstone, as we have seen, searched the colonial experience for ways to simplify the elaborate strict settlement of landed estates – an early example of local variation, competition if you will, among common law jurisdictions. After Independence, the interchange between periphery and center continued unabated. American courts kept in step with English cases restraining perpetuities, while the English cautiously followed the American lead concerning the property rights of married women.

3 1 Blackstone, *Commentaries* 70.
4 *Trial of John Peter Zenger* (1735) 67–68 (argument of defense counsel Andrew Hamilton).
5 Van Ness v. Packard, 27 U.S. (1 Pet.) 137, 144 (1829).
6 Kent, *Memoirs* 157–158. Kent served as Chancellor from 1814 to 1823.

In its new home, the common law encountered two new legal institutions that dramatically redirected its development: written constitutions and "new model" law schools, both of which had profound and sometimes unexpected implications. In addition, like its parent in England, the common law in America had to come to terms with the increasing volume of statutory production. Just as Blackstone presented legal fictions as a means of legal development and Lord Mansfield drew on the deep wells of equity for reform by judicial decision, statutes – strenuously promoted by Bentham and his followers – eventually became the principal means of legal adjustment, first in England, then in America.

Perhaps the most momentous change of conditions faced by the common law was the profound innovation in basic political organization. Rather than flowing down from the Crown, sovereignty welled up from the people. Promptly on Independence in 1776, colonies became states, most with freshly minted constitutions, organizing the government and declaring rights. Written constitutions with embedded bills of rights were novelties in the common law tradition and created new and unforeseen tensions. No sooner were the newly constituted states independent than they confederated into a new nation, the United States of America. After a brief and unhappy experience under the Articles of Confederation, the people of the United States famously constituted themselves anew in 1788, adopting the still operational Federal Constitution with its associated Bill of Rights, adding yet another layer of fundamental law.

James Iredell, by then a U.S. Supreme Court Justice, raced ahead of his generation in thinking through the implications of adding written constitutions to the common law tradition. No longer could law be based simply on reason and natural law (plus the occasional statute). "The ideas of natural justice are regulated by no fixed standard," he told his fellow justices: "The ablest and purest men have differed upon the subject."[7] The reduction of fundamental law to writing provided the necessary "fixed standard," obviating the need to resort to first principles. Forever after, American constitutional law has remained tethered, however loosely, to the text of the U.S. Constitution.

Experience of oppression, English and colonial, taught the colonists what problems needed to be addressed by their constitutions, while the common law supplied the legal vocabulary and means to deal with them. Not only did the common law help shape the constitutions, it also influenced the way American judges used the constitutional guarantees, increasingly over the years developing them by the traditional common law method of reasoning from case to case – defensible so long as the linkages are reasonably sound.

In turn, the new constitutional order profoundly shaped the common law tradition. The union of states, each with some residual sovereignty under the

7 Calder v. Bull, 3 U.S. (3 Dall.) 386, 388 (1798).

superintendence of the U.S. Supreme Court, meant that a variety of jurisdictions existed within the new American nation, allowing a variety of state constitutional provisions, statutes, and judicial decisions. Unlike the largely unitary legal system of England, where the commitment to *stare decisis* was steadily hardening, the American legal system allowed a "marketplace for laws" to develop, one that over time led to a lively jurisdictional competition among the states. More robust than the earlier jurisdictional competition within the British Empire, this competition produced an array of better, or at least more popular, legal alternatives. And it raised the question how to provide a (more or less) uniform law for a commercial republic composed of multiple jurisdictions.

Another distinctly American contribution to the development of the common law was a new model of legal education, a post-graduate professional school that produced the latest addition to the legal cast of characters, after judges and legislators: law professors. Freed from the daily demands of litigators, clients, and constituents, academic lawyers offered a new perspective. As Blackstone and his imitators refined academic statements of the law and the newly available law reports brought the judges' decisions out of the shadows, law professors initiated a rapid development of legal doctrine, replacing the law's traditional emphasis on property with a newfound commitment to contract, essential to the development of a capitalist economy. In an attempt to standardize American law, legal academics produced a growing body of treatises, eventually embarking on a project to "restate" the entire common law.

The common law was long familiar with statutes, but they were few and far between, usually concerned with land law or criminal law and procedure. For centuries, English lawyers had worked to assimilate statutes to the common law. Most statutes, they said, merely declared what was already (at least implicitly) the law or, at most, cleared up doubtful points. In time, with the rise of positivism, statutes supplanted cases as the most visible form of legal development, but in America, statute law and case law interacted in complex ways. Cases sometimes precipitated statutes, sometimes precluded them. The uniformity demanded in a nation of states led inevitably to professionally drafted codes presented to legislatures for adoption with little discussion or opportunity for amendment. In the event, the triumph of the legislature was often more apparent than real.

4

THE COMMON LAW AND THE CONSTITUTIONS

Near the beginning of his *Commentaries on the Laws of England*, Sir William Blackstone described the common law as *lex non scripta* (unwritten law).[1] By this he did not mean that the common law could not be reduced to writing. He himself wrote hundreds of pages about it. What he meant was that the common law was not found in an authoritative written source such as a code or statute (*lex scripta*) but was found in the decisions of the courts, accessible (to an extent) in reports and abridgments. Like the common law, the English constitution was unwritten. It still is. "Although the United Kingdom does not have a single document entitled 'The Constitution,'" Britain's highest court explained in 2019, "it nevertheless possesses a Constitution, established over the course of our history by common law, statutes, conventions and practices."[2] Blackstone had something similar in mind when he offered instruction to Oxford students on the "constitution of their own country."[3] So did Thomas Jefferson when he denounced King George in the Declaration of Independence for subjecting Americans to juryless admiralty courts, "a jurisdiction foreign to our constitution"[4] – this, before any American constitution in the modern sense. An unwritten constitution may even be better than a written one, or so it appears to British judges: "Since it has not been codified, it has developed pragmatically, and remains sufficiently flexible to be capable of further development."[5]

1 1 Blackstone, *Commentaries* 63.
2 R. (on the application of Miller) v. The Prime Minister, [2019] UKSC 41, [39].
3 Quoted in 12 Holdsworth, *History of English Law* 745–746 (App. IV-1).
4 *Declaration of Independence* para. 15.
5 R. (on the application of Miller) v. The Prime Minister, [2019] UKSC 41, [39].

DOI: 10.4324/9781003660859-6

The Americans who made the Revolution were not convinced. They were content, in general, to leave the common law as it was. Indeed, as we have seen, Jefferson warned that it would be "dangerous" to attempt to reduce the common law to a text. The political organization of the newly independent states, on the other hand, was another matter. It could not be an organic growth like the English constitution; it was inevitably the product of conscious design. First, the newly independent states needed to set up governments based on popular sovereignty, not royal fiat. As a former colonial-officer-turned-revolutionary explained: "At the time of our separation from Great Britain, we were thrown into a similar situation with a set of people shipwrecked and cast on a maroon'd island – without laws, without magistrates, without government, or any legal authority."[6] Like so many Robinson Crusoes, the ex-colonials had to establish their own individual commonwealths. Elections had to be held, voter qualifications established. There had to be legislators, a chief executive, and judges. But the machinery of government, however necessary, was not the most important thing.

Having experienced what they thought were unchecked abuses by colonial officials, the newly independent Americans were determined to guarantee the freedom they had fought for. No longer would the protection of their basic rights be left to unwritten law. Like the barons who forced King John to put his royal seal to Magna Carta, the Americans wanted it in writing – and not just in a statute. It had to be part of a new kind of document, a legally enforceable bill of rights embedded in a written constitution. Many states began their constitution-writing with a solemn declaration of rights. In the new state of North Carolina, the declaration was adopted *before* the "constitution," which established the machinery of government[7] – although the latter incorporated the former by reference. To put its importance to the new state beyond doubt, the constitution concluded with the imperative requirement that the declaration "ought never to be violated, on any pretence whatsoever."[8] Summarizing the lessons learned from the long history of English constitutional struggle and from the more recent colonial grievances, including abusive prosecutions, the declaration guaranteed fundamental rights such as freedom of religion and the press and also provided detailed protections for criminal defendants – from search and arrest through trial and punishment.

What makes constitutions so prominent in the American mind today are not the details of government, essential as they are, but the rights they guarantee – particularly in the first ten amendments to the Federal Constitution, known collectively as the Bill of Rights, many copied from the earlier state declarations

6 Den on the Dem. of Bayard v. Singleton, 1 N.C. 5, 6 (1 Mart. 42, 43) (1787) (Ashe, J.).

7 *The Colonial Records of North Carolina* 10: 973 (17 Dec. 1776) (Declaration of Rights); *Colonial Records* 10: 974 (18 Dec. 1776) (Constitution).

8 N.C. Const. of 1776, § 44.

of rights. While Blackstone made cautious use of the concept of a "social contract," and Bentham derided it as just another legal fiction, the Americans actually put it in writing. "With us," a Virginia judge pointed out in 1793, paraphrasing Tom Paine, "the constitution is not an 'ideal thing, but a real existence: it can be produced in a visible form.'"[9]

So attractive did the ex-colonials find the idea of written constitutions with declarations (or bills) of rights that almost all the newly independent colonies drafted one soon after Independence. (For complicated political reasons, Rhode Island continued to use its colonial charter for another half-century.) Today, there is a written constitution for each of the 50 states – creating, incidentally, the opportunity for a project of comparative constitutionalism reminiscent of one carried out in antiquity by Aristotle.[10] But so dominant has the U.S. Constitution become in the popular consciousness that many Americans think of it as *the* American constitution and find it odd to talk about "American constitutions" in the plural. Written constitutions in the American sense, arranging offices and guaranteeing rights, were an innovation in the common law tradition, soon to be widely copied. Indeed, one scholar has observed that the "basic form of the American Constitution, together with its underlying political theory, is comparable in its global influence to that of Roman law."[11]

American constitutions emerged from the common law world and were shaped by it. Many of the procedural protections – such as the privilege against self-incrimination, the prohibition of double jeopardy, and the right to a hearing – that are now enumerated in the constitutions began as common law practices. The texts presuppose the existence of the common law, using terms drawn from its vocabulary, such as *ex post facto* law, bill of attainder, and corruption of blood. Due process of law is guaranteed by all American constitutions. As a phrase, "due process" is as old as the seventeenth century[12]; as a concept, it is as old as Magna Carta's requirement of proceeding according to "the law of the land." (Indeed, some current state constitutions like North Carolina's still preserve the older phrase.) When the U.S. Supreme Court had to give the guarantee of due process operational meaning, it looked to the

9 Kamper v. Hawkins, 3 Va. (1 Va. Cas.) 20, 78 (Gen. Ct. 1793) (Tucker, J.). See Thomas Paine, *The Rights of Man* [1791], in *Collected Writings* 467 (1995) ("A constitution is not a thing in name only, but in fact. It has not an ideal, but a real existence; and wherever it cannot be produced in visible form, there is none.").

10 The only surviving product of Aristotle's project of comparing the constitutions of the Greek city states is the *Constitution of Athens*, reprinted in 2 *Complete Works of Aristotle: The Revised Oxford Translation* 2341 (Jonathan Barnes ed.; Benjamin Jowett trans. 2009).

11 Peter H. Russell, *Constitutional Odyssey: Can Canadians Become a Sovereign People?* 9 (3d ed. 2004).

12 Edward Coke, *Second Institute* 50 (1648). Coke derived the phrase from a statute in Law French, citing 25 Edw. 3, st. 5, c. 4 (1350) (*en due manere ou process fait sur brief original a la commune lei*). See 1 Holdsworth, *History of English Law* 59–63.

"settled usages and modes of proceeding existing in the common and statute law of England before the emigration of our ancestors."[13]

Trial by jury was a distinctive development of the common law, unknown to the law of Rome or the civil law systems derived from it; Americans were convinced of the jury's value and were determined to preserve it. The Sixth Amendment in the Federal Bill of Rights expressly guarantees an "impartial jury" in "all criminal prosecutions," while the Seventh Amendment guarantees trial by jury in civil cases "according to the rules of the common law." Because the Seventh Amendment is interpreted to guarantee whatever right was accorded at ratification in 1791, eighteenth-century English practice remains of more than historical interest.[14] The importance that constitution-writers, state and federal, attached to trial by jury has led American judges to go to extraordinary lengths to respect the deliberations of the jury. The North Carolina Supreme Court once held that it was reversible error for a trial judge to say that two opposing witnesses were both "gentlemen." The jury had to be free to decide without comment whether one or both were not.[15]

In the later history of the Republic, the guarantee of trial by jury has played a paradoxical role. Originally intended to protect defendants from oppressive judges, juries also protect judges from public anger. Even in the old days of monarchy, judges realized that, as Sir Thomas More once explained, "they may by the verdict of the jury cast off all quarrels from themselves."[16] This protective function is particularly attractive in a government based on popular sovereignty – even more so when American states began choosing judges by direct election. To this day, the consequences of electing judges are debated. In a final irony, jury trials are increasingly rare in modern America, replaced by "plea bargains" between prosecutors and criminal defendants.

In another, darker sense, the U.S. Constitution also bears witness to the omnipresence of the common law. Soon after Lord Mansfield ruled that slavery was so "odious" that it was irreconcilable with the common law, American constitution-makers had to confront the problem of constructing a union half slave and half free. How to recognize the enslaved population in a republic based on popular sovereignty? And what about slaves escaping into states without laws or customs recognizing the institution? While scrupulously avoiding the use of the words slave or slavery in deference to Northern sensitivities, the Framers nonetheless unmistakably referred to the condition. In the very first article of the Constitution, the "federal population" for purposes of representation was calculated by "adding to the whole Number of free Persons…,

13 Tumey v. Ohio, 273 U.S. 510, 523 (1928).
14 See, e.g., Markman v. Westview Instruments, Inc., 517 U.S. 370 (1996).
15 McRae v. Lawrence, 75 N.C. 289 (1876).
16 Quoted in *A Man of Singular Virtue being A Life of Sir Thomas More by his son-in-law William Roper* 63 (A.L. Rowse ed. 1980).

three-fifths of all other Persons" – in other words, enslaved persons.[17] The notorious fugitive slave clause made use of a different circumlocution: "No person held to service or labour in one state, under the laws thereof, escaping into another, shall, in consequence of any law or regulation therein, be discharged from such service or labour."[18] The laws or regulations that denied recognition to slavery were not only statutes in the free states but also and more fundamentally the common law itself.

After Independence, the common law in America would develop within the framework established by the constitutions, both state and federal. But American constitutionalism would also develop in ways shaped by the common law. In a world of texts, the common law is not a text but a process. When written constitutions were added to the common law tradition – or, more precisely, when written constitutions were incorporated into that tradition – it was without conscious recognition of the dynamic thereby established. Common law judges had long experience with documents – statutes and charters, deeds and wills, leases and mortgages, covenants and indentures – and they read the constitutions as they had read the documents, sometimes strictly, sometimes quite expansively. Furthermore, over time, the judges increasingly treated their constitutional decisions as precedents to be developed further in the traditional common law way of reasoning from case to case, adding a flexibility seemingly at odds with a written constitution.

Custody of the constitutions enhanced, if that were possible, the role of the judge in America's common law tradition. Scrutiny of legislative and executive action for possible constitutional violations gave judges exceptional power. And the recruitment of American judges from among the ranks of successful practitioners (and politicians) meant that too deferential an attitude was unlikely to prevail for long. More generally, as Justice Story once remarked: "The discussion of constitutional questions throws a lustre round the bar, and gives a dignity to its functions, which can rarely belong to the profession in any other country"[19] – including, he might have added, in the Mother Country herself.

At the apex of the federal judicial system is a single high court: "one supreme Court."[20] It is difficult today to appreciate how significant a break this represented with the English legal system. What seems an obvious institutional arrangement, in fact, meant that the federal legal system would not perpetuate the centuries-long separation of law and equity that existed in England until the 1870s, although some states did. (Indeed, Delaware still does.) The idea of combining law and equity was not new – perhaps nothing in the common law

17 U.S. Const. art. I, § 2.
18 U.S. Const. art. IV, § 2.
19 Story, *Miscellaneous Writings* 227.
20 U.S. Const. art. III, § 1.

tradition is. Francis Bacon reported on the English debate in the seventeenth century: "Some hold that the jurisdiction which decrees according to equity and conscience, and that which proceeds according to strict justice, ought to be deputed to the same courts; but others would have them kept separate." "I am clearly for keeping them separate," Bacon declared: "For if there be a mixture of jurisdictions, the distinction of cases will not be maintained, but discretion will in the end supersede the law."[21] Blackstone agreed, warning Lord Mansfield against "vague discretionary law."[22] As Bacon presciently foresaw, the merger of law and equity would not end competition between these ancient systems but simply move it into a single forum – and, perhaps, give the advantage to the one that maximized judicial discretion. How freely American judges should substitute their personal judgment for strict adherence to the letter of the law remains an open question.

One of the grievances of colonial Americans had been the insecurity of judicial tenure. Although English judges since 1701 no longer served merely at the pleasure of the Crown, colonial judges remained in that precarious position. As a Philadelphia lawyer tactlessly reminded one colonial judge, it is "a disagreeable tenure to any officer, but a dangerous one in the case of a judge."[23] Among the causes for revolution catalogued in the Declaration of Independence was that King George made colonial judges "dependent on his Will alone, for the tenure of their offices, and the amount and payment of their salaries."[24] In response, the U.S. Constitution provided for a life-tenured judiciary: "The Judges, both of the supreme and inferior Courts, shall hold their Offices during good Behaviour, and shall, at stated Times, receive for their Services, a Compensation, which shall not be diminished during their Continuance in Office."[25] Life tenure and a guaranteed income freed federal judges from politics; some would say it freed activist federal judges *for* politics.

Over the centuries, the English system had gradually separated the functions of government into legislative, executive, and judicial. In the seventeenth century, Sir Edward Coke had tried to use the courts to limit the power of an overreaching monarch: "The common law hath admeasured the King's prerogative,"[26] Coke solemnly declared. But by Blackstone's day, it was plain that parliament rather than the courts had gained supremacy. The French

21 Bacon's Aphorism 45 in *Examples of a Treatise on Universal Justice* (J. Stephen ed. 1889).

22 1 *A Collection of Tracts Relative to the Law of England* (Francis Hargrave ed. 1787), 489, 491, 496 (Blackstone's opinion in Perrin v. Blake).

23 *Trial of John Peter Zenger* (1735) 84 (argument for defendant by Andrew Hamilton).

24 *Declaration of Independence* para. 11.

25 U.S. Const. art. III, § 1. Tenure during good behavior is not a guarantee of continuance in office but a guarantee that removal from office may only be "for cause," not simply at will.

26 Quoted in Catherine Drinker Bowen, *The Lion and the Throne: The Life and Times of Sir Edward Coke* 484 (1956) (referring to Darnell's Case, 3 How. St. Tr. 1 (K.B. 1627) (The Five Knights Case)).

political philosopher Montesquieu, looking to the earlier era, idealized the separation of powers, and Americans incorporated it in their constitutions. It is implicit in the structure of the Federal Constitution. In state constitutions, the separation is often explicit, as in the Maryland Constitution of 1776: "The legislative, executive, and supreme judicial powers ought to be forever separate and distinct."[27] But the implications of separated powers for judicial law-making remained indistinct. American judges, state and federal, continued to develop the common law just as their English predecessors had before them. To rationalize the reality, one has either to find the creative function inherent in the common law concept of "judicial power" or to indulge the legal fiction that it has been delegated by the legislature – or, in the case of elected judges, by the people themselves. Or perhaps the Founders had not given it a thought, and the judges just kept doing what common law judges had always done.

But there is a judicial power that could not possibly have been delegated by the legislature: the power of the judges to declare acts of the legislature unconstitutional and *void*, the power known today as "judicial review" – the American refinement of the medieval barons' clumsy enforcement mechanism in Magna Carta. In England, the dawning recognition of what the logic of parliamentary supremacy demanded eventually led the judges there to reject the claim that the courts could invalidate acts of parliament – demonstrating that judicial review is not a necessary byproduct of the common law. In time, English courts even became reluctant to overrule their own precedents, preferring instead to leave legal change to parliament. Ironically, it was the country without a written constitution or express commitment to separation of powers that witnessed a more complete distinction between law-making and dispute resolution than the United States.

In America, written constitutions gave the judges the necessary opening. A constitution is a law, the U.S. Supreme Court early held in the celebrated case of *Marbury v. Madison* (1803),[28] a law in the sense that the judicial branch construes it but not in the sense that the law-making branch can amend or repeal it, making the judges the primary defenders of constitutional order. By contrast, case law, law that the judges make in their decisions of individual cases, is a law that the judiciary can distinguish or overrule – or, more candidly, amend or repeal. But while the common law in America remained largely unwritten, disclosed by the judges in the course of their decisions, the new American constitutions were there for all to see – and ready to be invoked by ordinary citizens. "In America," Tom Paine emphatically declared, "THE LAW IS KING."[29] But the restraints originally intended to limit the power of

27 Md. Const. of 1776, Declaration of Rights § 6.
28 5 U.S. (1 Cranch) 137 (1803).
29 Thomas Paine, *Common Sense* [1776], in *Collected Writings* 34 (1995) (capitalization in original).

a sovereign monarch also limit the power of the sovereign people – who sometimes, like the old kings, chafe at the restrictions.

Judicial review may have been inevitable in a legal system with a written constitution, but the new start offered by the formation of a new court also opened the door for innovations in traditional judicial procedure. In the first decade of the U.S. Supreme Court, the judges continued the time-hallowed English practice of delivering their opinions seriatim, one after another. English judges over the centuries had, of course, occasionally disagreed, but they registered their disagreement in their individual opinions, rendered not after the enunciation of the majority's opinion but in their proper turn to speak. In America, Justice James Iredell's lengthy opinion disagreeing with his fellow justices appeared first in 1793 in the report of *Chisholm v. Georgia*, which held a state liable on a contract between itself and a citizen of another state[30] – a decision overturned by a constitutional amendment that did not actually "amend" the constitution but instead instructed the justices on its proper construction.[31]

With the appointment of John Marshall as Chief Justice in 1801, the practice of seriatim opinions disappeared. Perhaps taking his cue from Lord Mansfield, who, as we have seen, had briefly managed to end seriatim opinions in King's Bench, Marshall pioneered the unitary "opinion of the court," beginning with the very first decision after his confirmation.[32] The "opinion of the court," now standard practice throughout the United States, emphasized the collective nature of the judgment and shielded individual judges from criticism – to the irritation of Jefferson, who thought the judges should be required to take individual responsibility for the result.[33] So familiar is the single "opinion of the court" today that American lawyers are startled to learn that common law practice for five hundred years was otherwise and that common law courts everywhere but in America continue the practice. Over the years, judicial unanimity proved increasingly difficult to maintain. The inevitable corollary of the unitary opinion of the court is the dissent, expressly so labelled – another distinctive American innovation in judicial practice, and one that necessarily gives rise to questions about the inescapable logic of legal reasoning. As Justice Oliver Wendell Holmes once remarked, a dissenter appears to be scolding the majority for "not doing their sums right."[34]

30 2 U.S. (2 Dall.) 419 (1793). For a comment about the substance of Iredell's dissent, see John V. Orth, "The Truth About Justice Iredell's Dissent in Chisholm v. Georgia," 73 *N.C. L. Rev.* 255 (1994).

31 See John V. Orth, "'Shall Not Be Construed': Reversal of Supreme Court Decisions by Constitutional Amendment," 72 *Fla. L. Rev. Online* 114 (2022).

32 Talbot v. Seeman, 5 U.S. (1 Cranch) 1 (1801).

33 Jefferson to William Johnson, 4 March 1823, in 12 *Works of Thomas Jefferson* 279–280 (P.L. Ford ed. 1905).

34 O.W. Holmes, "The Path of the Law," 10 *Harv. L. Rev.* 457, 465 (1897).

John Marshall and his generation of judges could recall the world before the U.S. Constitution, and they naturally construed that document in light of the wrongs it was intended to remedy (or prevent). As the years passed, the intention of the drafters and the particular mischiefs that inspired them receded. New problems were perceived, and the judges searched the text for guidance, just as they searched prior judicial reports for guidance in the decision of novel cases. And like the common law judges before them, they also appealed directly to reason. Parts of the text, particularly the pregnant common law phrase "due process of law," allowed ample scope for the exercise of discretion. Just as reason may be timeless and universal but conditions change, so the words remain the same but the judicial construction of them may vary, leading to the perennial and probably irresolvable debate about whether the judges are limited to the "original understanding," if indeed that understanding can be recovered today. What cannot be doubted is that each successive decision construing the text – in some cases amounting to an "informal amendment"[35] – widens the gap between the text and its meaning, just as the gap widens between the first case in a line of precedents and the last.

As the common law tradition shaped American constitutionalism, so the constitutional structure shaped the development of American common law. The Federal Constitution creates a union of states, but the states are united only at certain points. The national government is supreme with respect to the powers delegated to it and the rights protected by it, but the states retain – at least on paper – much of their original sovereignty. This elementary civics lesson has important consequences for the common law tradition in America.

In *Federalist Number 3*, John Jay made the case for national courts in terms of the new Republic's need to speak with a single voice in its relations with foreign powers: "Under the national government, treaties and articles of treaties, as well as the laws of nations, will always be expounded in one sense and executed in the same manner, whereas adjudications on the same points and questions in thirteen States… will not always accord or be consistent"[36] – another acknowledgement that reason may not necessarily lead all judges to the same result in every case. As Jay recognized, the federal system allows for variations among the states on many "points and questions," variations that only increased as the number of states inexorably grew. While uniformity was imperative for America's dealings with foreign nations, it was not necessarily so in other areas. State constitutions, state statutes, even state common law may vary considerably within wide limits.

35 See John V. Orth, John Gava, Arvind P. Bhanu, and Paul T. Babie, "Judges, 'Informal Amendment,' and the Evolution of Constitutional Meaning in the Federal Democracies of Australia, Canada, India, and the United States," 48 *Pepperdine L. Rev*. 1 (2021).

36 *Federalist Papers* No. 3, p. 98. Blackstone defined the "law of nations" as "a system of rules, deducible by natural reason, and established by universal consent among the civilized inhabitants of the world." 4 Blackstone, *Commentaries* 66. The law of nations, today more commonly called international law, is particularly important in international trade.

Justice Louis Brandeis once claimed that "one of the happy incidents of the federal system" is "that a single courageous State may, if its citizens choose, serve as a laboratory; and try novel social and economic experiments without risk to the rest of the country."[37] If they pass muster under the Federal Constitution, the results of these legal experiments are guaranteed a degree of acceptance throughout the Union: "Full Faith and Credit shall be given in each State to the public Acts, Records, and judicial Proceedings of every other State."[38] Successful (or, at least, popular) experiments are quickly repeated elsewhere, illustrating a general phenomenon of legal development that led one modern legal scholar to gloss the famous aphorism that "reason is the life of the law" and Holmes's just as famous rejoinder that "the life of the law has not been logic: it has been experience," by insisting that, in fact, "the life of the law has not been logic and it has not been experience. It has been borrowing."[39]

Jurisdictional competition in America is constant and robust, making the country in some instances resemble an archipelago of competing jurisdictions rather than a unitary nation. Whether this competition is good or bad depends on one's point of view. The results of the "social experiments" conducted by the states may be hailed for providing greater scope for individual initiative and a wider range of personal and economic choices, sometimes described as a "release of energy."[40] Alternatively, they may be blamed for degrading legal standards, in which case they are commonly characterized as a "race to the bottom" – more candidly, competition to get to a destination we do not wish to reach.

State and federal constitutions interact in complex ways. In an important early case, the U.S. Supreme Court held that the general prohibition of *ex post facto* laws in the Federal Bill of Rights applied only to criminal, not to civil laws – in part because the similar clauses in state constitutions were explicitly so limited.[41] And just as the Federal Bill of Rights copied many provisions found in prior state constitutions, so later state constitutions copied provisions in the Federal Constitution. The similar (or identical) wording of some provisions has led to a lively debate whether state courts should follow federal precedents or develop their own interpretations (always within the limits set by the federal courts). When the U.S. Supreme Court decided that a city could, without violating the Federal Bill of Rights, take one person's private property and turn it over to another private person[42] – once considered the paradigmatic

37 New State Ice Co. v. Liebmann, 285 U.S. 262, 280, 311 (1932) (Brandeis, J., dissenting).

38 U.S. Const. art. IV, § 1.

39 Watson, *Spirit of Roman Law* 111, 205.

40 See John V. Orth, "The Release of Energy: Reflections on a Legal History Trope," 34 *Adelaide L. Rev.* 159 (2013).

41 Calder v. Bull, 3 U.S. (3 Dall.) 386, 396–397 (1798) (citing constitutions of Massachusetts, Delaware, Maryland, and North Carolina).

42 *Kelo v. City of New London*, 545 U.S. 469 (2005).

violation of due process[43] – some states reacted by amending their own constitutions, placing express limits on the power of condemnation in order to prevent similar judgments in state courts. Conversely, when the U.S. Supreme Court held that due process (or was it equal protection?) forbids the denial of marriage licenses to same-sex couples,[44] it was following in the footsteps of Massachusetts' highest court which had earlier reached the same conclusion based on the state constitution.[45]

Statutes provide the most obvious opportunity for variation. Exploiting their residual sovereignty, states can use their law-making power in ways that distinguish them from their neighbors. A form of competition among states was bound to break out, creating a marketplace for laws, so to speak. In 1867, the Dakota territorial legislature reduced the residency requirement for obtaining a divorce to 90 days, at the time the quickest route to end a marital deadlock. When Dakota eventually raised the residency requirement, attention switched to Nevada where relaxed standards made it the destination of choice for those seeking rapid release from the bonds of matrimony. Despite reluctance in other states, popular demand led to increasingly lower thresholds for divorce, until in 1969 California became the first state to experiment with "no-fault divorce," a permissive regime that eventually spread throughout the country – effectively putting an end to the concept of marriage as a contract. Legalized gambling, another Nevada innovation, similarly spread widely, although legalized prostitution remains confined to certain Nevada counties.

Travel is obviously necessary if physical presence is required to enjoy the benefit of local law, but some advantages can be accessed remotely. Since money passes freely within the United States, well-endowed individuals can take advantage of attractive opportunities without leaving home. A lively competition has broken out among the states to secure the trust business of the wealthy by offering better (that is, less restrictive) trust law; today, it is even possible in certain cases for settlors to protect their assets from the claims of their own creditors. There had long been competition for trust business between American states, on the one hand, and foreign nations (particularly small island nations) on the other. What foreign nations could not offer, however, was the stability and security of American law.

Sometimes new ideas originated abroad. Beginning in the 1920s, Latin American countries authorized condominiums as a form of property ownership. Experience with the arrangement in Puerto Rico, an unincorporated territory of the United States, demonstrated its appeal. Putting common law building blocks together in a novel way – attaching inseverable easements to fee

43 See John V. Orth, "Taking from A and Giving to B: Substantive Due Process and the Case of the Shifting Paradigm," 14 *Constitutional Commentary* 337 (1997).
44 Obergefell v. Hodges, 576 U.S. 644 (2015).
45 Goodridge v. Department of Public Health, 798 N.E.2d 941 (Mass. 2003).

simple estates – and adding legislative schemes for self-government, the "condo" is now a feature of real estate development throughout the United States. Community property, whereby married couples each benefit from the earnings of either spouse, is another innovation borrowed from civil law. Its availability in Western states with Spanish or French backgrounds demonstrated its appeal and has led to ingenious attempts to secure a similar benefit in states that continue to adhere to the traditional common law "separate property" regime.

Not all foreign imports thrived in the United States. In 1857, Robert Torrens, an imaginative legal reformer in the Australian colony of South Australia, developed an improved system for establishing title to land by registration with the state. The benefits of Torrens registration were obvious: the owner got a secure title subject only to encumbrances listed on the certificate of registration. Once in the Torrens system, title could be conveyed simply by filing with the registrar an instrument of transfer executed by the seller and the certificate of title. "Torrens title," as it came to be called, spread rapidly throughout the Australian colonies and in time became nearly universal in the common law world – but not in the United States.[46] Although a significant number of American states experimented with the system of "registered titles" in the late nineteenth and early twentieth centuries, with few exceptions the system failed in competition with the cumbersome but established system of "title searching" plus warranties of title and title insurance – demonstrating that "survival of the fittest" means no more than that whatever survives is the fittest.

Residual state sovereignty also permits states to bid against one another for economic advantage. Starting in the 1890s, New Jersey and Delaware competed for the privilege of chartering corporations (and reaping the associated benefits). The states engaged in a sort of Dutch auction, progressively offering better and better (that is, lower and lower) terms in their standard-form corporate charters. Eventually, New Jersey dropped out of the running, and Delaware won the race – which is why today one of the nation's smallest states hosts the "headquarters" of so many large corporations and why Delaware's equity court is one of the world's most important business courts. Seeking investment to provide jobs and increase tax revenue, states regularly compete with one another by unseemly offers of "incentives" in the form of tax reductions or gifts of property. In a unitary nation like England, central administrative control limits such competition; local authorities there have little reason to engage in bidding for business. And in Europe as a whole, the construction of a continental common market has led to restrictions on "state aids" that distort economic decision-making.

Judicial development of the common law, too, has varied from state to state since the founding of the Republic. Recognizing slavery where permitted by

46 See John V. Orth, "Where Torrens Failed," 46 *Adelaide L. Rev.* 112 (2025).

statutes or local custom while denying it recognition at common law, as Lord Mansfield had done for the British Empire, became increasingly unworkable in the American Union. In slave states, statutes or custom failed to address every issue raised by the region's "peculiar institution," and the common law was necessarily called upon to adapt traditional rules and procedures, leading to chilling actions like "trover for a slave."[47] As one candid judge in a slave state put it: "It is the common law, cut down by statute or custom, so as to tolerate slavery."[48]

If written constitutions were America's greatest contribution to the common law tradition, its worst was the creation of a common law of slavery. Because the common law had never abandoned its vague connection with natural law, the attempt to integrate slavery created for many lawyers and ordinary citizens an unbearable tension. Ralph Waldo Emerson, transcendental philosopher and poet, called the Fugitive Slave Act of 1850 a "filthy enactment." Shocked that it was adopted "by people who could read and write," he vowed: "I will not obey it, by God!"[49] As pressure for resolution increased, Walt Whitman apostrophized the states: "Were you looking to be held together by the lawyers? By an agreement on a paper? Or by arms?"[50] The final answer was given on the great battlefields of the Civil War – and subsequently written into the United States Constitution in a series of amendments that abolished slavery and created a national citizenship, redefining the relationship between state and federal governments – effectively a "second American Revolution."

Common law rules not freighted with such high moral concerns also varied among states, leading to the law school game of "majority and minority rules" – as if the choices were binary. Variations among states also meant that a court confronting a novel question could search jurisdictions near and far for solutions, often comparing and contrasting the results, demonstrating the value of competition in the legal marketplace – at the expense of multiple and conflicting rules. One scholar has suggested that the resulting complexity of the common law in America explains the remarkable prominence of lawyers in the nation's economy: "Far more than in any other civilized country is it necessary in the United States on account of the multiplicity of laws, for men engaged in business to have the constant advice of lawyers."[51]

While the drafters of the Federal Constitution had foreseen the need to protect the common market by protecting interstate commerce from legislative

47 E.g., Barwick v. Barwick, 33 N.C. (11 Ired.) 80 (1850).

48 State v. Reed, 9 N.C. (2 Hawks) 454, 457 (1823) (Henderson, J.). See Joseph L. Hyde, "The Common Law Cut Down: Homicide and Human Property in Post-Colonial North Carolina," 36 *Australia Bar Rev.* 1 (2012).

49 Quoted in 1 Samuel Morison et al., *The Growth of the American Republic* 567 (1980) (citing Emerson's journal).

50 Walt Whitman, "States," Calamus 5, *Leaves of Grass* 30 (1860–1861).

51 John Maxcy Zane, *The Story of Law* [1927] 376 (1998).

barriers to trade, they had not foreseen that the common law of states could diverge and endanger that market. National courts offered one solution. In the United States, the federal system gave litigants a choice of federal or state courts in many civil cases, at least when the parties were not citizens of the same state. In the early nineteenth century, a New York case demonstrated the disruptive potential of variations among the states. Divergence on an obscure point of commercial law threatened to interfere with the smooth functioning of the national credit market.

In 1842, in a ringing opinion in Swift v. Tyson,[52] Justice Joseph Story – just then completing a massive "commentary" on bills of exchange – asserted the power of federal courts, in the absence of state statutes, to decide the case as a matter of "general common law." "The law respecting negotiable instruments," Story declared, echoing a decision by Lord Mansfield, is "not the law of a single country only, but of the commercial world"[53] – the law, in other words, "of nations." The effect of the decision in favor of independent determination by federal courts was the creation of a national commercial law, albeit at the expense of allowing inconsistent results in cases brought in state and federal courts – "forum-shopping" reminiscent of that among the old common law courts. For almost a century afterwards, federal judges exploited their "diversity jurisdiction" to offer litigants a better, or at least a national, brand of commercial law.

Only in 1938 did the U.S. Supreme Court put an end to this jurisdictional competition. In Erie Railroad v. Tompkins,[54] the court forcefully repudiated the rule in *Swift*, contradicting Story and roundly declaring: "There is no general federal common law." Ironically, the opinion of the court was authored by Justice Brandeis, who only a few years earlier had lauded "social experiments" conducted in different jurisdictions. Quoting from opinions by the late Justice Holmes, Brandeis described the "fallacy" underlying *Swift* as the assumption that there is a "transcendental body of law" existing outside any particular jurisdiction. In starkly positivist terms, Brandeis, again quoting Holmes, denied that the common law derives its authority from reason and natural law, independent of the state – whatever may have been the law, as he said, "in England or anywhere else." "The authority and only authority is the State, and if that be so, the voice adopted by the State as its own (whether it be of its Legislature or of its Supreme Court) should utter the last word."[55] – offering an answer to the lingering question how to reconcile judge-made case law with the constitutional requirement of separation of powers. (Incidentally, the common

52 41 U.S. (16 Pet.) 1, 19 (1842).

53 Luke v. Lyde, 2 Burr. 883, 887, 97 Eng. Rep. 614, 617 (K.B. 1765).

54 304 U.S. 64 (1938).

55 304 U.S. at 79 (quoting Kuhn v. Fairmont Coal, 215 U.S. 349, 370–372 (1910); Black & White Taxicab & Transfer Co. v. Brown & Yellow Taxicab & Transfer Co., 276 U.S. 518, 532–536 (1928) (Holmes, J., dissenting)).

law was not so easily banished from federal courts: federal judges continued to appeal to common law principles in cases concerning federal contracts or torts or to fill gaps in federal statutes.)

Without a general commercial law developed and enforced by federal courts, how was the national market to be preserved from the emergence of variations among the several states? Luckily, the other major forces acting on the common law in America – "new model" law schools and increased legislative activity – provided an answer. National law schools graduated cadres of elite lawyers trained in the "fundamental principles" of the common law, not local particularities. Through their work in practice, on the bench, and in the academy, they fostered the homogenization once provided by federal courts. Systematic "restatements of the law" sought to standardize the common law as applied by state courts, while "uniform laws" on a multitude of topics were proposed for adoption unchanged in every jurisdiction. The law professors were there to help.

5

THE COMMON LAW AND THE LAW SCHOOLS

In 1882, Albert Venn Dicey, the newly elected Vinerian Professor of English Law at Oxford – the seventh since Blackstone – chose a surprising question as the topic for his inaugural lecture: "Can English law be taught at the universities?"[1] He meant at the *English* universities. The fact that the question was still worth asking more than a hundred years after Blackstone had delivered the first Vinerian lectures, the lectures that resulted in his *Commentaries on the Laws of England*, reveals the extraordinary slowness of the common law to accept domestication in the academy. Blackstone's successors as Vinerian Professors, including his own son James, had done little to render the question moot.

To no one's surprise, Dicey, who had been chosen expressly to re-invigorate the Vinerian professorship, answered his question in the affirmative: "Yes, English law *can* be taught at English universities." After candidly acknowledging certain strengths of the traditional method of learning law by apprenticeship, Dicey insisted upon the benefits to be gained in perspective, analysis, and definition from university instruction. Cases, Dicey explained, give "inordinate attention to anomalies and exceptions"; "every reported case… is the record of some exception to a general rule." In consequence, traditionally trained lawyers, he said, are "forced to go a good deal on what an eminent lawyer has termed 'law taken for granted.'" University education can supply the rules that the exceptions "prove."

More surprising, though for a different reason, were Professor Dicey's reflections 16 years later concerning "the teaching of English law at Harvard,"

1 A.V. Dicey, *Can English Law Be Taught at the Universities? An Inaugural Lecture* (1883).

DOI: 10.4324/9781003660859-7

a byproduct of an invitation to deliver a series of lectures there.[2] That common law, English in origin, formed the basis of instruction at the Harvard Law School, as it formed the basis of law in every American state except Louisiana (where French law had put down deep roots) demonstrates its hardiness and adaptability to the new conditions in America. But that it could still be thought of, at least by an Englishman, as other than American after well over a century of development in an independent republic is remarkable. Admittedly, American public law was different – republican government, written constitutions, and accumulating legislation made it so – but private law, which constituted the largest part of instruction at Harvard, as at all American law schools, remained to a surprising degree recognizably "English." Of course, the British Empire was then at the height of its power and prestige, and throughout the nineteenth century, American higher education had presented English, rather than American, history as the proper subject of study for the sons of the elite.[3] Like the English language, English common law kept America culturally, if not politically, associated with the Mother Country.

Even as Dicey was lecturing at Harvard, Yale law students were still being taught property, tort, and criminal law by reference to Blackstone's *Commentaries*, aided by charts prepared by their professor.[4] And the dean at Duke (then Trinity) Law School in North Carolina based his classes on the *Commentaries* well into the twentieth century.[5] In many states, Blackstone remained required reading for the bar examination. Of even more consequence, the common law way of doing business continued to affect the way American constitutions and statutes were interpreted and everyday disputes resolved. One reason that "English law" persisted in America was historical: the American Revolutionaries had fought *for* the common law, not against it. The pre-Revolutionary Continental Congress in 1774 expressly laid claim to "the rights of life, liberty, and property, *and the common law of England*."[6] But what kept the

2 A.V. Dicey, "The Teaching of English Law at Harvard," 13 *Harv. L. Rev.* 422 (1900) (reprinted from 76 *The Contemporary Rev.* 742 (Nov. 1899)). Dicey's lectures on the "development of English law in the nineteenth century" were "reconsidered and rewritten for publication" in 1905 as *Lectures on the Relation Between Law and Public Opinion in England During the Nineteenth Century*. For the development of Dicey's thinking on the subject between his Harvard lectures and their final publication, see John V. Orth, "English Law and Striking Workmen: The Molestation of Workmen Act, 1859," 2 *Journal of Legal History* 238 (1981).

3 See George H. Callcott, *History in the United States, 1800–1860: Its Practice and Purpose* 88 (1970).

4 William C. Robinson, *Common Law Charts to Accompany Blackstone's Commentaries* (1872). Robinson taught law at Yale from 1869 to 1891.

5 S.F. Mordecai, *Law Lectures: A Treatise from a North Carolina Standpoint on Those Portions of the First and Second Books of the Commentaries of Sir William Blackstone Which Have Not Become Obsolete in the United States* (2 vols., 2d ed., 1916). Samuel Fox Mordecai was dean of the Trinity College School of Law from 1905 to 1927.

6 *Journal of Congress*, 14 Oct. 1774 (italics added).

common law on both sides of the Atlantic united was that it was based on an Anglo-American conception of reason. History and reason are hard to escape.

One of the common law's most elaborate creations was the Rule Against Perpetuities, a rule designed to limit the period within which a person could control the disposition of property after death, generally no longer than a lifetime plus 21 years. Although integral to the orderly transfer of wealth from generation to generation, this important area of law remained almost completely judge-made, largely uninfluenced by statute either in England or in America. On foundations laid down long before the American Revolution, the Rule Against Perpetuities reached final form only in the nineteenth century through a remarkable collaboration between English and American judges and an indefatigable American academic lawyer. After the courts had exhaustively explored the logical ramifications of the Rule, Professor John Chipman Gray, among Dicey's hosts at Harvard, systematized the results in an exhaustive treatise, first published in 1886. Throughout the nineteenth and most of the twentieth century, American law schools taught the common law Rule, and American courts almost without exception applied this "English law." When one state court, led by an unusually strong-willed chief justice, refused to accept a particularly strict application of the Rule, Professor Gray was vehement in his denunciation and warned the judge that it was "a serious thing deliberately to break away from the consensus of the English-speaking world."[7]

The history of American legal education exhibits its English roots as well as its American branches. A few colonial Americans, mostly scions of wealthy families, had actually made the pilgrimage across the Atlantic to experience the refinements of the metropolis and to eat their terms at the Inns of Court – for what that was worth in terms of legal education. Of the 55 delegates at the Constitutional Convention in Philadelphia in 1787 four had enrolled at the Inner Temple and five at Middle Temple (Blackstone's Inn). Of course, the large majority of American lawyers learned their legal skills closer to home, in apprenticeships in lawyers' offices. "Reading law" it was called and often was simply that: the unassisted reading of legal classics, such as Sir Edward Coke's seventeenth-century *Commentary* on Sir Thomas Littleton's fifteenth-century *Treatise on Tenures*, the foundational work on English property law. Joseph Story remembered being told by his mentor to read *Coke on Littleton*:

> It was a very large folio, with Hargrave and Butler's notes, which I was required to read also.... I took it up, and after trying it day after day with very little success, I sat myself down and wept bitterly. My tears dropped upon the book, and stained its pages.[8]

7 John Chipman Gray, *The Rule Against Perpetuities* 756 (4th ed. by Roland Gray, 1942) (commenting on Edgerly v. Barker, 32 A. 766 (N.H. 1893) (Doe, C.J.) (reforming a grant to comply with the Rule rather than voiding it for violation of the Rule)). See John Phillip Reid, *Chief Justice: The Judicial World of Charles Doe* 128–132 (1967).

8 Story, *Miscellaneous Writings* 20.

Thomas Jefferson, who admired Coke for his principled opposition to the pretensions of the Stuart kings – "a sounder Whig never wrote," Jefferson said[9] – advised students to read Coke rather than Blackstone, the enemy of American Independence. Jefferson himself was fortunate to read law under the tutelage of the conscientious lawyer and mentor, George Wythe, who took the task of instruction seriously. A scattering of American states still allow law office study as an alternative to law school.[10]

University teaching of law got off to a promising start in the new Republic. As we have seen, when Jefferson was governor of Virginia, he used his influence to create a professorship of law at the College of William & Mary – in imitation of Blackstone's Vinerian professorship – and secured the appointment of his former teacher George Wythe as its first incumbent. After the Revolution, John Marshall, future Chief Justice of the U.S. Supreme Court, attended a six-week lecture course there, although his surviving notebooks show that his attention wandered from the professor's learned lectures to thoughts of his sweetheart and future wife Polly Ambler. At other colleges, similar courses were begun. James Wilson, one of the first justices of the U.S. Supreme Court, lectured on law at the College of Philadelphia (later the University of Pennsylvania), and James Kent, "the American Blackstone," was briefly professor of law at Columbia College (later Columbia University). Kent was the last to attempt a wide-ranging "commentary" on American law – all the law (except criminal law), including the proliferating varieties of English common law in the several states. But in America, professorships in law barely outlasted their initial incumbents.

A somewhat longer-lived experiment in American legal education took place away from a university setting, in a law office in rural Connecticut. Tapping Reeve, a Litchfield lawyer, discovered that his talent for teaching offered an opportunity for profit and turned his law office "apprentices" into "law students." The Litchfield Law School was formally established in 1784, a year after the Treaty of Paris officially recognized American Independence. For many years the only professor at his school, Reeve lectured on the common law, drawing largely on Blackstone and faithfully communicating the traditionalism of his English predecessor. Reeve's own book reflected this emphasis on tradition and private law. Dealing with the various personal relationships discussed in the first volume of Blackstone's *Commentaries* – husband and wife, parent and child, guardian and ward, master and servant – Reeve actually outdid the conservative Englishman by reverting in his title to the archaic French label for husband and wife, "baron et femme," a phrase even the

9 Jefferson to James Madison, 17 Feb. 1826, in 12 *Works of Thomas Jefferson* 456 (P.L. Ford ed. 1905).

10 See National Conference of Bar Examiners & American Bar Association Section of Legal Education and Admission to the Bar, *Comprehensive Guide to Bar Admission Requirements, 2021*, at 10 (listing California, Maine, New York, Vermont, Virginia, Washington, and West Virginia).

traditionalist Blackstone thought belonged to the "elder law books."[11] Unlike the short-lived college professorships, the Litchfield Law School lasted several decades, but it, too, had shallow roots. When Reeve's assistant and successor, James Gould, retired in 1833, the school closed.

Institutional support was needed; the solo practitioner could not create a law school that would last. If it was to escape apprenticeship, legal education eventually had to return to the university. Perhaps influenced by Blackstone's professorship at Oxford, Isaac Royall, a wealthy Tory merchant and slave owner, left money to Harvard in 1781 to endow a professorship of law (or of "physic and anatomy"). Litigation concerning the disposition of confiscated royalist property delayed its implementation, but at last in 1815 Isaac Parker, Chief Justice of the Massachusetts Supreme Judicial Court, accepted appointment as the first Royall Professor of Law, and in 1817 the Harvard Law School was founded. Over two hundred years later, sensitivities about the source of the benefactor's wealth led Harvard to "retire" the professorship.

In 1829, a second professorship was added, supported by a gift from Nathan Dane, the author of an eight-volume *General Abridgment and Digest of American Law* (1823) – a direct imitation of Viner's massive *General Abridgment of Law and Equity*, as his gift to Harvard was a direct imitation of Viner's to Oxford. Joseph Story, by then a justice of the U.S. Supreme Court, was persuaded – in part, perhaps, by his own unhappy experience as a legal apprentice – to add teaching to his judicial duties and become the first Dane Professor. In contrast to Reeve, Story, who began his publishing career a decade or two later, picked topics more suitable to an expanding commercial republic: bailments (1832), agency (1839), partnership (1841), bills of exchange (1843), and promissory notes (1845), among others. Although also called by the hallowed name "commentaries," Story's books were not surveys of all the law on the order of Blackstone and Kent but treatises on individual topics, systematic summaries of cases – mostly English. For a few years, the Harvard Law School flourished, but Story's death in 1845 (probably from overwork) showed how much it, too, depended on one individual. A university setting alone was not enough without a sustained institutional commitment.

In 1870, Harvard's reform-minded president, Charles Eliot, determined on a new beginning and picked a little-known lawyer, Christopher Columbus Langdell, to serve as dean with the charge of remaking the law school. Langdell had been a law student at Harvard during the years of decline following Story's death but had educated himself by assisting Professor Theophilus Parsons in preparing his book on contract law. Contract was only then gaining attention as a body of law comparable to property. The earliest book on the subject, John Joseph Powell's *Essay upon the Law of Contracts and Agreements*, was

11 Tapping Reeve, *The Law of Baron & Femme; of Parent & Child; of Guardian & Ward; of Master & Servant; and of the Powers of the Court of Chancery* (1816); 1 Blackstone, *Commentaries* 421.

published in 1790, three hundred years after Littleton's foundational work on property law and ten years after Blackstone's death.

Joseph Story, as we have seen, candidly admitted that "the common law was an *utter stranger* to the principles of commercial jurisprudence." "Almost all the principles that regulate our commercial concerns," he continued, "are of modern growth, and have been engrafted into the old stock of the law."[12] Not surprisingly, Story took Lord Mansfield as his judicial hero. Yet apparently it never occurred to him to add to his collection of commentaries on commercial topics a commentary on contracts. That was left to his son, the lawyer and artist William Wetmore Story, whose book on contracts, more candidly labelled a "treatise" rather than a "commentary," was published in 1844, the year before his father's death.[13] A revised and expanded second edition appeared three years later but was soon overshadowed by *Parsons on Contracts*, published in two volumes in 1853–1855, which became the standard reference.

Over the course of his 25-year deanship from 1870 to 1895, Langdell was to transform the Harvard Law School and make it into the model for legal education in America. No longer the subject of an isolated lecture course for college students, as in Blackstone's day, or a semi-detached school within the undergraduate curriculum, as in Story's day, law would be taught as a distinct professional discipline, eventually requiring three years of study after college – incidentally restricting access to the profession to those who could afford such prolonged education. Proclaiming that "law is a science," Langdell disengaged legal education from day-to-day legal practice. He even disengaged it from the particularities of the law in any given jurisdiction, encouraging its homogenization. Harvard advertised itself as providing training in "the fundamental principles of English and American law," preparing students for practice "in any place where that system of law prevails."[14] Central to Harvard's prestige was its national, even international, focus; state law was irrelevant.

Not only would law no longer be learned by apprenticeship in a lawyer's office, it would no longer be taught by practicing lawyers or sitting judges. Langdell found the prototype of the new-model law professor in James Barr Ames, his brilliant student and eventual successor as dean, who was hired as a Harvard law professor immediately on graduation, without any experience in practice. "What qualifies a person… to teach law," Langdell explained, "is not experience in the work of a lawyer's office, not experience in dealing with men, not experience in the trial or argument of causes, not experience, in short in using law, but experience in learning law"[15] – perhaps a direct *riposte* to Holmes'

12 Story, *Miscellaneous Writings* 269, 272 (italics in original).

13 William Wetmore Story, *Treatise on the Law of Contracts not under Seal* (1844). Contracts "under seal" (technically "covenants"), unlike the more familiar contracts, did not require consideration for their effectiveness. Covenants are now rarely encountered, although the name is still used to refer to promises in deeds and leases.

14 Harvard Law School catalogue, 1878–1879.

15 C.C. Langdell, "Teaching Law as a Science," 21 *Am. L. Rev*. 123, 124 (1887).

aphorism a few years earlier that "the life of the law has not been logic: it has been experience."[16] The tension between academic legal education and the actual experience of legal practice continues to this day.

Confident of his intellectual brilliance, Ames like his mentor, displayed the independence and, indeed, the arrogance of a legal academic. As we have seen, Langdell had dismissed Mansfield's goal of "doing substantial justice" as "irrelevant," and Ames had charged "the great Mansfield" with confounding equity and law. Ames's object in his classes, as reported by Louis Brandeis, was "to convince us that nine-tenths of the Judges who have sat on the English Bench and about ninety-nine-hundredths of the American Judges 'did not know what they were talking about' – that the great majority of Judges were illogical, inconsistent, and unreasonable."[17]

Convinced that law is a "science," Langdell – like Blackstone before him – aspired to make its study worthy of a university. "If law be not a science," the dean said, "a university will consult its own dignity in declining to teach it."[18] Langdell admired the rigor of legal education offered at continental European universities and aspired to reproduce it in America – "as far as differences of circumstances would permit." But the circumstance that would inevitably make Langdell's Harvard Law School different from the great law faculties at Berlin and elsewhere in Europe was that the law of continental nations was civil law, based on national codes modelled on the Corpus Juris Civilis, which naturally lent itself to instruction by lecture. By contrast, the common law was derived from cases, not a code, so Langdell made the fateful decision to base legal education at Harvard on the intensive study of reported cases.

Determined to teach from cases, Langdell prepared the first "casebook" – ever after the characteristic educational vehicle for American legal education, even for subjects that did not naturally lend themselves to instruction from cases. Dispensing with lecturing, Langdell adopted the question-and-answer approach to instruction, later dignified as "the Socratic method" – bringing the method of the courtroom into the classroom. Coming as it did at the moment when statutes were about to threaten continued common law development, Langdell's new model of legal education helped to maintain the primacy of the common law in America and preserve its traditional method of casuistic reasoning, reasoning from case to case. By putting judicial decisions at the center, the case method of instruction reduced the apparent role of statutes. Indeed, Professor Gray, Langdell's coadjutor at Harvard, suggested that law is, in fact, nothing more than the rule laid down by a court. "Statutes are to be dealt with as sources of Law," he said, "not as part of the Law itself." "All the Law is judge-made law"[19] – an insight that helps to explain the American anomaly of

16 Holmes, *The Common Law* 1 (1881).

17 Brandeis to Otto Wehle, 12 Nov. 1876, in 1 Brandeis, *Letters*.

18 Langdell, "Teaching Law as a Science," 21 *Am. L. Rev*. 123.

19 Gray, *Nature and Sources of Law* 125.

formally adopted and enrolled statutes that are, despite the appearance of "law," unenforceable in court if found to be unconstitutional.

Law schools on the Harvard model – and eventually they were everywhere – redirected legal teaching and scholarship. Whereas once Blackstone and Kent lectured on all the law and turned their notes into comprehensive commentaries, the compartmentalism of academic instruction inevitably produced a kaleidoscopic view of the law – one of the reasons law students find legal education so frustrating. With the end of formal lectures, the legal professoriate rushed to produce the casebooks required for classroom use. And the preparation of treatises restricted to individual subjects further obstructed a view of the law as a whole. The founding, in 1887, of the *Harvard Law Review*, the model for all others, created a growing market for specialized academic legal articles.

Langdell's chosen law school subject was contract law, which he had studied with Professor Parsons. So the first law school casebook was *Langdell's Cases on Contracts* (1871), assembling cases that formerly were scattered among distinct forms of action with distinct entries in the abridgments: *covenant* for breach of a promise under seal, *debt* for breach of a promise given in exchange for consideration, *assumpsit* for the nonperformance of a promise (often fictional) on which the plaintiff had relied. In his casebook and classroom, Langdell was developing the set of principles that would become "general contract law." No longer was primacy accorded to the form of the promise but to the intention of the parties as expressed in their agreement. In time, the commitment to effectuating intention was to spread beyond contract and to undermine many traditional rules, particularly in the law of property.

Probably without being consciously aware of it, the dean was responding to (and hastening on) a fundamental reorientation taking place in the common law. For centuries, that law was largely concerned with property, particularly with property in land. Consequently, traditional lawyers tended to think about legal rights and arrangements in property terms. Magna Carta, the "great charter of liberties," took the form of a grant of land. In the seventeenth century, Sir Edward Coke described the law as "the golden metwand" – a tool used by surveyors – "whereby all men's causes are justly and evenly measured."[20] For good measure, he added that royal power too was bounded by the law: "The common law hath admeasured the king's prerogative."[21]

All sorts of things, even those recognized as "incorporeal" – without physical existence – were "owned," giving them the advantages of the protections accorded property. In the Middle Ages, a right to care in old age, called a corody, could be purchased from an abbey; failure to provide the service

20 Edward Coke, *Fourth Institute* 240 (1641).

21 Quoted in Catherine Drinker Bowen, *The Lion and the Throne: The Life and Times of Sir Edward Coke* 484 (1956) (referring to Darnell's Case, 3 How. St. Tr. 1 (K.B. 1627) (The Five Knights Case)).

amounted to an "ejectment," remedied by the same action as a wrongful eviction from land. Today, of course, similar protection would be acquired by a contract with a nursing home, backed by a contract of insurance, the breach of either giving rise to an action for damages.

As we have seen, Blackstone thought a master had a "property... in the service of his domestics; acquired by the contract of hiring and purchased by giving them wages"; in consequence, he could sue anyone who enticed them away by offering better terms, just as he could sue anyone who took anything else belonging to him.[22] Likewise, a husband acquired by marriage a "property in the company, care or assistance" of his wife and could recover damages from anyone who injured her, thereby depriving him of his rights.[23] (Unfortunately, as we will see, the converse was not true: a wife acquired no "property" in her husband and had therefore no cause of action for injury to him.) Even an office, treated by Blackstone as just one of many items of property, was "a right to exercise a public or private employment, and the fees and emoluments thereunto belonging."[24] The concept was not finally abandoned in America until early in the twentieth century.[25]

Property arrangements, even those extending over time like the lease, the mortgage, and the real estate contract, were originally understood solely in property terms. The lease was a conveyance of an estate in land; rent, an interest in the land "reserved" by the landlord in the grant. If a tenant assigned the lease, the assignee became liable for the rent, even though the tenant remained liable as well. This double liability followed from the fact that the obligation was based not only on contract (the tenant's promise to pay) but also on property (the assignee's possession of the land subject to the obligation) – to the bewilderment of modern law students. A lease to commence in the future created an *interesse termini* (interest in a term), a present property right protected from interference, not a contract promising future performance.

Eventually, the lease would become a "rental agreement," to be treated "like any other contract" – with, as we will see, dramatic consequences for tenants. The mortgage, today often in the form of a deed of trust, was first cast as a conditional conveyance of land – that is, a conveyance that would become void on condition that the loan was repaid – not a contract of indebtedness. (Today, mortgage financing involves a promissory note, in addition to a mortgage of the land.) The long history of the law of mortgages is the story of the slow recasting of the transaction as a debt with land pledged as security, known to property students today as the transition from the "title theory" of mortgages to the "lien theory."

22 1 Blackstone, *Commentaries* 417.

23 3 Blackstone, *Commentaries* 142–143.

24 2 Blackstone, *Commentaries* 37.

25 Mial v. Ellington, 134 N.C. 131, 43 S.E. 961 (1903), reversing Hoke v. Henderson, 15 N.C. 1 (1834).

The contract for the sale of land was – and, given the conservatism of property lawyers, still is – understood not as an agreement to convey title in the future but as a conveyance of a title immediately enforceable in equity. By a process known as "equitable conversion," a purchaser "under contract" becomes in effect an owner. In time, the recognition of an equitable title in the purchaser has come to seem anomalous – it was abolished in England in 1925 – as the law shifted from an emphasis on the protection of vested rights (property) to an emphasis on contract and intention. With respect to restrictive covenants in deeds, the shift is not yet complete: they may be characterized as either property or contract, with serious consequences when choosing the correct statute of limitations in case of violation.

Equity's greatest creation, the trust, was (and, to a large extent, still is) created by a gratuitous conveyance of property by a settlor to a trustee to hold on behalf of a beneficiary. So understood, the conveyance results in the separation of legal title, given to the trustee, from equitable title, given to the beneficiary. The modern trust often includes detailed – sometimes very detailed – directions to the trustee about how to handle the property and under what conditions to deliver some or all of it to the beneficiary, who has the right to insist on proper performance. Having parted with title, the settlor retains no interest in the property, but increasingly settlors and their lawyers are seeking legal means to enforce the terms of the trust by recharacterizing the relationship between settlor and trustee, not as a conveyance but as a contract. (Even simple deeds are sometimes today loosely referred to as contracts rather than conveyances.)

The old law, as we have seen, treated agreements as the gateway to status. The contract of purchase created the status of owner; the contract of marriage created the status of husband and wife; the contract of labor created the status of master and servant. These contracts became effective (executed) immediately. Thereafter the law, not the agreement of the parties, governed their relationship. But increasingly, the potential of contract to set the terms of a relationship over time gained recognition. Contracts could remain "executory" (not fully performed) for years. The agreement to work for another, rather than create a status, was now understood as a contract setting the terms of the relationship for the duration, allowing the master to dictate many of the conditions of labor, such as long working hours[26] or whether to join a union.[27] As if to signal this change, a new terminology was adopted: the old "servant" became the new "employee" – or, as it was spelled at first, "employé," usage that prevailed into the twentieth century. Even marriage, where the rights of the parties had been set by law (usually to the advantage of the husband), became subject to variation by prenuptial agreements; lately, postnuptial agreements have been recognized.

26 Lochner v. New York, 198 U.S. 45 (1905).

27 Adair v. United States, 208 U.S. 161 (1908); Coppage v. Kansas, 236 U.S. 1 (1915).

The very nature of the common law and the judicial process ensured that the developing law embodied then-current social and political assumptions. Just as property law reflected the ethos of the feudal world in which it developed, so the new law of contract reflected the ethos of individualism that flourished in the nineteenth century. Only a few years before Langdell assumed the deanship at Harvard, Sir Henry Maine, a professor at the University of Cambridge, had concluded a lecture on "ancient law" with the emphatic declaration: "The movement of the progressive societies has hitherto been a movement *from Status to Contract*."[28] Taken out of context and redirected, Maine's observation was turned from a summary of the past into a signpost to the future. Contract was the way forward. For a while in the late nineteenth and early twentieth centuries, "freedom of contract" was even treated as a constitutional right comparable to life, liberty, and property – until in the 1930s the U.S. Supreme Court, belatedly recognizing a new political and social reality, ruefully acknowledged that, in fact, "the Constitution does not speak of freedom of contract," and overturned many of its precedents.[29]

28 Maine, *Ancient Law* 100 (1861) (italics in original).
29 West Coast Hotel v. Parrish, 300 U.S.379, 391 (1937).

6

THE COMMON LAW AND THE STATUTES

Among the pilgrims in Geoffrey Chaucer's fourteenth-century *Canterbury Tales* was a bustling Man of Law. "*In termes hadde he caas and doomes alle / That from the tyme of kyng William were falle..../And every statut koude he pleyn by rote*."[1] That is, he knew word-for-word every case and judgment rendered since the time of William the Conqueror in 1066 and could recite every statute from memory. The cases come first, then the statutes. This is no accident or literary convention. The common law was prior to all statutes. When King Henry II instructed his judges to go out and do justice in the twelfth century, they went with no rule book to guide them. As Frederick Pollock and Frederic William Maitland observed in their magisterial *History of English Law Before the Time of Edward I*: "It was rather as an organizer and governor than as a legislator that Henry was active."[2] Unlike Hammurabi, Justinian, and Napoleon, King Henry gave his name to no code. The historians even doubt whether the king established "any one new rule which we should call a rule of substantive law." Instead, they say, Henry was "for ever busy with new devices for enforcing the law," the law that came from the recognition of common customs as legally binding.

Edward I, whose accession in 1272 marks the end of Pollock and Maitland's *History of English Law*, was a lawgiver, described by Gibbon (with considerable exaggeration) as "our national Justinian,"[3] but he too left his mark not with an imperial code but with a series of loosely related landmark statutes.

1 *The Canterbury Tales* (late 14th century), I (A) 323–324, 327, in *The Works of Geoffrey Chaucer* 20 (2d ed., ed. F.N. Robinson, 1957).

2 1 Pollock & Maitland, *History of English Law* 136.

3 4 Edward Gibbon, *Decline and Fall of the Roman Empire* 470 n. 2 (J.B. Bury ed. 1909).

DOI: 10.4324/9781003660859-8

Despite the absence of a foundational code, the common law has endured as well as, if not better than, code-based legal systems and has spread with English settlers around the world. The fact of the matter is that courts and "devices for enforcing the law" wear better than rules, which have a tendency to outlast their usefulness. A great "organizer and governor" rivals or excels a great legislator.

In the Latin treatise attributed to Henry de Bracton, *De Legibus et Consuetudinibus Angliae (On the Laws and Customs of England)*, written about a century before Chaucer, few statutes are mentioned. Nor had many been added in the years between Bracton and Chaucer. While no small feat of memorization – medieval statutes, done up in a form of Latin, were no simpler than modern ones – the Man of Law's claim that he could recite every statute "*by rote*" is not quite as impressive as it sounds. As Maitland observed of English legislation in the early twentieth century: "The writings of Bentham and his school and the example of foreign nations have called forth the desire for comprehensive and symmetrical legislation." "Every year has produced a volume of statutes," some of which "exceed in bulk the whole legislation of a mediaeval reign."[4] And the common lawyers steadfastly minimized the effect of most early statutes, including Magna Carta, by insisting that they merely restated the common law. Even King Edward agreed, as we have seen, confirming the "great charter of liberties" and ordering his officers to recognize it as common law. Three hundred years later, Richard Hooker could still assume that what statutes there were, only declared or clarified what was already common law.[5]

Most of the statutes that Chaucer's Man of Law could recite, and certainly the ones he was most interested in, concerned property, specifically land; he seemed to be an expert in real estate transactions. According to the pilgrims' host on the journey to Canterbury: "*Al was fee symple to him in effect*," referring to the basic legal estate in land, what Blackstone called "property in its highest degree,"[6] suggesting that he was a drafter of deeds and perhaps even himself a purchaser, like many contemporary lawyers. One of the earliest statutes in the English lawbook, the Statute De Donis Conditionalibus (1285),[7] an exception to the general deference of the barons to the judges, concerned an important (to the barons) point of property law: whether land could be tied up in one family from generation to generation. Enacted a hundred years before the *Canterbury Tales*, De Donis, the root of the entailed estate, was actually intended to counteract a line of judicial decisions that had threatened to frustrate dynastic intent. To legislative interventions, the judges sometimes responded with ingenious fictions nullifying the effect of the legislation, as was the eventual fate of the Statute De Donis.

4 Frederic W. Maitland & Francis C. Montague, *A Sketch of English Legal History* 161–62 (1915).
5 Richard Hooker, *Of the Laws of Ecclesiastical Polity* 95 (Arthur Stephen McGrade ed. 1989).
6 2 Blackstone, *Commentaries* 105.
7 13 Edw. I, c. 1 (1285).

Dialogue between case and statute was to be a constant feature of the common law tradition. To some extent, courts treated early statutes like judicial decisions. The modern law of criminal conspiracy has its roots in an early fourteenth-century statute, entitled "Who be Conspiritours."[8] Although originally limited to those who agreed "falsely and maliciously to indite [indict]" an innocent person, by the eighteenth century the statutory crime had become an expansive common law crime that swept up all those who agreed to perform any unlawful act (or a lawful act by unlawful means). In the heated conflicts between capital and labor in the nineteenth and twentieth centuries, indictment for conspiracy became a legal (and lethal) weapon against labor organizations.[9]

Capital, too, was constrained (more or less) by the interaction of statute and case. Almost six hundred years after the medieval statute on conspiracy, the Sherman Anti-Trust Act (1890) declared illegal "every contract, combination in the form of trust or otherwise, or conspiracy, in restraint of trade."[10] Lacking clear definitions, the Act constituted a direction to the courts to develop the law case-by-case, the common law way. The process continues to this day.

Just as the higher courts declared the common law in the form of precedents, so the highest court of all, "the high court of parliament," declared it in the form of statutes. The logic of this view was not exhausted by the time of Blackstone and explains the otherwise baffling rule of statutory construction that he recited: "If a statute that repeals another is itself repealed afterwards, the first statute is thereby revived, without any formal words for that purpose"[11] – just as a judicial decision that overrules a prior decision restores the *status quo ante*. The abandonment of this rule in the mid-nineteenth century in both England and America,[12] ironically by statute, is an indicator of the extent to which common law and statute had by then parted company.

Common law remained "reason," its judicial discernment subject to occasional human error and eventual correction by the courts, while statute law came to be seen as an act of will and in that sense arbitrary. By statute, parliament could do unreasonable things, like make a man a judge in his own case (as Blackstone reluctantly acknowledged) or make one man the property of another (as Lord Mansfield regretfully admitted). Statutes were different and, by virtue of the supremacy of parliament, were the supreme law of the land. "Where the common law and a statute differ," Blackstone conceded in another canon of statutory construction, "the common law gives place to the statute."[13] And, in America though not in England, a statute yields to the constitution.

8 33 Edw. I, st. 2 (1304).
9 See Orth, *Combination and Conspiracy* 25–27, 37–40 (1991).
10 Act of 2 July 1890, ch. 647, 26 Stat. 209.
11 1 Blackstone, *Commentaries* 90.
12 E.g., 13 & 14 Vict. c. 21, § 5 (1850); La. Civ. Code, art 8.
13 1 Blackstone, *Commentaries* 89.

Yet, to the extent that some rules of the common law are incorporated in American constitutions, they trump a statute – a realization of Sir Edward Coke's claim that law can qualify legislative supremacy.

Statutes declared the common law or clarified it – or changed it. But they were, in turn, "construed" and applied by the judges. Action and reaction created a dynamic that became a persistent feature of the common law tradition. While accepting the effectiveness of legislation, the judges were at first rarely welcoming. "Statutes in derogation of the common law will not be extended by construction" was a common law maxim, still sometimes recited.[14] Moreover, the judges were of the decided opinion that statutes often did more harm than good. Blackstone, as we have seen, cautioned his readers that "whenever a standing rule of law" – he meant a rule of the common law – "of which the reason perhaps could not be remembered or discerned, hath been wantonly broke in upon by statutes or new resolutions, the wisdom of the rule hath in the end appeared from the inconveniences that have followed the innovation."[15] Even Lord Mansfield, as we have also seen, had argued while solicitor general that since "a statute can seldom take in all cases…, the common law that works itself pure by rules drawn from the fountain of justice, is for that reason superior to an Act of Parliament,"[16] drawing upon him the predictable scorn of Jeremy Bentham.[17] Judicial "distortion" of statutory texts has been denounced – even in the highest circles – as "undemocratic."[18]

Into the nineteenth century, English appellate courts were still making important decisions in developing areas of law, such as contract and tort, and American courts tended to follow their lead. (Occasionally, as we will see, the reverse was also true.) But as time passed and the logic of parliamentary supremacy became clear, the creative impulse of the common law "at home" waned, and statute gradually became the preferred means of legal change. Thus, it took Lord Campbell's Act (1846) – the pattern of American wrongful death statutes – to overturn the rule that a cause of action in tort did not survive the life of the victim, a rule with the scandalous consequence that it was cheaper if a defendant's negligence led to death rather than injury.

English appellate courts were becoming less a forum for the development of new law and more a guarantor that the lower courts had applied existing law correctly – in contrast to America, where the creative function of the higher courts became steadily more important. As Mansfield's demand for systematic and accurate law reporting was realized – the Incorporated Council on Law

14 See, e.g., Gray v. Gray, 947 So.2d 1045, 1048 (Ala. 2006).

15 1 Blackstone, *Commentaries* 70.

16 Omychund v. Barker, 1 Atk. 22, 33, 26 Eng. Rep. 15, 23 (Ch. 1744).

17 Bentham, 7 *Works* 311.

18 Antonin Scalia & Bryan A. Garner, *Reading Law: The Interpretation of Legal Texts* 3 (2012). Scalia was a justice of the U.S. Supreme Court from 1986 to 2016.

Reporting was established in England in 1865 – precedents became harder for English courts to disregard. Eventually, as we have seen, it even came to be conceded in England that the courts could no longer overrule their own precedents, a resolution only slightly modified in the mid-twentieth century.[19]

By the time of American Independence, a modest set of English statutes had accumulated, although even after six hundred years the then-current Statutes at Large (that is, those statutes still in effect and set out at full length) occupied only 31 modest volumes. Having separated themselves from England, the new American states, while claiming the common law as their birthright, had to decide which English statutes to accept, either because they were so fundamental or because they had become over the centuries part and parcel of the common law itself. But the reception of statutes, unlike the reception of the common law, was a complicated business. Statutes are jurisdiction-specific; the common law is universal. While the common law could be adopted at a stroke, whether by a simple statute or simply by judicial decision, the English statutes to be retained (or readopted) had to be carefully screened. Thomas Jefferson labored on the project in Virginia.[20] In North Carolina, commissioners appointed in 1817 specified which statutes remained in force in the state.[21] A bare handful of fundamental laws such as the Statute of Tenures (1660), the Statute of Frauds (1677), and the Habeas Corpus Act (1679) qualified for retention.

While the supremacy of statutes over the common law was firmly established, the fact of the common law's omnipresence has been of continuing significance. For one thing, the federal structure of the new Republic meant that in America, unlike in England, there was no national legislature with authority to undertake wholesale legal reform. As we have seen, each state was left to develop the law for itself. In the nineteenth century, state legislatures passed very little general legislation. Their relatively brief sessions were largely devoted to taxes, law enforcement, and education – and to adopting an extraordinary number of local, private, and special acts: chartering corporations, changing the names of towns, granting divorces, legitimating children. The development of the common law was generally left to the courts, one reason Blackstone's *Commentaries* remained evergreen in America.

The common law's omnipresence also allowed what may be called "common law statutes," that is, statutes that assume or incorporate the common law – just as the U.S. Constitution does. Sweeping away common law cobwebs in the law of property, a statute may simply provide: "The rule of property

19 See Practice Direction (Judicial Precedent), [1966] 1 W.L.R. 1234 (H.L.).

20 Jefferson, *Notes on the State of Virginia* 137.

21 "Statutes and Parts of Statutes of Great Britain, Reported as Being in Force in This State, by the Commissioners Appointed Under the Act of 1817, Entitled, 'An Act for the Revision of the Acts of the General Assembly,'" in 1 *Laws of the State of North Carolina* 85 (1821).

known as the Rule in Shelley's case is abolished."[22] Notice that the statute does not state the Rule; it simply abolishes it. The definition is incorporated by reference to the common law. A distinguished property law scholar recalled that although the Rule in Shelley's Case had been abolished in England a quarter-century before he studied property law at Oxford, "we still had to know what it was, since otherwise, it was argued with perverse but yet compelling logic, we could not understand what precisely had been abolished."[23] The same scholar, recognizing the afterlife of repealed property rules, conceded that the Rule in Shelley's Case, whatever it was, still applied in England "to instruments executed before 1 January 1926," the effective date of the statute.

Lawyers trained in the civil law system of continental Europe would be shocked that a statute fails to define an essential term. But lawyers trained in the common law system find nothing unusual about it. The common law is always there in the background. An extraordinary example from the period after the American Civil War illustrates the point. The victorious Northern states were willing to allow Southern states to continue to disqualify felons from voting but feared that expansive definitions of felony could be used to disenfranchise formerly enslaved persons. So readmission to representation in Congress in 1868 was on condition that Southern state constitutions never be amended to deny the vote to felons, "except as punishment for such crimes as are now felonies at common law."[24] No attempt was made to list the specific crimes referred to; they were simply to be determined by reference to the common law as it then was.

Even in modern criminal law, the common law still plays a role, albeit a diminishing one. In states that continue to recognize common law crimes, criminals are punished for crimes that are not defined by statute. To this day, there is no statutory definition of murder, assault, or conspiracy in North Carolina. As to the crimes of burglary and arson, the statutory offences remain "as defined at the common law."[25] Here the common law is incorporated by reference – not to abolish but to affirm. Whatever the elements of the offences were at common law, they still are. It might be difficult to pin them down in a statute. Perhaps that is what Jefferson had in mind when he said that it might even be "dangerous" to do so. Something might be left out, leaving an opening for a criminal to escape punishment. A criminal statute may even direct the courts to be guided by "the principles of common law as they may be applied

22 N.C. Gen. Stat. § 41-6.3.

23 A.W. Brian Simpson, *Leading Cases in the Common Law* 41 (1995).

24 An Act to Admit the States of North Carolina, South Carolina, Georgia, Alabama, and Florida to Representation in Congress, ch. 70, 15 Stat. 73, 73 (1868). I am indebted to W. Bryson Penley for this example.

25 N.C. Gen. Stat. §§ 14–51 (burglary), 14–58 (arson).

in the light of reason and experience"[26] – "reason and experience," the life of the common law.

The interaction between caselaw and statute is even more complicated. In 1973, the Massachusetts Supreme Judicial Court confronted the question whether a wife had a claim for loss of consortium (that is, companionship and sex) arising from injury to her husband caused by the negligence of a third party. Clear precedent in Massachusetts, well rooted in the common law, indicated that the answer was No. Blackstone had unhelpfully explained that, although a husband could maintain an action for injuries sustained by his wife, a wife could not maintain an action for injuries sustained by her husband, because – in keeping with the marriage-as-conveyance concept – "the inferior hath no kind of property in the company, care or assistance of the superior..., and therefore the inferior can suffer no loss or injury."[27] Only two years earlier, the Massachusetts court had stood by the rule and indicated that change, if any, should come from the legislature, not the court.

But then there was a change of personnel on the court – or maybe the justices just lost patience with the legislative process – and they overruled the recent precedent and allowed the action to proceed. As explained by Justice Benjamin Kaplan, a Harvard Law School professor newly appointed to the court: "In a field long left to the common law, change may well come about by the same medium of development."[28] Another ex-academic, the influential Chief Justice of New Jersey, Arthur T. Vanderbilt, emphatically agreed: "The courts are under as great an obligation to revise an outmoded rule of the common law as the legislatures are to abolish or modernize an archaic statute."[29] Revision of the common law, in the professors' view, is the province of the courts; repeal or amendment of statutes is for the legislatures. Having made a rule in the first place, the judges can change it. The ex-Harvard professor went even further, suggesting that "the Legislature may rationally prefer to act, if it acts at all, after rather than before the common law has fulfilled itself in its own way."[30] Once the court "revised" the common law of Massachusetts, there was no need for legislative action.

Recognition of a wife's action for loss of consortium was only one of many adjustments of traditional law in response to changing attitudes toward women and marriage. A century earlier, a more fundamental adjustment was demanded: that the legal disability of married women to control

26 N.C. Gen. Stat. § 130A-26.1(e).

27 3 Blackstone, *Commentaries* 143.

28 Diaz v. Eli Lilly & Co., 302 N.E.2d 555, 563 (Mass. 1973).

29 Reimann v. Monmouth Consol. Water Co., 87 A.2d 325, 332 (N.J. 1952) (Vanderbilt, C.J., dissenting). Vanderbilt was dean of New York University Law School from 1943 to 1948.

30 Diaz v. Eli Lilly & Co., 302 N.E.2d 555, 563 (Mass. 1973).

their own property be eliminated. The problem had long troubled wealthy fathers who feared that a wayward son-in-law would dissipate family assets. Invoking the powers of equity, creative lawyers devised the trust "for the sole and separate use" of a married woman, circumventing the male-dominated common law and preserving an heiress's property from her husband and his creditors.

Statute law eventually followed equity's lead. Married women's property acts, adopted in American states beginning in the 1840s, eventually democratized the benefits, making them available to all married women. In 1868, North Carolina made it a constitutional right:

> The real and personal property of any female in this State acquired before marriage, and all property, real and personal, to which she may, after marriage, become in any manner entitled, shall be and remain the sole and separate estate and property of such female, and shall not be liable for any debts, obligations, or engagements of her husband.[31]

Demonstration to male law-makers in England that women could safely be trusted to manage their own property reassured parliament that the experiment could be safely tried, leading to a series of ever more liberal parliamentary acts, beginning in 1870.

Sometimes, in our federal system, the signal for legislative change is sent long-distance. In 1970, the United States Court of Appeals for the District of Columbia decided to abandon the centuries-old common law conception of the lease as a conveyance, at least insofar as residential tenancies are concerned, and adopt the civil law concept of the lease as a contract. According to Judge J. Skelly Wright, who had trained in civil law in Louisiana, "leases should be interpreted and construed like any other contract."[32] Since purchasers of ordinary consumer goods were by then protected by an implied warranty of fitness for use, Judge Wright reasoned that residential leases should be interpreted to include an implied warranty of habitability. That decision triggered a nationwide re-thinking of traditional law on landlord and tenant – a re-thinking that has not yet reached a final conclusion. Although many state courts followed Judge Wright's lead, other courts hesitated, awaiting legislation, eventually forthcoming. Something similar happened with Judge Wright's decision a few years later prohibiting eviction in retaliation for exercising the rights created by the warranty

31 Current version in N.C. Const. art. X, § 4.

32 Javins v. First Nat'l Realty Co., 428 F.2d 1071, 1075 n. 13 (D.C. Cir. App. 1970). See La. Civ. Code art. 2669.

of habitability.[33] In these cases, the statute law in one jurisdiction caught up with the caselaw in another.

Whether a tenant's right to habitable premises came from case or statute, it came from the law, not the agreement of the parties. Residential landlords could not use their superior bargaining power to extract a waiver of this right from their contracting tenants. Paradoxically, the recognition of the lease as a contract did not mark progress from status to contract. In fact, it marked the reverse. Once categorized as the relationship of landlord-and-tenant, many of the rights and obligations of the parties derive from their status. Terms imposed by statute in other relationships also contracted the scope of contract. Legislation, state and federal, imposed nonwaivable terms in certain contracts, many of them the most important for ordinary Americans. Although the terms have been characterized as "fictitious," they are quite real; what is fictitious is that the parties agreed to them. Vulnerable classes came to be protected by implied terms dependent not on their agreement – other than their agreement to rent, work, or buy – but on the statutory law of landlord and tenant, labor law, or consumer law. In these areas, once again what mattered was not what they had agreed to but who they were – tenant, employee, consumer – in other words, their status.

To standardize statute law across the multiple jurisdictions of the United States, standard statutes were required. In 1892, the American Bar Association, then a relatively new organization of elite lawyers, sponsored the formation of the National Conference of Commissioners on Uniform State Law, known since 2007 as the Uniform Law Commission. Over the years, the Commission – usually relying on law professors as "reporters" – has proposed hundreds of "uniform laws," many of them dealing with basic common law issues. Although the impetus was the need to standardize laws that affected national business interests, the Commission has increasingly ventured into areas that are purely local, such as real property law, allowing law professors to put their preferred rules in statutory form. None of the proposed uniform laws has been enacted unchanged in all jurisdictions; others have been periodically revised by the Commissioners, sometimes substantially, seriously compromising the goal of uniformity as states have adopted different iterations.

To become an actual law, of course, a proposed "uniform law" must be adopted by a state legislature; to be uniform throughout the United States, it must be adopted by all state legislatures without local variations. The ideal had been demonstrated two hundred years ago when England began the statutory reform of land law, previously largely left to common law development. Lord Campbell, one of the sponsors of the legislation, described the process:

33 Edwards v. Habib, 397 F.2d 687 (D.C. Cir. App. 1968), cert. denied, 393 U.S. 1016 (1969).

bills drafted by experts "quietly passed through both Houses of Parliament without one single syllable being altered in any of them." "A mixed and numerous deliberative assembly," his lordship explained, "is wholly unfit for such work."[34] As in the English example, "uniform law-making" is not really a job for legislators, the hard choices having been made by the Commissioners – complicated in America by the fact of the multiple "deliberative assemblies." Drafted by law professors, uniform laws are presented on a take-it-or-leave-it basis; the legislature's role is simply to make it official. If the triumph of contract was in many cases more apparent than real, so too was the triumph of the legislature.

34 2 *Life of John, Lord Campbell* 29 (2d ed. by his daughter, Mrs. Hardcastle 1881).

PART 3

The Common Law in America

Theme & Variations

Introduction

In 1918, when the eminent English biographer Lytton Strachey was writing sketches of Victorian worthies, he declared that the history of the then recently concluded Victorian Age could never be written. "We know too much about it," he said.

> It is not by the direct method of a scrupulous narration that the explorer of the past can hope to depict that singular epoch. If he is wise, he will adopt a subtler strategy.... He will row out over that great ocean of material, and lower down into it, here and there, a little bucket, which will bring up to the light of day some characteristic specimen, from those far depths, to be examined with a careful curiosity.[1]

Like the Victorian Age, the common law tradition in America is too vast a subject for a comprehensive history. There is too much of it. Yet without an examination of legal details, the peculiar dynamic of the common law in America – the continuing interaction of tradition, innovation, and criticism – will be missed. So the method adopted here is reminiscent of Strachey's: "little buckets" will be lowered into the depths, bringing up for detailed examination some specimens of the variations that developed on the leading common law themes.

1 Lytton Strachey, *Eminent Victorians* vii (1918).

DOI: 10.4324/9781003660859-9

A few of the specimens dredged up will be very odd indeed: for example, the Rule in Shelley's Case, a "living fossil" like the coelacanth, nearly extinct, that tells us something about how traditional elements of the common law were created and why they survived into the modern world. Not only do ancient rules, particularly in property law, tend to linger, but the traditional common law method of development by judicial decision continues to operate, albeit often out of sight. While legal fictions may seem quaint today, mutated into other forms – constructions, equities, etc. – they permit the creation of new law by the extension of old rules to new cases, demonstrating yet again the legislative (i.e., law-making) role of the courts.

Technological developments, particularly the rapid growth of railroads in the nineteenth century, generated legal problems – some new, some familiar but arising with unprecedented frequency – that demanded immediate resolution. In response, the judges rapidly developed the law of contract and tort, which soon challenged the traditional primacy of property law. But judicial innovation was ultimately unable to provide acceptable solutions to many of the problems affecting ordinary people. Statutorily imposed terms in contracts, as we have seen, were needed in areas like landlord-and-tenant and consumer protection. Industrial accidents, increasingly common as the new technology sparked a revolution in the means of production, posed problems particularly difficult of resolution. With casualties mounting in the newly dangerous workplaces, English and American courts traded ideas about legal solutions. But the amalgam of contract and tort that they developed, with its emphasis on individual disputes, proved inadequate to solve the social problem of widespread injuries. In this area, statutory terms in labor contracts would not suffice; to spread the cost of accidents over an entire industry required a new institutional structure, representative of the coming administrative systems.

As American states in the early twentieth century sought to replace the Anglo-American case-by-case adjudication of industrial accidents with industrial commissions, they encountered two characteristic American obstacles. Unlike the common law, whose constitutionality normally goes unquestioned, statutes had to survive demanding judicial review under state and federal constitutions. And unlike legal precedents, which spread naturally from one jurisdiction to another (even back and forth across the Atlantic), statutes had to be adopted in each of the multiple jurisdictions of the federal republic if there was to be a more or less uniform system throughout the United States.

The rise of the legal professoriate created by the new law schools produced a chorus, knowledgeable in the law but largely free of the client-counseling that occupies the time (and pays the bills) of practicing lawyers or the daily grind of dispute resolution that occupies the judges. At first supportive of tradition, even celebratory in the manner of Blackstone, academic lawyers soon demanded greater analytical rigor in the law. Eventually, they tended to become constant critics after the order of Bentham, introducing a new dynamic into the common law. Indeed, modern American law schools generally reward not the Blackstonian preservation of traditional doctrine but the Benthamite project of constant challenge.

As law professors cogitated about ways to improve the law, some claimed the role of unacknowledged legislators, leaders in the drafting and re-drafting of "uniform laws." Others sought to direct the course of judicial decision with "restatements of the law." Still others used their classrooms for the subtle (and sometimes not so subtle) inculcation of novel, even radical, approaches to the law. Unfortunately, conclusory labels sometimes precluded reasoned analysis of traditional rules or bizarre hypothetical cases ridiculed them. The rule of law itself was subjected to searching inquiry, as the underlying structures of the common law were exposed. Meanwhile, the perennial dispute about whether to insist on strict rules strictly applied or to allow discretionary justice in each individual case continued unabated, with the preference increasingly given in favor of greater discretion.

7

THE FORCE OF TRADITION

At the Parliament of Merton in 1235, it was proposed to adopt the rule that the subsequent marriage of a man and a woman who had already begotten a child would eliminate the stigma of bastardy and make their child legitimate. This would have changed the common law and brought English law into conformity with canon law and the developing law of Continental Europe. With one voice the barons replied: "*Nolumus leges Angliae mutare*" (We do not wish to change the laws of England),[1] and the principle of legitimization *per subsequens matrimonium* did not enter English law for almost seven hundred years, until introduced by statute in 1925. As a practical matter, the barons were probably more concerned with the uncertainty that the change would introduce into the law of succession to property than with the morality of the proposition, but their reply can also stand for the traditional attachment to the law as it is, whatever it is. As one wise legal historian has observed, "The role of inertia in inhibiting law reform has been grossly underestimated."[2]

Tradition certainly remains a force to be reckoned with in the common law. For one thing, it is easier to do again what we have done before. As the Victorian essayist Walter Bagehot once observed: "The active voluntary part of a man is very small, and if it were not economised by a sleepy kind of habit, its results would be null." "We could not do every day out of our own heads all we have to do."[3] For judges, it means not having to solve every problem anew – and reduces the risk of reversal by a higher court. But following precedent also has positive value. It conforms to society's sense of fairness that if a similar

1 20 Hen. III. The Statute of Merton is generally considered to be the earliest English statute.
2 Watson, *Making of Civil Law* 185.
3 Walter Bagehot, *The English Constitution*, chap. 1 (1867).

DOI: 10.4324/9781003660859-10

controversy arises, a similar result should follow. "Like cases should be decided alike" has been a common law maxim since before the time of Coke, still repeated today.[4] As we have seen, legal experts from Mansfield to Brandeis have even gone so far as to say that in certain cases it is more important that a rule be settled than that it be settled right. Frequent change diminishes respect for the law, as thinkers from Aristotle to Aquinas have stressed; Dante even made the point in the *Divine Comedy*. And lending predictability to judicial action makes legal counseling more reliable. Lawyers can advise their clients about the likely consequences of their actions. It also endows the law with a certain venerability, connecting the present with the past, sometimes with the remote past.

Many of the oldest entries in the common law rulebook concern property law. Before the rise of the modern economy, land was the principal source of wealth and the only source of dependable income. The fee simple and the life estate may have arisen in the days of feudalism, but they remain the basic building blocks of modern property law, having spread from real property to personal property, particularly through the law of trusts. The joint tenancy with its associated right of survivorship originated to serve feudal purposes yet endures long after the decline of the society that called it into being, adapted to forms of property, such as bank and brokerage accounts, unknown to the Middle Ages. Similarly, the form of ownership in which married couples in many states take title to real property, tenancy by the entirety, dates to a time when married women had few rights. Male domination obviously had to go, but the golden opportunity the tenancy offered for asset protection and probate avoidance made it too attractive to lose. A hardy survivor, tenancy by the entirety easily accommodated the modern recognition of same-sex marriage.

The Rule in Shelley's Case, one of the hoariest remnants from long ago, tells us something about the dynamics of common law development, but it tells us even more about later law and the eventual triumph of statutes. The rule ever after known as the Rule in Shelley's Case gained its name and fame from Sir Edward Coke's elaborate report of the sixteenth-century case of Wolfe v. Shelley,[5] although the rule was actually much older. Coke's 13 thick volumes of Reports, like his *Commentaries on Littleton*, became canonical sources of the common law. Just as Aristotle was known in the Middle Ages simply as The Philosopher, so Coke's Reports came to be cited simply as The Reports. Some of the cases Coke included, like Shelley's, became part of every lawyer's mental repertory, much as cases in modern law school casebooks linger in the minds of lawyers long after graduation.

4 See, e.g., June Medical Serv. v. Russo, 591 U.S. 299, 345 (2020) ("The legal doctrine of *stare decisis* requires us, absent special circumstances, to treat like cases alike.") (Roberts, C.J., concurring).
5 1 Co. Rep. 93b, 76 Eng. Rep. 206 (C.P. 1581).

A comprehensive statement of the Rule is not necessary for present purposes.[6] It is sufficient to say that the Rule concerns the words necessary to create the estate of fee simple, the estate that preoccupied the Man of Law in the *Canterbury Tales*, what today we generally call ownership. Hallowed by long usage, the phrase "to John Doe and his heirs" was (and still is) the standard formula to grant a fee simple. But what if, instead of giving John an estate in fee simple, John is given an interest in the property for his life (a "life estate") and those people who will eventually turn out to be his heirs are given the right to the fee simple after his death (a "remainder in fee simple")? In other words, what if the grant ran: "to John Doe for life, *then* to his heirs"? The answer, according to the Rule in Shelley's Case, is that John gets the fee simple anyway, free to dispose of during his life by sale or gift, as he sees fit. Only if he dies still owning it without a will, would his heirs receive it – and even then, not by virtue of being named in the original grant but by the law of inheritance. In other words, the effect of the Rule is to make a grant "to John Doe for life, then to his heirs" functionally the same as a grant "to John Doe *and* his heirs."

However seemingly arcane the Rule itself, the reason it was formulated is explainable in terms of dollars and cents – or, rather, shillings and pence – and is as understandable as the reason for modern tax planning. In the feudal world in which the Rule arose, a charge called a "relief" was due on inheritance. (King John's attempt to increase the amount of the relief came high on the barons' list of grievances in Magna Carta.) But medieval lawyers, anticipating modern estate planners, tried to structure their clients' transfers of wealth to avoid the need to pay this "inheritance tax." If an heir could take by some means other than by inheritance, no relief would be owed. To close this loophole, the judges on their own motion simply restated the common law: "then to his heirs" means the same thing as "and his heirs," they held. The grantor's intention was defeated, but public policy (as understood in the Middle Ages) was served. Over the centuries that followed, the Rule in Shelley's Case hardened into a highly technical rule and became a prized item of legal arcana, a test of the traditional lawyer's mastery of his trade. As judicial sympathy for individual volition increased at the expense of intention-defeating property rules, judges and lawyers often found means to evade the effect of the Rule – not, characteristically, by discarding it but by strict construction of its terms and liberal construction of the alternatives.

Today, of course, those who collect tolls in the form of inheritance or estate taxes –stigmatized as "death taxes" – have learned not to make payment depend on the form of the transfer. Succession by way of remainder or inheritance (or by will, right of survivorship, or any other "will substitute") are all treated by the tax collector more or less the same, and there is no longer any reason to unsettle the property lawyers' tidy system of estates and future interests. But it

6 An oft-cited statement of the Rule may be found at 4 Kent, *Commentaries* 215*.

is noteworthy that the attempted medieval tax avoidance was prevented not by statute or by extending the incidence of the relief but by the judges' creation of a new common law rule, the Rule in Shelley's Case: a life estate followed by a remainder to the life tenant's heirs is a fee simple (in effect).

Nowadays, we would generally expect that changes to the common law, especially those that affect the transfer of wealth from generation to generation, would be done by statute. Even the barons, as we have seen with the Statute De Donis, adopted in 1285, 50 years after the Parliament of Merton, were willing to change the laws of England if their dynastic interests were at stake. But it took an extraordinary effort. In the pre-modern world, parliaments were infrequent, and the radical separation of legislative and judicial powers was still unknown. The judges in their quotidian work of resolving disputes made the rules of the common law by doing what they thought reason and natural law required. Then, and far into the future, legislators largely left the judges alone as they went about their judicial duties.

The remarkable thing about the Rule in Shelley's Case is not what it was or why it came to be but why it stayed so long. In 1660, the Statute of Tenures[7] reformed the English system of landholding and in the process did away with the payment known as the relief. Why, once its reason for being had ceased, did the Rule linger? It was not because the common law had lost its vigor. In 1682, in the Duke of Norfolk's Case,[8] the Chancery Court laid the foundation for an even more famous and more important rule, the Rule Against Perpetuities, which (as we have seen) the judges on both sides of the Atlantic elaborated over the following 200 years. Nor did the Rule in Shelley's Case outlive its usefulness simply because nobody noticed or cared. Lord Mansfield, as we have also seen, tried to eliminate the Rule as part of his project to "construe instruments according to the intent of the parties."[9] No medieval anachronism should be allowed to stand in the way of clearly expressed intention. So momentous was Mansfield's decision that it was appealed to the extraordinary Court of Exchequer Chamber, which handed his lordship one of his rare reversals.[10]

Among the judges who overruled Mansfield was Sir William Blackstone, only a few years away from his Oxford professorship. Blackstone's defense of the Rule came as no surprise. For him, *stare decisis* (standing by prior decisions) was an article of faith: "What before was uncertain, and perhaps indifferent, is now become a permanent rule, which it is not in the breast of any

7 12 Car. 2, c. 24 (1660).

8 3 Ch. Cas. 1, 22 Eng. Rep. 931 (Ch. 1682).

9 Eaton v. Jacques, 2 Dougl. 455, 460, 99 Eng. Rep. 290, 292 (K.B. 1780).

10 Perrin v. Blake, 4 Burr. 2579, 98 Eng. Rep. 355; 1 Collectanea Juridica 283 (Exch. Ch. 1772). A writ of error, a proceeding in the nature of an appeal, lay from King's Bench to the Court of Exchequer Chamber, which consisted of the judges of the Court of Common Pleas and the barons of Exchequer.

subsequent judge to alter or vary from, according to his private sentiments."[11] Here, we can detect a growing countercurrent to the continued activism of the common law judges, an early indication of the idea of separation of powers: what the judges had made, only the legislature could unmake – demonstrating another feature of the developing common law tradition. The genius of the common law, it seemed, was better at adding than subtracting.

Maintaining the Rule in Shelley's Case could always be defended because, in the hands of experienced conveyancers, it could do little harm; there were always ways to approximate the desired result. In time, the Rule even acquired a new rationale, one suitable to a new state of things: to promote the transferability of land. The longer title to property remains in the form of life-estate-and-remainder, the longer it cannot, as a practical matter, be mortgaged or sold. Indeed, in a curious way, the medieval Rule in Shelley's Case fell in with a later judicial preference for the unencumbered fee simple. As one judge explained in the early twentieth century:

> The rule has been so beneficial… in making possible the transfer of land a generation earlier and subjecting it to liability for the debts of the first taker, that… it remains in force notwithstanding that often it may be contrary to the intent of the devisor or grantor to confer an estate for life only, on the first taker.[12]

Intention matters in the law of property…, until it doesn't.

In time, a newfound emphasis on effectuating intention – associated with the rise of "contract thinking" – doomed the Rule in Shelley's Case, but unless some modern Mansfield (or American law-professor-turned-judge) abrogates it by judicial fiat, the job is left to the uncertain attention of the legislature. Ironically, the triumph of the (distracted or inactive) legislature often had the practical effect of freezing the ancient rules in place. In future, judges would continue to apply the Rule and other relics of the common law until the lawmakers saw fit to alter or abolish them. Even then, abolition by statute could apply only to future grants. The constitutional guarantee of property means that interests, once vested, cannot simply be legislated away. And American federalism means that the fate of the Rule in Shelley's Case varies from state to state. In 1925, England abolished the Rule (prospectively) at a stroke.[13] In America, it is dying a lingering death.

The continuing force of tradition in American common law can be seen not only in the "stickiness" of basic property law but also (less obviously) in the

11 1 Blackstone, *Commentaries* 69–70 (excepting only rules "evidently contrary to reason" or to "divine law").

12 Crisp v. Biggs, 176 N.C. 1, 23, 96 S.E. 662, 663 (1918) (Clark, C.J.).

13 15 & 16 Geo. 5, c. 20, § 131 (1925).

continued use of legal fictions, the time-hallowed means of bringing in new law under cover of the old. Legal fictions – pretending one thing to be another in order to apply to the latter a rule that properly applies to the former – sounds like something from the Dark Ages, but for centuries they were the means by which judges kept the law responsive to the needs of a changing society. We have seen how the old actions of assumpsit, trover, and ejectment were stretched to accommodate new causes of action; how the fiction of the lost grant was used for the purpose of "quieting the possession," in the words of Lord Mansfield[14]; and how bizarre fictions enlarged the jurisdiction of the common law courts. The traditionalist Blackstone, while acknowledging that fictions "may startle the student," defended them as harmless since every educated lawyer knew how things really were.[15] Bentham, on the contrary, thought they were a dishonest power-grab by the judges. They certainly compromise the *elegantia juris* – the simplicity, clarity, and coherence of the law – and complicate the efforts of code-drafters, particularly in the academy.

Despite Bentham's strictures, legal fictions remain, albeit under new names, such as judicial "constructions." A standard legal dictionary defines "constructive," when used to modify a legal concept, as "legally imputed; existing by virtue of legal fiction though not existing in fact," and includes a non-exhaustive list of 56 "constructive" things.[16] They can be found throughout the modern common law. The law concerning gifts of personal property has long required actual delivery of the donated item, but some gifts, actually undelivered, may nonetheless be upheld in the event of "constructive delivery," delivery of something else instead. Bailment, the intentional transfer of property for safekeeping, is now commonly understood to be based on a contract between two parties, but "constructive bailment" may be found where a finder simply takes possession of a lost item. A landlord may be found guilty of "constructive eviction" and denied recovery of rent without actually evicting a tenant if conditions on the premises became so intolerable that the tenant voluntarily left. The government may take private property for public use so long as it pays just compensation, a legal procedure known as condemnation or taking by eminent domain. But if the government simply takes the property without legal process, "constructive condemnation" may be recognized. The deprived landowner's remedy in such case is an action colloquially known as "inverse condemnation": rather than be sued by the government, the landowner sues the government for compensation, inverting the usual parties.

The modern system for recording titles to land could not function without the doctrine of "constructive notice." The record exists to allow anyone dealing with land – purchasing it or taking it as security for the repayment of

14 Eldridge v. Knott, 1 Cowp. 214, 215, 98 Eng. Rep. 1050, 1051 (K.B. 1774).

15 3 Blackstone, *Commentaries* 42–43.

16 *Black's Law Dictionary* 380–381.

a loan – to know exactly who owns it. So everyone is treated as if they actually knew what they could have known if they had consulted the record. They have "record notice" whether they looked at the record or not. A court may even find constructive notice from facts on the ground that would cause a reasonable person to make inquiries, "inquiry notice" – whether they asked any questions or not. Fraud in the law of tort is the intentional misrepresentation of a material fact, but "constructive fraud" may be found in case a fact is unintentionally misrepresented by a person who could know the truth.

Sometimes, legal title to land or other property ends up in the wrong hands. In such cases, a court may treat the person as "constructive trustee" for the rightful owner. An ordinary trust is intentionally created, but the constructive trust is a legal fiction – not really part of trust law at all but part of the law of remedies. Unlike the usual trustee who is charged with preserving the property for the beneficiaries, the constructive trustee has no duty except to get rid of it as quickly as possible by transferring legal title to the proper person. An elaborate fiction in the law of wills is sometimes used to effectuate presumed intention when a testator revokes a prior will in the mistaken belief that a subsequent will is valid. Under the doctrine unhelpfully labeled "dependent relative revocation," the revocation is said to be "dependent upon" and "relative to" the validity of the subsequent will. A revocation may be made expressly conditional; here the condition is supplied by legal fiction.

"Constructive contract" is, as a leading scholar explained, not actually a contract at all but "a legal fiction necessary to promote the ends of justice and, in particular, to prevent 'unjust enrichment'" by presuming a promise to pay for a benefit received.[17] Blackstone, of course, saw no difficulty with this, indulging the fiction that "every man hath engaged to perform what his duty or justice requires."[18] Constructions even appear in criminal law. A person may be convicted of illegal possession of a banned item despite the fact that it was not in the defendant's actual possession, if it was in the defendant's "constructive possession." Where actual presence at the scene of a crime is required for conviction, "constructive presence" may suffice if the defendant is close enough to have aided and abetted the crime's commission.

John Marshall knew a good fiction when he saw one. In a case reminiscent of the English fictions that extended a court's jurisdiction, Marshall announced that a corporation would be treated for purposes of suit in federal court as a citizen of the state of which all its stockholders were alleged to be citizens.[19] Professor Gray observed that thereafter the court went much further, holding that "the stockholders of a corporation will, for purposes of jurisdiction, be conclusively presumed to be all citizens of that State by which the corporation

17 Gilmore, *Death of Contract* 73.

18 3 Blackstone, *Commentaries* 161–166.

19 Bank of U.S. v. Devaux, 9 U.S. (5 Cranch) 61 (1809).

was established, no evidence to the contrary being admissible."[20] As Dean Wigmore, a leading expert on the law of evidence, explained: "'Conclusive presumptions' or 'irrebuttable presumptions' are usually mere fictions, to disguise a rule of substantive law."[21] Today, Marshall's fiction has been replaced with another, simpler fiction: that a corporation, which may colloquially be described as a "fake person," is nonetheless a "citizen" of its state of incorporation – at least for purposes of federal jurisdiction.

Of course, sometimes the stretch is just too far. As we have seen, Lord Mansfield thought that "constructive revocations" in the law of wills often defeated the intention of the testator and "brought a scandal upon the law."[22] Even John Marshall initially misspoke about the possibility of "constructive treasons" in American law but quickly corrected himself, recognizing that the Federal Constitution's strict definition of the crime excluded the possibility of construction in that case.[23]

Fictions can extend well beyond judicial constructions. Under the common law, whatever is affixed to land becomes land and therefore belongs to the landowner. Justice Story recognized that this rule, if applied to a commercial tenant, would discourage adapting rented premises to the needs of the tenant's business, an undesirable result in a developing country like the United States. So he restated the common law of fixtures; or, rather, he changed its substance, while keeping its form, by simply adding a qualifier – not, in this case, "constructive" but "trade." An item of personal property affixed by a commercial tenant in furtherance of a trade or business is a "trade fixture" – a fixture of a special kind, one that belongs to the tenant rather than to the landlord, if it can be removed before the end of the term without damage to the property.[24] As a legal dictionary tactfully puts it: "Despite its name, a trade fixture is not usually treated as a fixture"; or, more candidly, it is not really a fixture at all.[25]

Perhaps without intending it, Story's decision on trade fixtures began the slow-motion process of common law change. Judging from the latest restatement of the law of landlord and tenant, one may conclude that what Story held concerning trade fixtures – that a commercial tenant may remove them – is now true of all fixtures, including ordinary items of personal property affixed by a residential tenant.[26] Of course, the justification for allowing the removal of non-trade fixtures cannot be the same as the justification for allowing the removal of trade fixtures; affixing ordinary items of personal property to

20 Gray, *Nature and Sources of Law* 185.

21 John H. Wigmore, *A Students' Textbook of the Law of Evidence* 454 (1935).

22 Swift v. Roberts, 3 Burr. 1488, 1491, 97 Eng. Rep. 941, 942–943 (K.B. 1764).

23 United States v. Burr, 25 F. Cas. 59–80 (C.C.D. Va. 1807) (distinguishing Ex parte Bollman, 8 U.S. (4 Cranch) 75 (1807)); U.S. Const. art. III, § 3.

24 Van Ness v. Packard, 27 U.S. (2 Pet.) 137 (1829).

25 *Black's Law Dictionary* 755.

26 Restatement of Property (Second): Landlord and Tenant § 12.2(4) (1983).

residential tenancies does not have the same pro-developmental effect. But maybe the real reason for the exception is that tenants – all tenants, not just commercial tenants – should not be penalized for suiting the property to their own use, whether commercial or residential, if it would do no harm to the landlord. The trade-fixtures exception may be in the process of "swallowing the rule" – a characteristic way of common law development.

Something similar happened with the common law of waste. Originally, waste was any permanent physical change to property made by someone with only a limited interest in the property, such as a tenant, including a joint tenant or tenant for life. It gave the landowner the right to an injunction and damages and in extreme cases resulted in the forfeiture of the estate. But what if the change actually improved the property? Perhaps the principle behind the rule is not to protect the landowner against *any* change but to protect against one that causes harm. Too restrictive a law of waste, like too restrictive a law of fixtures, could inhibit a tenant from making a useful improvement. Viewed in this light, such a change by a tenant did not seem to merit the intervention of equity or the award of damages, let alone forfeiture. Still, it was a change and therefore waste under traditional law. So a new category of waste was recognized: "ameliorating waste." This is waste that does not trigger the remedies for ordinary waste. In other words, it is technical waste that is not legal waste. The law maintained a superficial consistency while preventing the uneconomic consequences by attaching a fancy Latin adjective. A little Latin has also been used to explain the denial of a legal remedy in case of actual harm, as where a national retail chain puts a local shopkeeper out of business. Admitting the damage but denying the remedy because of the economic benefits of competition, judges since Blackstone have dismissed the claim as a case of *damnum absque injuria* (damage without legal injury).[27]

In addition to proliferating constructions and transformative qualifiers are further fictions made possible by invoking the powers of equity, a possibility made even more likely when law and equity are administered by the same court. Under the name of "equitable this-or-that," legal rules thought to lead to unjust results may be nullified. Where a child is raised by persons other than the natural parents who did not follow the statutory procedures for legal adoption, it might be equitable (in the general sense of "fair") to treat the child as adopted; thus was born the concept of "equitable adoption," not a legal adoption but treated like one, creating the legal status of parent and child.

Transfers of title to land are specially affected by the powers of equity. Although the Statute of Frauds requires evidence of a signed writing for enforcement of a contract for the sale of land, most courts nonetheless allow enforcement in the absence of a writing if there are some elements of "part performance," the equitable principle that reliance on an oral promise is

27 See, e.g., 3 Blackstone, *Commentaries* 219.

objective evidence of intent, comparable to the written word. And "equitable conversion," as we have seen, "converts" a contract for the sale of land into a conveyance of an equitable title (what really matters). Promises in deeds binding on future owners, a common feature of modern real estate development, which is ordinarily accomplished by "covenants running with the land," occasionally cannot be recognized for technical reasons, so "equitable servitudes" with the same effect have been recognized.

Financing the purchase of property with a mortgage is also subject to special equitable rules. Although originally structured as a defeasible transfer of title – that is, a transfer that would become void on the repayment of a debt – the mortgage has been hedged about over the years with an elaborate series of protections for the borrower's "equity" (ownership interest in the property). But distressed borrowers might succumb to the lenders' demand that they waive these protections or that they allow the transaction's true nature to be disguised as an outright sale or as an installment contract. In such cases, equity will "pierce the veil" and look through to the reality – doing justice by means of a fiction, the "equitable mortgage," not a legal mortgage but treated like one.

Fictions may be inherent in all legal systems, particularly in the early stages of development. Even Roman law, eventually crystalized in the Corpus Juris Civilis, seems to have begun with ad hoc adjustments of old legal rules.[28] Lecturing on *Ancient Law* in 1861, Sir Henry Maine modestly advanced what he called "a general proposition of some value… with respect to the agencies by which Law is brought into harmony with society." "These instrumentalities," he said, "seem to me to be three in number, Legal Fictions, Equity, and Legislation" – a trio which, incidentally, may be associated respectively with Blackstone, Mansfield, and Bentham. "Their historical order," he added, "is that in which I have placed them."[29] While the sequential emergence of these means of legal change may be as Maine indicated, all remain active in modern law. Their effect is cumulative, not successive.

28 Watson, *Spirit of Roman Law* 80.
29 Maine, *Ancient Law* 15.

8

THE POWER OF INNOVATION

Reminiscing in old age, Felix Frankfurter, then a Justice of the U.S. Supreme Court, recalled his days as a Harvard Law School professor: "I used to ask my classes, 'Who was the most important law reformer of the Eighteenth and Nineteenth Centuries?' They'd guess, 'Blackstone, or Mansfield, or Jeremy Bentham,' and after I'd get all their guesses I'd say, 'Watt, the inventor of the steam engine.'"[1] James Watt's discovery of a practical means for harnessing steam power, patented in 1769 even as Blackstone was completing his *Commentaries*, revolutionized the economy. As applied to transportation (by water and later by rail) and to industrial production (in mines and factories), the steam engine powered more than ships and mills; it also powered rapid legal development.

Judges are often the first legal agents to confront novel problems thrown up by economic and social upheaval. Given their charge to resolve disputes, they are required to decide the cases for which there are no ready answers in existing social and legal arrangements. Just as improvements in finance and international shipping had demonstrated the need for a new law of international trade, so improvements in industrial technology demonstrated the need for a new law of labor. And just as Lord Mansfield worked to meet the legal needs of merchants engaged in moving commodities from one point on the globe to another, so judges throughout the common law world struggled to address the legal problems that were generated by the new means of production.

Railroads, the greatest technological development of the early nineteenth century, brought enormous economic benefits to passengers and shippers and

1 *Felix Frankfurter Reminisces* 233 (recorded by Harlan B. Phillips, 1962). Frankfurter (1882–1965) taught law at Harvard from 1914 until appointed to the Supreme Court in 1938.

DOI: 10.4324/9781003660859-11

new employment opportunities to workers, but they also blazed a trail marked by damage to adjacent property and littered with the mangled bodies of injured workers. In consequence, as one legal historian put it, "The railroad created the law of torts."[2] In what became the leading case on industrial accidents, Farwell v. Boston & Worcester RR (1842),[3] Chief Justice Lemuel Shaw of the Massachusetts Supreme Judicial Court confronted a claim against a railroad by an "engine driver" whose right hand had been crushed when the locomotive he was driving derailed because of a mistake by the "switch-tender." "The question is," Shaw said, "whether, for damages sustained by one of the persons so employed, by means of the carelessness and negligence of another, the party injured has a remedy against the common employer." Describing the case as "an action of new impression in our courts," one involving "a principle of great importance," Shaw considered the claim under the developing law of contract as well as the developing law of torts – not yet clearly distinguished.

As we have seen, in the steady shift from status to contract, the old law of master and servant was being replaced by the new law of work: the contract of employment that fixed the terms of service. Accordingly, Shaw first asked whether the worker's contract obligated the railroad to compensate him in case of injury. Finding no express agreement concerning the allocation of risk, Shaw quickly concluded that there was no implied "contract of indemnity" either. Just as contemporary residential tenants who sought fit premises had to negotiate with the landlord for an express covenant of habitability, so workers who sought protection against loss from injury had to negotiate with the employer for an express promise of compensation. In neither case – tenants or workers – were they likely to have the necessary bargaining power.

Having concluded that the injured worker in *Farwell* had no claim under contract, express or implied, Shaw held that he had voluntarily agreed to assume "the natural and ordinary risks and perils" of the employment. In a striking display of legal fiction, Shaw confidently asserted that the worker's wages must have reflected this reality: "In legal presumption," he said, "the compensation is adjusted accordingly." The precedent thus created spread rapidly through the American states, even crossing the Atlantic. In 1869, the learned editor of John Austin's *Lectures on Jurisprudence* recognized that the principle, "first distinctly laid down by Shaw, C.J. in an American case," had subsequently been adopted in similar cases in England.[4] Although commonly referred to as "assumption of the risk," a phrase normally associated today with torts, its original basis lay in contract.

Turning to torts, Shaw first acknowledged that the railroad would be liable to a passenger who was injured through the negligence of a worker or to a

2 Lawrence Friedman, *American Law* 144 (1984).
3 Farwell v. Boston & Worcester RR, 35 Mass. (4 Metc.) 49 (1842).
4 Austin, *Lectures* 514 n.18 (note by Robert Campbell).

shipper whose goods were lost in transit. Likewise, an innkeeper would be responsible for the loss of a guest's baggage. The employer's liability in such cases was too well established to be denied. "It is laid down by Blackstone," Shaw intoned, "that if a servant, by his negligence, does any damage to a stranger, the master shall be answerable for his neglect."[5] The rule, Shaw explained, is encapsulated in the legal maxim *respondeat superior* (the superior shall answer). In these cases, Shaw accepted the employers' liability, which he said was supported not only by tradition but also by "general considerations of policy and security." But taking Blackstone at his word, he limited the employers' liability to injuries to a *stranger* caused by a servant. Treating passengers, shippers, and guests at an inn as "strangers" to the employer, Shaw – knowingly or not – ignored the fact that Blackstone elsewhere described the relationship between those parties as based on contract: "There is also in law always an implied contract with a common inn-keeper, to secure his guest's goods in his inn; with a common carrier or bargemaster, to be answerable for the goods he carries."[6]

Refusing to allow an injured worker to recover from the employer if the injury was caused by another worker, Shaw maintained that workers, unlike passengers, shippers, and guests, were able to protect themselves:

> Where several persons are employed in the conduct of one common enterprise or undertaking, and the safety of each depends much on the care and skill with which each other shall perform his appropriate duty, each is an observer of the conduct of the others.

Rather than run the risk of injury, a worker could report unsafe conditions to the employer and, if the situation did not improve, could simply "leave the service"; that is, could quit. (This is, of course, to ignore the possibility that passengers, shippers, and guests could investigate the safety record of the respective businesses and decide whether or not to assume the risk of dealing with them.) But for workers, the developing law of torts meant that unless an employer was "actually in default," a worker's loss from injury "must rest where it first fell." "No liability without fault" was the new maxim, qualifying the old *respondeat superior*. Just as property law reflected the ethos of the pre-industrial world, so the new law of torts reflected the nineteenth-century values of "rugged individualism."

Because Shaw did not acknowledge – or perhaps even recognize – that the new law of labor had only recently emerged from the old law of master and servant, he found it significant that there were no reported cases in which *respondeat superior* had been applied to the case of an injured worker, ignoring

5 Citing 1 Blackstone, *Commentaries* 431 [418 in 1st ed.].
6 3 Blackstone, *Commentaries* 164.

the facts that injuries must have occurred even in the pre-industrial world and that passengers, shippers, and guests were more likely than workers to seek legal redress. If it were "a rule of frequent and familiar occurrence," he reasoned, "its existence and application, with all its qualifications and restrictions, would be settled by judicial precedents." Instead, Shaw set the baseline of no liability from which "qualifications and restrictions," some quite dramatic, would eventually be established – until the whole elaborate structure was demolished.

Shaw did take notice of a recent English case, Priestley v. Fowler (1837),[7] which also emphasized that there was no precedent for an action by a worker against an employer for an injury caused by the fault of another worker. Justifying the result in terms familiar from the old-style master and servant, the English court explained that allowing a servant to recover from the master for the tort of another servant would lead to the "absurdity" that "the footman… who rides behind the carriage, may have an action against his master for… drunkenness, neglect, or want of skill in the coachman." Although Farwell's employer was a for-profit corporation, not a carriage-riding gentleman, Shaw adopted the reasoning of the English court – another example of trans-Atlantic exchange, this time from the Old Country to the New. The rule, ever after known as the "fellow servant rule," incidentally showed that the new terminology of employment did not yet extend to the worker – not an employee (or employé), still a servant. Between them, the twin doctrines of assumption of the risk (by contract) and the fellow servant rule (in torts) exempted employers from liability for industrial accidents through most of the nineteenth century.

In the new legal paradigm, contract with its emphasis on agreement and torts with its emphasis on fault joined property with its emphasis on vested rights as organizing principles. Property, inherited or acquired, remained inviolable. Only through an act of will (sale or gift) or through fault (tort or crime) could an owner lose title. Even the government, invoking its sovereign power of eminent domain, took property under the form of a sale, albeit an involuntary one. The old law of torts, Blackstone's "private wrongs," largely concerned with protecting property from injury (as with trespass, nuisance, and waste), was overshadowed by the new law of torts as the legal means of allocating the cost of accidents (as with negligence). Legal scholarship struggled to catch up. The first book on modern tort law, Francis Hilliard's *Law of Torts*, did not appear until 1859, seventy years after the first book on modern contract law and almost four hundred years after the foundational treatise on property law.

The new emphasis on fault as the basis of liability in tort led in time to a reconceptualization of the old rule of *respondeat superior*. Advanced legal thinkers like John Austin had insisted that where the maxim still applied, it was

7 3 Mees. & Welsb. 1, 150 Eng. Rep. 1030 (Exch. 1837).

not merely because of tradition and policy but because the employer was actually at fault – for hiring an improper person. "I am liable for injuries done by persons whom I employ, because it is generally in my power not to employ persons of such a character, or to form them by discipline and education so as to be incapable of the commission of wrong."[8] Years later, Austin's editor added the qualification – from the law of contract – that liability did not extend to an injured worker: "The distinction that obtains in the case where the injured party is also a servant rests upon the contract express or implied between the master and the latter, who is held to undertake the risks incident to the service."[9]

Just as the railroads drove development of the law of torts, so the imperative need to manage industrial labor forced the growth of contract law. What had developed in the eighteenth century, largely under the superintendence of Lord Mansfield, to manage commercial transactions, was now extended to all elements of the new economy. Mansfield, ever precocious, had anticipated the development: a century earlier, he had declared that "everyman may work at what price he pleases" – a proposition not then widely accepted, when justices of the peace were still setting the wages of agricultural laborers.[10] By the mid-nineteenth century, the triumph of contract over status was apparently complete, allowing maximum scope to individual volition. In the words of a contemporary English statesman: "There is no sound distinction between contracts to buy and sell labour and contracts to sell any other commodity, and the sooner this absolute equality between all persons contracting irrespective of the subject matter of the contract is recognized, the better."[11] Contract permitted individuals to make their own enforceable legal rules, tailor-made to their unique situations, just as voters made general laws through representative democracy. "Freedom of contract" was triumphantly proclaimed – as if contract itself could have rights.

The rule of law meant equal law for everyone, regardless of subject matter or relative bargaining power. The new paradigm, however effective in the market for commodities, proved unsustainable when applied to many of the most common transactions affecting the lives of ordinary people. As we have seen with respect to the law of landlord and tenant, legal remedies eventually qualified the "absolute equality between all persons," depending precisely on the "subject matter of the contract." As a matter of law, not of agreement,

8 Austin, *Lectures* 514.

9 Austin, *Lectures* 514 n.18 (note by Robert Campbell).

10 R. v. Eccles, 1 Leach 274, 276–277, 168 Eng. Rep. 240, 241 (1783). See Orth, *Combination and Conspiracy* 32–33 (1991).

11 Robert Lowe quoted in Jonathan Spain, "Trade Unionists, Gladstonian Liberals and the Labour Law Reforms of 1875," in *Currents of Radicalism: Popular Radicalism, Organized Labour and Party Politics in Britain, 1850–1914*, at 124 (Eugenio F. Biagini & Alastair J. Reid eds. 1991). Lowe was successively Chancellor of the Exchequer (1868–1873) and Home Secretary (1873–1874).

residential tenants came to be protected by an implied warranty of habitability. In like case, consumers were provided an implied warranty of fitness for use. In both cases, the "contractual protections" were nonwaivable.

As industrial accidents accumulated, assumption of the risk and the fellow servant rule came under increasing pressure. Shaw's rationale that workers could police one another, not very persuasive even in the early days of railroading, was obviously unrealistic in the new conditions of mass production in the late nineteenth and early twentieth centuries. In his 1915 bestseller, *Spoon River Anthology*, lawyer-poet Edgar Lee Masters held the law up to ridicule. Denied recovery from his employer, an injured worker, when told by the Circuit Judge that "whoever did it was a fellow servant of mine," responded by "saying over and over, 'I didn't know him at all.'"[12]

In the decades that followed the Farwell Case, the rigor of the rules was steadily eroded by "qualifications and restrictions," as lawyers for injured workers came up with ingenious arguments, some so common that they acquired labels included in legal dictionaries. The servant who was at fault was not a fellow servant but was engaged in a separate service (the "different-department rule") or was part of the management (the "superior-servant rule"). Or the employer was actually the "person in default" for failing to supply proper equipment (the "safe-tool rule"). Juries, constitutionally guaranteed as a protection against oppression, often ignored a judge's instructions. In 1897, Oliver Wendell Holmes, then a justice of the Massachusetts Supreme Judicial Court and soon to become one of Shaw's successors as chief justice of that court, asked rhetorically: "Why does a judge instruct a jury that an employer is not liable to an employee for an injury received in the course of his employment unless he is negligent, and why do the jury generally find for the plaintiff if the case is allowed to go to them?"[13]

The common law rules, the legal system's first response to a problem that ballooned in importance as the pace of industrial development quickened and the risk of accidents increased, were in obvious need of repair or replacement. Widely adopted by the courts and fortified by the doctrine of *stare decisis*, the rules were resistant to change by judicial decision. In any event, the common law method of case-by-case development could not produce the administrative system that seemed to be called for. Holmes puckishly suggested that "it is conceivable that some day in certain cases we may find ourselves imitating, on a higher plane, the tariff for life and limb which we see in the Leges Barbarorum." The learned reference was to the collection of laws from the Dark Ages, literally the "laws of the barbarians," that imposed a duty to pay the victim a fixed

12 "Butch Weldy," in Edgar Lee Masters, *Spoon River Anthology* (1915). Masters (1868–1950) had a distinguished legal practice before his literary career. See John V. Orth, "The Law in Spoon River," 16 *Legal Studies Forum* 301 (1992).

13 O.W. Holmes, "The Path of the Law," 10 *Harv. L. Rev*. 457, 467 (1897).

amount – so much for an eye, a hand, a foot, and so on. Holmes was highlighting the resemblance between barbaric law and progressive proposals to establish a compulsory system of insurance to compensate injured workers – so much for an eye, a hand, a foot, and so on – the system first known as workmen's compensation, now by the gender-neutral name workers' compensation.

The common law spreads naturally from jurisdiction to jurisdiction, even (as we have seen) back and forth across the Atlantic. But only a statute could establish the new system. England, the home of the common law and the world's first industrial nation, responded with a series of ever more comprehensive statutes beginning in 1880. Rather than allocate the risk of loss by searching for who was "actually in default," the new system spread the cost over all employers in the industry, who could treat it as a cost of doing business – just as the implied covenant of habitability in leases allocated the cost of repairs to the landlords, who could treat it as another item of overhead, and as the implied warranty of fitness in consumer products allocated the cost of accidents to the producers, who could treat it as part of the cost of production. As Holmes put it, "such wrongful acts as by ordinary human laws are likely to happen in the course of the service are imputable to the service" – or, more pithily, "there ought to be a remedy against someone who can pay the damages."[14] But legislation on industrial accidents confronted two specifically American obstacles: challenges under state and federal constitutions and the federal system of multiple jurisdictions.

Common law rules are generally presumed to be constitutional: after all, the judges who make and apply the rules are themselves the custodians of the constitutions.[15] In addition, the American concept of unconstitutionality seems to presuppose the existence of written (rather than unwritten) law, which is not surprising since it developed as a way to resolve conflicts between statutes and constitutions. And statutes that dramatically change the common law are often subjected to harsh scrutiny. In 1911, New York's highest court declared the state's pioneering workmen's compensation act unconstitutional under both state and federal constitutions.[16] "The statute, judged by our common-law standards, is plainly revolutionary." In a dubious excursion into legal history, the court declared: "When our Constitutions were adopted it was the law of the land that no man who was without fault or negligence could be held liable in damages for injuries sustained by another." To change that principle by imposing "upon an employer, who has omitted no legal duty and has committed no wrong, a liability based solely upon a legislative fiat is," the court held,

14 Holmes, *The Common Law* 9.

15 For further discussion of this point, see John V. Orth, "Can the Common Law be Unconstitutional?" in *How Many Judges Does It Take to Make a Supreme Court? And Other Essays on Law and the Constitution* 53 (2006).

16 Ives v. South Buffalo Ry. Co., 201 N.Y. 271, 94 N.E. 431 (N.Y. 1911).

"a taking of property without due process of law." The problem, as the court saw it, was not that the statute took property without compensation but that it took property at all from someone who had done nothing wrong – a violation of what would later be described as substantive due process. To overturn that decision required an amendment to the state constitution and a new statute – as well as favorable decisions by New York's court and the U.S. Supreme Court.[17]

Once grudgingly accepted as constitutional, the workers' compensation system then confronted the fact of American federalism. Just as repeal of old property laws like the Rule in Shelley's Case required legislation in each state, so the new insurance system required separate state statutes – and encountered the same fragmented and slow-motion response. Delayed by inertia and opposition by business interests, adoption of workers' compensation acts proceeded at a glacial pace, state-by-state, the final adoption not achieved until the mid-twentieth century.

The common law met technological innovation with legal innovation: a renovated law of contracts and torts. But the new maxims of "freedom of contract" and "no liability without fault," when applied to industrial accidents, were first subjected to rigorous testing by imaginative legal challenges, often aided by sympathetic juries. Just as the rigor of the traditional law of fixtures and waste was undermined by the grudging recognition of exceptions, so the new amalgam of contract and tort was qualified and restricted – until it was finally overthrown and replaced by a statutory system. Bentham would have approved.

Socializing the cost of accidents by spreading it over a larger group shocked traditionally minded scholars, who convinced themselves that contemporary ideas of liability were of ancient pedigree. As we have seen, Langdell dismissed arguments based on "substantial justice" as "irrelevant."[18] And legal logicians were blinded to the unequal consequences of "freedom of contract" when the contracting parties were of grossly unequal bargaining power. In his lectures at Harvard, Professor Dicey denounced the new system as "collectivism," depriving the individual worker of the right, as Dicey bluntly put it, "to bargain away his claim to compensation" for injury. As the lecturer ruefully admitted, compensation for accidents had become "a matter not of contract, but of status,"[19] reversing the supposed movement of "progressive societies."

Innovation is never ceasing. New technologies follow one another with increasing rapidity, generating new legal problems, which in turn demand legal innovation. At first, judicial decisions resolve individual disputes and hazard

17 Jensen v. Southern Pac. Co., 215 N.Y. 514, 109 N.E. 600 (1916); New York Central RR v. White, 243 U.S. 188 (1917).

18 O.W. Holmes, Review of *Langdell's A Selection of Cases on the Law of Contracts* (2d ed. 1880), 14 *Am. L. Rev*. 233, 234 (1880).

19 A.V. Dicey, *Law and Opinion* 201.

rules of general application. In some instances, the rules endure – as with Mansfield's commercial decisions, still widely accepted. In other instances, the rules are qualified at first by exceptions, later by the imposition of statutory terms in contracts – as with landlord-and-tenant and consumer protection – or rejected and replaced by statutes creating an administrative system – as with assumption of the risk and the fellow servant rule. The complex interaction of case and statute seems destined to continue, a perennial feature of the common law tradition in America.

9

THE CHALLENGE OF CRITICISM

Among Blackstone's successors as Vinerian professor at Oxford was his son James, the incumbent from 1793 to 1824. Unlike his distinguished father, James Blackstone published nothing during his long tenure and, so far as we can see, gave no lectures. The terrified reaction of English authorities to the excesses of the French Revolution, at its height when James was chosen, and the long war against Napoleon that followed made just about any criticism of English law dangerous. It was probably safest to say nothing at all. As the learned historian of the Vinerian Chair commented in defense of the younger Blackstone: "The study of law without the cogitation of ideas for its improvement is indeed jejune."[1] In other words, teaching law by merely reciting the rules is boring.

Because of Dean Langdell's determination to view law as a purely objective science and his insistence on intellectual rigor in its teaching, the Harvard-style law professor had no hesitation about speaking up. As we have seen, James Barr Ames, Langdell's protégé and successor as dean, denounced Lord Mansfield as a "fraud" – and added, for good measure, that most of the judges, on both sides of the Atlantic, were "illogical, inconsistent, and unreasonable."[2] Conservative legal scholars like Professor Dicey thought legal development was moving in the wrong direction (and said so), while progressives advocated rapid change. Today a law professor might be criticized for not cogitating about ways to improve the law and, indeed, might earn tenure precisely for the most telling critique of existing law.

The Harvard model of legal education helped to keep critical attention focused on judicial decisions, even as statutes multiplied. For every subject,

1 H.G. Hanbury, *The Vinerian Chair and Legal Education* 83 (1958).

2 Brandeis to Otto Wehle, 12 Nov. 1876, in 1 Brandeis, *Letters*.

DOI: 10.4324/9781003660859-12

there was a collection of cases, a "casebook" – the title eventually expanded from "Cases on" to "Cases and Materials on," a concession to the need to place the cases in a broader context. Statutes, both state and federal, rarely made it into the casebooks – the form itself seemed to preclude their inclusion – and the national focus of legal education discouraged parochialism. Capping their education, law students demonstrated their skills (and tried to attract the attention of employers) by publishing "case notes" in their schools' law review or journal; "statute notes" rarely appeared. Common law was the ideal subject for instruction because it was just that, "common" – shared by all American states (except Louisiana) and other English-speaking countries.

At first, law professors busied themselves with the systematic exposition of traditional doctrine in treatises and law review articles: resolving inconsistencies, tying up loose ends, analyzing legal concepts. Perhaps the most rigorous exponent of the close analysis of fundamental legal concepts was Ames's younger contemporary, Yale law professor Wesley Newcomb Hohfeld, intellectual descendant of John Austin and Jeremy Bentham. Under his analysis, for example, the old common law "right of re-entry for condition broken" (the interest that followed a fee simple subject to condition subsequent) was recognized to be not a *right* at all but a *power*: the "power of termination." As with other attempts to reform legal terminology, the new label never fully displaced the old, to the bafflement of law students. Hohfeld and legal logicians like him in the early twentieth century inspired the movement that resulted in the "restatements of the law," a massive set of volumes offering orderly statements – or, rather, curated re-statements – of American common law, particularly the branches still primarily composed of case law.

Unlike "uniform laws," the other great academic project to homogenize American law, which are legally binding only in states where enacted and uniform only when enacted unchanged by all states, the restatements are intended to standardize the law the old common law way, through judicial decisions, which (as we have seen) can easily cross jurisdictional boundaries. A purely private compilation, the restatements are reminiscent of the early "nominative" law reports, their persuasiveness dependent on the clarity of their presentation and the prestige of their reporters. Prepared mainly by law professors at elite law schools, the restatements were originally described as their authors' "considered opinion… of the way in which the law would be decided in the light of decisions by the courts."[3] Formulated as a series of propositions like the articles of a code, the restatements demonstrate the academic preference for neat authoritative systems rather than ad hoc judicial development.

The first set of restatements had barely reached completion in the 1940s, when a second set was commenced; lately, a third and even a fourth set on selected topics have been undertaken. In 1973, one scholar mischievously asked

3 Restatement in the Courts 8 (4th ed. 1939).

why there should be a second (or further) series of restatements: "There can be little or no doubt that the first generation of Restaters implicitly assumed that they were reducing to black letter text what we like to call the 'fundamental principles of the common law'"[4] – the subject matter, as we have seen, of instruction at the new Langdellian law schools.

Whether residential landlords had a duty to provide their tenants with fit and habitable premises was firmly answered in the negative in the first restatement of property. Tenants were still understood, as they had been for centuries, as grantees of an estate in land; landlords generally had no duties respecting the condition of the premises. *Caveat lessee*: "Let the tenant beware." In the (unlikely) event that tenants had sufficient bargaining power, they could secure further rights by express promises in the lease, known as "covenants." Like the old promises under seal – the original meaning of "covenant" – which were enforceable without regard to consideration, these covenants were treated as "independent," that is, not dependent on reciprocal performance by the other party. Breach of a landlord's covenant gave rise to an action for damages but did not relieve the tenant of any duties under the lease, including the duty to pay rent.

After the reconceptualization of the residential lease as a contract, the relationship between the parties had to be re-thought. In some states, it took a statute to recognize what had become obvious: "The tenant's obligation to pay rent under the rental agreement…and the landlord's obligation…shall be mutually dependent."[5] A second restatement of landlord and tenant was obviously needed. Not only were leases contracts, but a "covenant of habitability" – comparable to the warranty of fitness in consumer contracts – was now implied (by law) in all residential leases. The judges, as we have repeatedly seen, cannot always agree about "fundamental principles"; neither, it seems, can the law professors.

Once embarked on "restating" the law, the reporters began to venture beyond the mere prediction of the likely result "in the light of decisions by the courts" and to "codify" their preferred view of what the law should be. The second restatement of wills, as we will see, endorsed a significant change in the Rule Against Perpetuities, despite the conceded fact that it had been adopted by only a bare majority of jurisdictions – in most cases by statute, not by judicial decision.[6] And the third restatement of servitudes allows the relocation of easements by burdened landowners without the consent of the easement owners.[7] Although the reporter acknowledged that the "weight of authority in the United States" does not support the new rule, the restatement nonetheless

4 Gilmore, *Death of Contract* 67.
5 N.C. Gen. Stat. § 42–41.
6 Restatement (Second) of Property: Donative Transfers viii (1983).
7 Restatement (Third) of Property: Servitudes § 4.8(3) (2000).

adopts it, preferring the "civil-law rule" in effect in Louisiana – just as the concept of the lease as a contract was borrowed from civil law.

Recently, restatements have begun to converge with uniform laws, advocating the judicial adoption of rules that are also proposed for legislative adoption – revealing (again) the uncertain boundary in the common law tradition between case and statute. The third restatement of wills urges relaxed application of the statutory requirements for the execution of wills – "the harmless error rule," imported from criminal procedure – despite the fact that judges are normally bound to apply statutes as written. Perhaps for this reason, the change is also proposed for statutory adoption in the Uniform Probate Code.[8] Latterly, the judges have been encouraged to "dispense" with the statutory requirements altogether in the interest of effectuating intention, the universal solvent of strict rules of law.

It is a common observation that what goes on in law school classrooms forms the minds of the next generation of lawyers and judges. Indeed, it is hard to see how it could be otherwise since legal education is intended to induct law students into what Sir Edward Coke long ago called "the artificiall reason and judgment of law,"[9] now better known as "thinking like a lawyer." Overt advocacy of reform, or at least change, by law professors is now generally expected. Even the conservative Blackstone made modest suggestions for improvement. A more covert form of advocacy is often difficult to recognize. Editors of the ubiquitous casebooks can inculcate their preferred view of the law by their selection of appellate opinions that challenge or reject traditional rules. And as we have seen, the very name of a legal rule can incorporate a particular social outlook: the "fellow servant rule" once encoded a traditional view of the worker as servant not employee.

Today, preferred results may be concealed in conclusory labels, rather like the "persuasive definitions" described by the philosopher C.L. Stevenson.[10] Competitive reduction in legal restrictions is a "race to the bottom," not a welcome "release of energy" or useful "social experiment," as it would be if the destination was thought to be desirable. Competition between courts with concurrent jurisdiction is "forum shopping," regardless of whether it is likely to produce better results. Inheritance laws that allow succession to property by remote kindred benefit only "laughing heirs," those who feel no pang of sorrow at the death of the decedent, implicitly suggesting that escheat to the government would result in the money being put to a better use.[11] Torts that protect

8 Restatement (Third) of Property: Wills and Other Donative Transfers § 3.3; Uniform Probate Code § 2–503.

9 Case of the Prohibitions, 12 Co. Rep. 65, 77 Eng. Rep. 1343 (1607).

10 C.L. Stevenson, "Persuasive Definitions," 47 *MIND* 331 (1938).

11 Compare David F. Cavers, "Change in the American Family and the 'Laughing Heir'," 20 *Iowa L. Rev*. 203 (1935) with John V. Orth, "'The Laughing Heir': What's So Funny?" 48 *Real Property, Trust & Estate L. J*. 321 (2013).

the marital relation – criminal conversation and alienation of affections – are dismissed as "heartbalm actions." The bad name for intention that seeks to extend its reach too far in the future is control by the "dead hand." Estate and inheritance taxes are condemned as "death taxes." Who would want a will to fail because of a "harmless error" in execution?

Harvard Law Professor W. Barton Leach once acknowledged that "items of jargon" can be "usefully argumentative" by highlighting "the absurdity of the designated doctrines."[12] That is, colloquial labels can be used to stigmatize traditional rules. Perhaps the most dramatic use of "argumentative jargon" to undercut existing law is the way law professors made the common law Rule Against Perpetuities ridiculous as part of their project to reform it. The Rule, which began to take shape in the seventeenth century, reached its classic expression in the formulation of John Chipman Gray in the nineteenth century: "No interest is good unless it must vest, if at all, not later than twenty-one years after some life in being at the creation of the interest."[13] The Rule, which is applied as of the "creation of the interest," voids any interest that is not certain to vest within the "perpetuities period."

When Professor Leach wanted to point out the "absurdity" of requiring prospective application of the Rule Against Perpetuities – what he called the "might-have-been rule" – he made up ridiculous labels for hypothetical cases. One of the Rule's greatest strengths, the certainty provided by immediately voiding remote interests, was also one of its potential weaknesses. Because any possibility of remote vesting was fatal, bizarre and unlikely eventualities could cause the failure of benign interests. The possibility that a beneficiary might marry a woman not alive at the creation of the interest who might then outlive him (and all others alive at the creation of the interest) was caricatured as the "unborn widow rule," making invalid any interest contingent on surviving the widow. The common law's conclusive presumption of fertility until death, regardless of age or sex, a source of certainty in applying the Rule, was ridiculed as the "fertile octogenarian rule" – despite the fact that legal adoption is now possible at any age.

Having made prospective application of the Rule ("at the creation of the interest") a source of amusement, Professor Leach's proposed solution was simply to allow retrospective application; that is, to restate the Rule – "No interest is good unless it vests [not 'must vest'] not later than twenty-one years after some life in being at the creation of the interest" – in other words, to await the expiration of the perpetuities period and see if the interest actually vests in time. This "wait-and-see" version of the Rule was adopted by the second restatement of property and adopted by a number of states.

12 W. Barton Leach, "Perpetuities: The Nutshell Revisited," 78 *Harv. L. Rev*. 973, 991 n.78 (1965).

13 Gray, *Rule Against Perpetuities* § 201, p. 191 (capital letters in original).

Having demonstrated the "absurdity" of the traditional Rule and the ease of its modification, Professor Leach had, perhaps unwittingly, illustrated that the Rule was subject not only to modification but even to repeal. Since then, lobbied by lawyers and bankers competing for the business of establishing and servicing well-funded trusts, many states have weakened the Rule or simply eliminated it. The result is to permit perpetual trusts. Popularly known as "dynasty trusts," such trusts can preserve property for the benefit of a settlor's descendants from generation to generation forever – a modern form of the medieval entailed estate, the legal foundation of the English aristocracy. The example suggests that what begins as a classroom joke can have unexpected consequences and that what law professors ridicule might be a predictor of legal change, if not reform.

Law has always been close to politics; indeed, in the early days of the common law, before the separation of powers, the distinction between adjudicating and legislating was not clear. Medieval judges unapologetically made law, as they made the Rule in Shelley's Case; the impulse is not exhausted yet. The judicial recognition of a common law covenant of habitability in leases was obviously intended to rectify a medieval bias in favor of "lords," in this case landlords. And legal fictions today continue to stretch old rules to fit new cases.

In America, constitutional law comes closest to politics. This has always been so. Judicial review means that supreme courts, state and federal, sometime seem to be part of the legislative process. James Bradley Thayer, one of Langdell's professors at Harvard, prefaced the first casebook on "con law" with the observation: "The study of Constitutional Law is allied not merely with history, but with statecraft, and with the political problems of our great and complex national life."[14] In contrast to Langdell's belief that experts can discern the right answer to legal problems, political problems in a democracy are more likely to be solved by votes. There is a story, probably apocryphal, that Dean Langdell was reluctant to have constitutional law taught at his law school because he thought it was politics, not science.

There is a way of thinking about law that makes it seem just about the most important thing in society, a point of view that appeals (not surprisingly) to lawyers, especially academic lawyers. Law students who want "to change the world" are also drawn to this view. Because laws, usually nowadays in the form of statutes, regulate marriage, parentage, property, and just about everything else, it is tempting to think that such things would not exist without laws. Indeed, Bentham said just that: "Before laws were made, there was no property: take away laws, and property ceases."[15] This way of thinking about law leads naturally to the idea that all that is needed to change the world is to change the law. Law, in a phrase that sounds scientific, might be a grand form

14 James Bradley Thayer, *Cases on Constitutional Law* v (1895).
15 Jeremy Bentham, *A Theory of Legislation* 113 (4th ed. 1882).

of "social engineering." From this point of view, law is hardly distinguishable from statecraft.

The common law was founded and to a large extent still functions on an entirely different premise, that the business of law is not the design (or re-design) of society at large but the resolution of specific disputes. Until a plaintiff or prosecutor brings a case to court, there is strictly speaking no legal problem, and even then, the only problem is the one presented – not what is to be done in general but what is to be done in particular, as between these parties. The common law judges did not think that they had created marriage, parentage, property, and so on, but only that they needed to resolve any disputes that were brought to them concerning these human institutions – to resolve them in a manner that was fair, just, and reasonable and that, in consequence, would be accepted by society at large.

Not only are traditional rules re-examined today in the academy, but the rule of law itself has been subjected to scrutiny. In the transition from status to contract, equality before the law was regarded as the distinguishing mark of a progressive society, and the legal fiction was indulged of the "absolute equality between all persons." In a popular Victorian poem, Tennyson described "unequal laws" as fit only for a "savage race."[16] But equal laws applied to an unequal society inevitably produce unequal results, as captured by the famous quip: "The rich as well as the poor are forbidden to sleep under the bridges of Paris."[17] Undeviating adherence to equality before the law prevents unequal laws that promote substantive equality. Today, specialized bodies of law, as we have seen, have developed to protect various classes perceived to be at a disadvantage in the marketplace: tenants against landlords, consumers against producers, workers against employers. Groups victimized by past (and present) discrimination may benefit from programs giving them preferential treatment – to the alarm of critics, convinced that "any policy aiming directly at a substantive ideal of distributive justice must lead to the destruction of the Rule of Law."[18]

Beyond the concern that equal laws produce unequal results lies the concern that rules themselves are a form of hegemony – that is, that rules subtly incorporate values that are made to seem necessary, even desirable, and that are consequently difficult to isolate and challenge. There can be hardly any doubt that the common law has always prioritized property and that the modern law of contract and tort incorporates a spirit of individualism. The procedural demands of due process offer decided advantages to the wealthy, the educated, and the well counseled, who can be sure to obtain all the protections afforded by law (and more). Law's proverbial delay not only penalizes those in need of a remedy but also benefits those seeking escape from the legal consequences of

16 Alfred Lord Tennyson, "Ulysses" (1833).
17 Anatole France, *Le Lys Rouge* chap. 7 (1894).
18 F.A. Hayek, *The Road to Serfdom* 87–88 (1944).

their actions. The "deep structures" of the law may privilege specific values of race, class, and sex. But exposing the values implicit in the common law, while useful in itself, has so far not resulted in any serious alternative to the present system.

As a practical matter, the contest between strict and discretionary application of the law – a contest as old as that between Blackstone and Mansfield (and even older) – is of more consequence than radical re-examination of the law's foundational assumptions. The modern commitment to recognizing presumed intention at the expense of formal requirements has particularly affected property law, where adherence to strict rules has been traditional. Inevitably, the relaxation of the rules has the effect of increasing judicial discretion. Today, Blackstone's emphasis on rigid rules, both in the *Commentaries* and in his judicial decisions, can be dismissed as legalistic, exalting the letter over the spirit of the law. And his faith in legal rules, at least if rigorously enforced, to protect individuals from the abuse of power may often seem naïve. But his warnings about discretionary justice, which would de-legitimate equitable resolutions by enlightened judges, sound more persuasive when judges are perceived to be oppressive or politicized.

AFTERWORD

Legal History, Legal Future

To begin at the end: Of the future we know nothing. All we have are guesses based on what has gone before. One of the few guesses that can be hazarded on that basis with any confidence is that law will continue to grow – or, at least, to change. This is not necessarily the lesson that all legal historians have drawn from their studies of the past. In lectures scheduled for delivery at the Harvard Law School in 1905, James C. Carter, eminent lawyer and lifelong critic of the Benthamite project of universal codification, traced the different stages of legal development up to what he called "the last stage…., the stage of full enlightenment, such as is exhibited in Europe and the United States at the present day."[1] It is an occupational hazard of historians to assume that history exhibits constant change, progress, or development – until, that is, the present moment, when history stops, having reached its climax. After describing the common law's "rise, progress, and gradual improvements,"[2] Blackstone too believed that relatively little remained to be done. He would probably have agreed with Carter that the "stage of full enlightenment" had been reached, although Blackstone dated the arrival at that happy destination a full century and a half earlier than Carter.

Such massive complacency is hard to find today. The *ignis fatuus* of "full enlightenment" continues to elude us and most likely always will. Old certainties are too often unsettled, and novel problems too frequently encountered. The law is under seemingly constant criticism – not just from those outside the legal profession. Without engaging in a fruitless search for the "lessons of

1 James C. Carter, *Law: Its Origin, Growth and Function* 66 (1907). Because of Carter's untimely death, the lectures were never actually delivered.

2 4 Blackstone, *Commentaries* chap. 33 (title).

DOI: 10.4324/9781003660859-13

history," one can at least search for a pattern in the past, which – if continued – will shape future developments. The difficulty, perhaps insuperable, is that no single pattern emerges from a study of the past. Too many patterns emerge, and it is impossible to know which will prevail at any particular time and on any particular issue.

Rules tend to linger, sometimes well past their usefulness; interests may have vested, harms may be perceived to be minimal, or a new rationale for an old rule may be discovered. Tradition, or at least inertia, will likely remain a force in the future. Judges will continue to apply common law rules, outdated or not, until the legislature provides otherwise (which it often will not). In rare cases, judges in the mode of Lord Mansfield – several have been named in these pages – will break through the crust of precedent and radically redirect the law, to the consternation of traditionalists like Blackstone. In any system based on precedent, the past is ever-present. But a system that claims to be guided by the past cannot rest content with the past as it was. The past must somehow be made to do the work of the present. In defiance of the concept of separation of powers, incremental judicial law-making will continue, often out of sight, as with legal fictions.

Of more importance, the common law way of doing things seems set to continue, shaping the way disputes are resolved, usually one at a time. Courts and judges will remain at the center, as they have been ever since Magna Carta. Although the day may be long past when judges routinely discount the significance of statutes by saying that they merely restate the common law, courts will not necessarily be welcoming of legislative initiatives and may counter with strict "constructions." In any event, the judges will regularly be called upon to resolve conflicts and fill gaps left by ambiguous drafting – often by reference to the common law. And they will probably continue to develop constitutional provisions in ways similar to their treatment of common law precedents.

Statute and common law will continue to interact in ways unseen in other countries, including other common law countries, where parliaments reign supreme. Legislatures, now seemingly in constant session, will produce large numbers of statutes – sometimes codifying common law rules, sometimes modifying them, sometimes upending them altogether. In cases of widespread public concern, statutes will qualify the extent of "freedom of contract," as with statutorily imposed terms; sometimes administrative bodies will be created to bypass traditional litigation and mitigate the impact of social and economic inequality, as with workers' compensation.

In the many-constitutioned United States, variations in local law will continue to appear, frustrating easy generalizations. Without a unitary national legislature able to adopt comprehensive statutes, the common law in America will continue to fragment. In response, a lengthening series of uniform laws will be proposed for adoption state by state; few (if any) will be adopted everywhere unchanged, and frequent revisions will only complicate matters. Without a national civil code, successive restatements will continue to attempt the standardization of common law but will be frustrated by its ongoing development. Law schools will be sources of change as well as of continuity. Driven by their institutional culture, law professors will continue to propose ideas for the law's improvement, some of which will be adopted.

The Benthamite project of comprehensive codification will likely never be realized, if it is even possible. Instead, specialized codes will proliferate. But whatever the fate of codification, Bentham's legal positivism will affect the way law is thought about – and taught. The state will increasingly be seen as the sole source of law, and statute law will increasingly predominate over case law. Utilitarianism will generally prevail over appeals to natural law, risking loss of a perceived connection to morality and jeopardizing public recognition of legal legitimacy.

The life of the law will, if we are fortunate, continue to be reason *and* experience *and* borrowing. Clues to the legal future may be found in an understanding of the dynamics that drive legal development, like jurisdictional competition and judicial activism. And clues to the direction of that development may come from a grasp of the deep tendencies that drive it, like the growing emphasis on the primacy of individual intention over strict rules and the consequent willingness to tolerate ever greater scope for judicial discretion.

Certainty about the future will ever elude us. As we are reminded by the standard investment disclaimer, "past performance is no guarantee of future results." Discontinuities are only to be expected. Legal development seems to proceed in fits and starts, creative bursts followed by consolidation and eventual correction. Tensions that may disrupt smooth development build unobserved by those raised within the system – for whom the contradictions are ignored, subsumed, or internalized. Even when these tensions are recognized, it will be impossible to predict the form the response will assume, which strand of the common law tradition will be uppermost at any given moment. Thoughtfulness about the past and present is the best guide to what lies ahead – at least until war, revolution, political upheaval, or some other powerful extraneous and unexpected force upends our assumptions. But then history has already alerted us to that possibility.

INDEX

Pages followed by "n" refer to notes.

For Product Safety Concerns and Information please contact our EU
representative GPSR@taylorandfrancis.com
Taylor & Francis Verlag GmbH, Kaufingerstraße 24, 80331 München, Germany

www.ingramcontent.com/pod-product-compliance
Ingram Content Group UK Ltd.
Pitfield, Milton Keynes, MK11 3LW, UK
UKHW020000200926
475702UK00015B/2400
9781041116219